Medicine, Health and Being Human

Medicine, Health and Being Human begins a conversation to explore how the medical has defined us: that is, the ways in which perspectives of medicine and health have affected cultural understandings of what it means to be human.

With chapters that span from the early modern period through to the contemporary world, and are drawn from a range of disciplines, this volume holds that incremental historical and cultural influences have brought about an understanding of humanity in which the medical is ingrained, consciously or unconsciously, usually as a mode of legitimisation. Divided into three parts, the book follows a narrative path from the integrity of the human soul, through to the integrity of the material human body, then finally brought together through engaging with end-of-life responses. Part I examines the move from spirituality to psychiatry in terms of the way medical science has influenced cultural understandings of the mind. Part II interrogates the role that medicine has played in the nineteenth and twentieth centuries in constructing and deconstructing the self and other, including the fusion of visual objectivity and the scientific gaze in constructing perceptions of humanity. Part III looks at the limits of medicine when the integrity of one body breaks down. It contends with the ultimate question of the extent to which humanity is confined within the integrity of the human body, and how medicine and the humanities work together towards responding to the finality of death.

This is a valuable contribution for all those interested in the medical humanities, history of medicine, history of ideas and the social approaches to health and illness.

Lesa Scholl teaches in the School of Communication and Arts, University of Queensland, Australia.

Routledge Advances in the Medical Humanities

For more information about this series, please visit www.routledge.com/Routledge-Advances-in-Disability-Studies/book-series/RADS

Medicine, Health and Being Human

Edited by Lesa Scholl

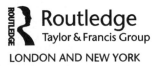

Routledge
Taylor & Francis Group

LONDON AND NEW YORK

First published 2018
by Routledge

2 Park Square, Milton Park, Abingdon, Oxfordshire OX14 4RN
52 Vanderbilt Avenue, New York, NY 10017

Routledge is an imprint of the Taylor & Francis Group, an informa business

First issued in paperback 2019

British Library Cataloguing-in-Publication Data
A catalogue record for this book is available from the British Library

Library of Congress Cataloging-in-Publication Data
Names: Scholl, Lesa, editor.
Title: Medicine, health and being human / edited by Lesa Scholl.
Other titles: Routledge advances in the medical humanities.
Description: Abingdon, Oxon ; New York, NY : Routledge, 2018. |
Series: Routledge advances in the medical humanities | Includes
bibliographical references and index.
Identifiers: LCCN 2018002001 | ISBN 9781138301184 (hbk) |
ISBN 9780203732700 (ebk)
Subjects: | MESH: Medicine | Philosophy, Medical | Health | Human Body
| Medicine in Literature
Classification: LCC R733 | NLM WB 300 | DDC 610–dc23
LC record available at https://lccn.loc.gov/2018002001

ISBN: 978-1-138-30118-4 (hbk)
ISBN: 978-0-367-45752-5 (pbk)

Typeset in Times New Roman
by Wearset Ltd, Boldon, Tyne and Wear

This volume is dedicated to Dr Des McGuckin, a doctor who understood and relished both the humanness of life and the precision of medicine

Contents

Figures

Contributors

M. Renee Benham is a Postdoctoral Teaching Fellow at Ohio University, where she received her PhD in 2017 for her interdisciplinary dissertation, *Beyond Nightingale: The Transformation of Nursing in Victorian and World War I Literature*. Her research interests include the history of British nursing and its representation in literature, as well as women's role in the development of sanitary reform in Victorian England.

Kathryn Bird is an Associate Lecturer at Edge Hill University in the Department of English, History and Creative Writing. She has a PhD in English from the University of Leeds and an MA in Contemporary Literature and Culture from the University of Manchester. Her research interests are in modern and contemporary literature, Gothic and detective fiction, and the interdisciplinary fields of biopolitics, animal studies and medical humanities. Her publications include book chapters and journal articles in *The Routledge Handbook to the Ghost Story*, *Landscapes of Liminality: Between Space and Place* and *Neo-Victorian Studies*, and she is currently working on a monograph from her PhD dissertation, "Undeath and Bare Life: Biopolitics and the Gothic in Contemporary British Fiction."

Uzo Dibia is a poet and consultant in acute and general medicine with the Metro-North Hospital and health service, based at Caboolture Hospital, where he heads the hospital in the home (HITH) unit. He is also Senior Lecturer with the University of Queensland medical school. After graduating with a bachelor of medicine and surgery degree from the University of Ibadan, Nigeria, he commenced his postgraduate training in the United Kingdom and then moved to Australia where he completed a fellowship in acute and general medicine. He holds master's degrees in public health and health management from the University of New South Wales, Sydney, and his interests are in the treatment of soft tissue infections in the home setting, clinical governance and the use of literature as a means to understanding the patient's experience.

Xavier Escribano (Barcelona, 1970) obtained his doctoral degree in philosophy at the Universitat de Barcelona (2003). Currently a lecturer in philosophical anthropology at the Universitat Internacional de Catalunya (UIC), his main research interests concern theories and concepts of human embodiment, especially in contemporary thought, and the relationship between humanism and health. He is a member of the Phenomenological Studies Group of the Catalan Philosophical Association, as well as of the Spanish Society for Phenomenology. He is currently the director of the research project *Anthropology of Corporeality/Interdisciplinary Studies in Embodied Subjectivity* (UIC 2012–2015) and the coordinator of the SARX research group on the anthropology of corporeality.

Ian Frazer is a clinician scientist, trained as a clinical immunologist in Scotland. As a professor at the University of Queensland, he leads a research group working at TRI in Brisbane, Australia on the immunobiology of epithelial cancers. He is recognised as co-inventor of the technology enabling the HPV vaccines, currently used worldwide to help prevent cervical cancer. He heads a biotechnology company, Admedus Vaccines, working on new vaccine technologies, and is a board member of several companies and not-for-profit organisations. He is the current president of the Australian Academy of Health and Medical Sciences, and a member of the Commonwealth Science Council, and was most recently appointed chair of the federal government's Medical Research Future Fund. Professor Frazer was recognised as Australian of the Year in 2006. He was recipient of the Prime Minister's Prize for Science, and of the Balzan Prize, in 2008, and was elected Fellow of the Royal Society of London in 2012. He was appointed Companion of the Order of Australia in the Queen's Birthday Honours list in 2013.

Anna Gasperini received her PhD from the National University of Ireland Galway, where she completed a thesis on discourses of ethics, monstrosity and medicine in the Victorian penny blood. She co-edited for Palgrave Macmillan the collection of essays *Media and Print Culture Consumption in Nineteenth-Century Britain: The Victorian Reading Experience* (2016), and she is the current Membership Secretary of the Victorian Popular Fiction Association (VPFA). Her research interests include Victorian cheap serialised fiction, popular culture and popular fiction, and the relationship between Victorian literature and medicine.

Jennifer Greenwood trained as a nurse, midwife and teacher before training as a philosopher. She was awarded a PhD in Education from the University of Leeds in 2000 and she held a variety of positions in the operational and strategic management of health services in the UK before emigrating to Australia. In Australia, she was a Professor of Nursing for eight years at the University of Western Sydney prior to moving to Canada. Her special interests as a nurse were evidence-based practice development and qualitative research methodology. Jennifer spent five years in Canada training as a philosopher and returned to Australia to research for her PhD (2013) at the University of Queensland. Her special interests in philosophy are the philosophy of emotion and mind. She is currently researching the philosophy of pain. Jennifer teaches philosophy at the University of Queensland and tutors in nursing, in education and in philosophy at Emmanuel College, University of Queensland.

Catherine Jenkins holds a PhD in Communication and Culture from Ryerson-York Universities in Toronto, Canada. Fostered by her experience teaching communication skills to healthcare students and professionals at the University of Toronto, her research explores the impact of healthcare technologies on patient-practitioner communication. She currently teaches Professional Communication at Ryerson University. Her article "Curing Venice's Plagues: Pharmacology and Witchcraft" was published in the journal *Postmedieval*'s special medical humanities issue (2017). She has published book chapters in the peer-reviewed anthologies *Finding McLuhan* (2015) and *The Power of Death* (2014) and has several other book chapters forthcoming. Her current research interests remain in medical humanities and cultural studies, including the medicalisation of comic book superheroes.

Hannah Lesshafft is a Research and Teaching Fellow at the Medical School, University of Edinburgh and a member of the Edinburgh Centre for Medical Anthropology. She trained and worked as a medical doctor and obtained a research doctorate degree from the Charité School of Medicine, Berlin, before she completed an MSc degree in Medical Anthropology and a PhD in Social Anthropology at the University of Edinburgh. Hannah has conducted research in Brazil on the social exclusion of leprosy patients, cutaneous larva migrans (a poverty-associated parasitic skin disease), and on healing and the notion of care in the Afro-Brazilian religion Candomblé. Currently, she works on a mixed-methods study on video consultations in primary care in Scotland and teaches social aspects of medicine. Her main research interests include ritual practice in biomedicine and traditional healing, the placebo effect, social movements, practices of care and most recently environmental medical anthropology.

Bonnie Millar is the Musculoskeletal Project Manager within the NIHR Nottingham Biomedical Research Centre in the School of Medicine, University of Nottingham. She has authored a critical study of the "Siege of Jerusalem," and has published extensively on alliterative poetry, medieval romances, gender theory, disability studies, medical humanities and sound studies. Recent publications include a paper entitled "Hero or Jester: Gawain in Middle English Romances and Ballads" in *Le Personnage de Gauvain dans la literature européenne de Moyen Âge*, a chapter on "Key Critics, Concepts & Topics" in the *Continuum Handbook of Medieval British Literature*, "A Measure of Courtliness: Sir Gawain and the Carl of Carlisle" in *Cultures Courtoises en Mouvement: Proceedings of the Thirteenth Congress of the International Society of Courtly Literature* and "Naming and Un-naming: Cynewulf's Runic Signatures" in *La constucció d'identitats imaginades*.

Current projects include the analysis of Tinnitus narratives, an exploration of the language of Tinnitus and a full-length study of Gawain in Middle English and Early Modern English romances and ballads.

Hazel Morrison most recently held the post of Research Associate at Durham University, on the Volkswagen Foundation-funded project "Wandering Minds: Interdisciplinary Experiments on Self-generated Thought," 2016–2017. Before this, she graduated in 2014 from the University of Glasgow with a PhD in historical human geography, specialising in the history of psychiatry. Her specialism is the study of the dynamic, or psychobiological, approach to psychiatry as employed by early twentieth-century Scottish psychiatrist Dr David Kennedy Henderson. An in-depth hermeneutic engagement with the patient case note records of Gartnavel, Glasgow's Royal Mental Hospital (1921–1932), enabled her work to explore the development of psychiatric knowledges from *within* clinical encounters. Taking methodological and theoretical influence from research emerging in the interdisciplinary spheres of the medical humanities, her aim is to understand the agency of both patient and psychiatrist in shaping the history of psychiatry.

April Patrick is the Director of the University Honors Program and faculty in Literature at Fairleigh Dickinson University's Florham Campus. Her work and reviews have appeared in *Victorian Periodicals Review* and *Victorian Review*. She is one of three Co-Directors of *Periodical Poetry*, an index of poetry published in nineteenth-century periodicals, and is currently working on a project about nineteenth-century breast cancer narratives.

Michelle Pfeffer is a PhD candidate at the University of Queensland's Institute for Advanced Studies in the Humanities and is concurrently completing a Master of Science in History of Science, Medicine and Technology at the University of Oxford. Her research explores the multifaceted discussions about the human soul in the seventeenth and eighteenth centuries, which embraced scientific, philosophical, medical, theological and historical discourses. Her particular interests lie in the contentious debates over the immortal and immaterial nature of the human soul. Other research interests include early modern medicine, the history of scholarship and religiously motivated responses to contemporary "materialist" science.

Andrea Rodríguez-Prat (Barcelona, 1988) obtained a degree in humanities (2010) and a master's in nursing and health research (2014). She is currently a lecturer in philosophical anthropology at the Universitat Internacional de Catalunya (UIC). As a research member of the *WeCare Chair: End-of-life Care* at the UIC she brings her humanistic background (and especially a philosophical/anthropological perspective) to the biomedical and experimental sphere. Currently her main research interests are focused on the concepts of dignity, autonomy and the wish to hasten death in the end-of-life context. She is also interested in the phenomenology of embodiment and illness, and in the experience of suffering, death and dying from the perspective of the history of mental illness, cultural anthropology and qualitative analysis.

Patrick Seniuk is a doctoral student at the Centre for Studies in Practical Knowledge at Södertörns University in Stockholm. His background in philosophy and bioethics has led him to specialise in existential-phenomenology and philosophy of psychiatry. His dissertation addresses the way in which clinical psychiatry conceptualises selfhood in depression. The dissertation is part of a larger project entitled "Phenomenology of Suffering in Medicine in the Baltic Sea Region," which encompasses topics such as teaching of medical ethics, bioethics and personhood, and the nature of empathy in medicine.

Carmen Voinea is a PhD student at the Faculty of Sociology and Social Work, University of Bucharest. Her research is exploring the plastic surgery phenomenon in Romania, concentrating on the negotiation of the surgical change between the patient and the aesthetic surgeon as reflexive actors in the context of a consumer society. She has a bachelor's degree in political sciences from the University of Bucharest and a master's degree from the Faculty of Sociology and Social Work, University of Bucharest.

Corinna Wagner is Associate Professor in Literature and Visual Culture at the University of Exeter. Her research interests include Victorian art, architecture and photography, and the relationship between medicine and the arts. Her books include *Pathological Bodies: Medicine and Political Culture* (California UP, 2013) and with Joanne Parker, *Art and Soul: Victorians and the Gothic* (Sansom, 2014). She has also edited *A Body of Work: An Anthology of Poetry and Medicine* (with Andy Brown, Bloomsbury, 2015) and *Gothic Evolutions: Poetry, Tales, Context, Theory* (Broadview, 2014). She is completing a monograph titled *Art and Anatomy: The Body and Visual Culture*.

Foreword

Medicine, health and being human

Ian Frazer

We live in an increasingly technology-led, business-oriented and time-poor age, in which the *art* of medicine, and the essential humanity of the interaction between patient and doctor, is at risk of being relegated to second place behind the science of "precision medicine." While the practice of medicine is, appropriately, increasingly assisted by new technologies which are giving new insights into diagnosis and management of disease, these technologies have tended to separate the health care practitioner from direct contact with the patient seeking help. The collection of essays that make up this book serve to remind us of the complexity of the relationships between body and mind and between health and disease and draw the distinction between the patient as a human being and as an object to be examined and managed. The reader of these essays should enjoy and benefit from the insights provided by the various essayists, who have drawn on a diverse selection of perspectives on this topic. Hopefully, they will come away a wiser and more thoughtful person from their reading, whether they approach the topic of health and disease as a patient, a caregiver or a philosopher.

Acknowledgements

Within 36 hours of my birth, I was rushed interstate for a seven-hour life-saving operation. This operation was performed by Dr Des McGuckin and his team at the Mater Hospital in Brisbane. Throughout my childhood I would return to Dr McGuckin for consultations on my progress. He was the only doctor I looked forward to seeing, perhaps partly because of the adventure of travelling away from home to do so, but also because he was kind and had a funny beard. In general, though, with the excess of doctors in my young life, I didn't like them; at best, the relationship was fraught. Doctors were associated with pain, with my childhood inability to understand why they couldn't make everything better, and my frustration that they didn't seem to understand what my feelings were. By the time I was a precocious 10-year old, I felt like I knew more about medicine than they did – at least about my own health.

In a lot of ways, that childhood experience undergirds my interest in the themes of this book: the relationship between the doctor's and the patient's humanity; the capacity to communicate; angst regarding the medical profession; and the willingness to accept the doctor's limitations. I grew up with the unfair image of doctors as failed gods: they were meant to be able to fix everything, but inevitably didn't succeed in doing so. As an adult, of course, I look back with incredible gratitude, especially for that life-saving surgery and the kindness of my specialist, who was known for understanding how to treat sick children with compassion. But at the same time, I can appreciate the clinical distance that, as Jane Macnaughton observes, helps to maintain the dignity of the patient when in a position of vulnerability: it helps not to think of the doctor as a human being with thoughts, feelings and flaws as you are exposed before them. These tensions remain something to grapple with, a part of the complexities of human expectations.

In a practical sense, this volume began as a part of an interdisciplinary research group I ran, in which our conversations persistently returned to questions of health, well-being and ethics. Stewart Gill, Master of Queen's College, University of Melbourne, was particularly supportive of the project from the start, as were longstanding members of the group who didn't end up contributing chapters to the volume, but were instrumental in its formation: Charlotte Chambers, Myles Lawrence, Marissa Daniels, Prue Ahrens and Stephen Young each played a significant role in the shape of the volume, and contributed to the inter-disciplinary conversations that, most crucially, connected contemporary concerns regarding medical culture across historical frameworks and disciplinary boundaries. Anna Ritt was also of great assistance in drawing together the current state of the medical humanities from the perspective of a medical student.

I would also like to thank Katherine Inglis at the University of Edinburgh, and Jane Macnaughton and Angela Woods at Durham University's Centre for Medical Humanities for their support of this project, for their advice as well as helping me find the right contributors for this collection. In particular, I am grateful for Professor Ian Frazer's support of the project from its inception, and Shelley Templeman for helping to make it happen.

Each of my contributors has shown great patience and faith, agreeing to work on the project before publication was guaranteed. Their commitment to *Medicine, Health and Being Human* has been extraordinary, especially given the complications and difficulties some of them experienced through the process of writing. I'm so grateful for their willingness to work on this book, and for their vision to see an increased conversation between the medical sciences and various humanities and social science disciplines. At Routledge, I'd like to thank Grace McInnes for believing in this project, Carolina Antunes, for her friendly and helpful efficiency throughout, and the anonymous readers, whose feedback helped significantly in bringing the book together.

It would be remiss not to thank my adopted family – the team at the Armstrong Browning Library at Baylor University in Waco, Texas – for providing me with an amazing space to work, first with a one-month fellowship in 2017, and then on my ad hoc return visits. You always welcome me back with open arms. My parents continue to give me unwavering support in all of my endeavours. Finally, I would like to thank Professor Mike McGuckin, Dr Des McGuckin's son, who gave me more insight in the man behind the beard: a passionate, caring doctor who knew how to enjoy the diversity and beauty of life, with a deep love for music and the theatre. Having a window into the humanity of the man who saved my life gives me a profound sense of wholeness; and I hope that he would be pleased to know that his legacy is living on through both medicine and the humanities.

Introduction
Medicine and modernity

Lesa Scholl

Over the past decade in particular, the medical humanities have become a significant field for interdisciplinary study, drawing attention from the sciences in relation to "humanising" medical students, and from the humanities as a form of legitimisation and research impact. Yet such binaries are potentially reductive and unsatisfactory in addressing the role or importance of medical humanities in current scholarship, or its potential to impact future generations of society. Alan Bleakley has observed quite rightly that "Science study has ... progressively claimed and partially eroded the ground of a liberal education once thought to be an essential background for practicing medicine," arguing:

> The benefits of scientific and technological advances in medicine are clear and we might say that the erosion of the art of medicine is a small price to pay for advances in population health. However, this erosion of the human face of medicine is a symptom of a wider structural problem – that of the continuing dominance of hierarchical clinical teamwork that favours doctors and marginalizes other healthcare professionals and patients.
>
> (2015, 9)

Similarly, Sander Gilman has emphasised in *Illness and Image* (2015) that the medical humanities are crucial and intrinsic to all health sciences, including "nursing, public health, dentistry, disability studies, and all other fields that deal with human illness and wellness" (xi), deliberately extending the definition of medicine itself. Indeed, medicine is being challenged to broaden its concepts of wellness and illness. Des Fitzgerald and Felicity Callard suggest that "If the task is to think how practices of making, breaking and shifting boundaries constitute moments of illness and healing," the medical humanities have a role in defining those boundaries, and simultaneously the boundaries of what constitutes humanity: "we need to displace, if not significantly reimagine, how medical humanities has tended to figure the 'human' – an entity whose boundaries have commonly been understood to end at her skin" (2016, 43).

Indeed, given the growth of focus on mental wellness and illness, and its impact on physical health, questions arise regarding how wellness and illness can be identified in and through the body, primarily centred in sensory experience. In the 1960s, Georges Canguilhem evoked René Leriche's "life lived in the silence of the organs" to suggest that "[t]he state of health is a state of unawareness where the subject and his [*sic*] body are one. Conversely, the awareness of the body consists in a feeling of limits, threats, obstacles to health" (Canguilhem [1966] 1978, 46). Although Canguilhem acknowledges, as Leriche does, that "the silence of the organs does not necessarily equal the absence of disease, that there are functional lesions or perturbations which long remain imperceptible to those whose lives they endanger," he importantly draws attention to the role of sensory awareness in understanding disease, and the problems of the "invalidity of the sick man's judgement concerning the reality of his own illness" (46). Jo Winning asks fundamental questions regarding the relationship between the body, human identity and sensory experience: "What *is* a body? What are its boundaries and its contours? Can we ever really know the body in its entirety, or only ever in its parts? How do we come to know the body through the senses?" and finally, "what does it mean to *be* a body and to encounter the body of the Other?" (2016, 325) In a similar manner, sensory historians David Howes and Constance Classen have suggested that as "'gateways' to the body, the senses [seem] eminently suited to receive influences that could either benefit or injure the body" (Howes and Classen 2014, 38). Thus, interactions between the mind and body, including the mind's perceptions of the body, and therefore the interactions between science, social science and humanities, become central to understanding what it means to be human.

While the medical humanities began with pleas to incorporate and "make space" for the humanities in the training of doctors, as seen in articles, for example, in the longstanding medical journal *The Lancet* in the early 2000s, the field has developed to critique its own position, constituting a much broader stance and clearer definitions through the contributions of key scholars such as Angela Wood, Jane Macnaughton, Felicity Callard and William Viney. Macnaughton has observed that there are historical and political reasons for the characterisation of medical humanities as a field of studies designed to help doctors learn to "do what they are already doing in a more humane, empathetic way" while not interfering with "medicine itself" (2011, 928). Yet she also points towards the "much bolder intention" of current medical humanities (928), with "a compelling vision of human nature, informed by philosophy, illustrated and explored in literature and the other creative arts, assumed by the empirical enthnographic and qualitative methods of social science" (929). However, while Macnaughton goes on to say that medical humanities has failed to take its agenda "forward into collaborative discussion with those at the forefront of policy and research in medicine so that it can inform the basis of decision making about how medicine is practiced" (929–30), this failure is one aspect that *Medicine, Health and Being Human* seeks to address – not as a definitive project, but to open up conversations between medical practitioners and researchers, alongside humanities and social science scholars, from across the globe, who are concerned about the narrowing of medicine to medical science that has been occurring since the early modern period.

Unwieldy in its expanse, the medical humanities is now at once a critical force but also a field that struggles for clear territory within scholarly culture: it seems that everyone wants to get onto the medical humanities bandwagon. This volume could begin with the question as to why this bandwagon exists. What is it about the concept of medical humanities that is so appealing to the scholarly mind, regardless of fields of disciplinary training? Through tracing a history of medical thought, it is evident that medicine, in broad terms, has played a crucial role in the development of modernity, and therefore current understandings of culture, society and what it means to be human. With the growing body of material exploring medicine through humanist lenses, as well as the critical need to define a position within the field, this project specifically addresses the medi-calised body and the idea of the human being, through an historical trajectory. As Corinne Saunders suggests, it is crucial to understand that a "properly critical medical humanities is also a historically grounded medical humanities," yet this historical understanding needs to go beyond the established histories of disease, treatment and practice. Rather, it is necessary

> to trace the origins and development of the ideas that underpin medicine in its broadest sense – ideas concerning the most fundamental aspects of human existence: health and illness, body and mind, gender and family, care and community. Historical sources can only go so far in illuminating such topics; we must also look to other cultural texts, and in particular literary texts, which, through their imaginative worlds, provide crucial insights into cultural and intellectual attitudes, experience and creativity. Reading from a critical medical humanities perspective requires not only cultural archae-ology across a range of discourses, but also putting past and present into conversation, to discover continuities and contrasts with later perspectives.
>
> (Saunders 2016, 411)

Saunders' observations in relation to the incorporation of the types of history are at the heart of this project, hence the inclusion of cultural history, literary history, anthropology and philosophy, to name a few. The boundaries of the human body can be in conflict with the boundaries of the human being. Knowing the body and knowing the human, and understanding the differing boundaries of these two concepts, reflects in many ways the conflicting and expansive boundaries of medical humanities. Indeed, the latest research into critical medical humanities provides useful conceptual frameworks for understanding how human society has reached its current position. In their introduction to *The Edinburgh Compan-ion to the Critical Medical Humanities* (2016), Anne Whitehead and Angela Woods aptly reposition medical humanities by building on what they refer to as the three Es of the medical humanities (ethics, education and experience) with a fourth E, entanglement. Through the idea of entangling disciplines, Whitehead and Woods move away from the oppositional tradition of medical humanities to reflect more appropriately the base of the field in "mobility, fluidity, movement: a creative boundary-crossing in and through which new possibilities can emerge" (8).

This vision resonates with our project here, which brings together scholars and medical practitioners, as well as medical practitioners turned humanities and social science scholars; but it also speaks to the dislocation of human identity within the body – a feature of modernity that has roots in the rise of liberal capitalism as much as the medicalisation of both philosophy and science, both of which emerge in the early modern period.

The boundaries of being human

The fluid, mobile boundaries of the medical humanities speak figuratively to the boundaries of the human body/human being as well as the boundaries of medicine's remit. As much as questions arise about the role of the mind in defining humanity, the implications for differences and changes in the body, or even the humanity within the decomposing human body, these same questions can be applied to the changing nature of medicine. Yet it is just as important to realise that while the theoretical approach of medical humanities is new, the tensions regarding the remit of medicine are not. In the middle of the nineteenth century, the Canadian physician William Osler wrote, "The practice of medicine is an art, not a trade; a calling, not a business; a calling in which your heart will be exercised equally with your head" (qtd in Bleakley 2015, 10). More recently, Howes and Classen have observed, somewhat tongue-in-cheek:

> And while medicine may be referred to as an "art," aesthetics is not really considered to play any role in it. In fact, a library or internet search for discussions on the aesthetics of medicine is likely to simply turn up works on cosmetic surgery.
>
> (2014, 38)

The pressures of science and economics upon the humanising nature of the arts of medicine have clear historic precedence; and so, the rise of medical humanities emerges, as Claire Hooker suggests, from "concerns, often expressed by doctors as well as critics, that medical practice has become distanced from 'the human side of medicine' as it has become more technically accomplished" (Hooker 2014, 214). Yet, this volume reveals that the impact of technical advancement on medicine is not a twenty-first-century, or even twentieth-century development, but one that is tied inherently to the centuries-old project of modernity.

While the technical advances of medical science are certainly not to be regretted, the medical humanities provide an important critical role that maintains the necessary tension between science, economics and the human figure. As Viney (2015) suggests, this does not need to be an adversarial relationship, but one that, through entanglement, acknowledges the vital aspects of each field in speaking to the definition of how human wellness and illness ought to be considered. To return to our particular focus here, the identity of the human being in relationship to the human body is the critical arena for this entanglement. Deborah Bowman argues:

The confining effects of identity are felt too by those who become patients, from the mundane, but significant, dehumanisation that occurs when a person is distilled into a hospital number, test results, systemic pathologies or bed location to the existential crises to which illness and suffering give rise. Diseases too are telescoped into singular identities in which a particular narrative, often predicated on a reductive or mechanistic account, dominates discourse, leading to what Havi Carel describes as "epistemic injustice." The privileging of particular ways of describing illness or disease has significant implications for how we identify and respond to illness. It represents a clash of identities: the collision of personal, professional, individual, systemic and epistemological identities in which multiplicity of meaning may be unseen, disregarded, misunderstood or diminished.

(Bowman 2015, 1)

With this context in mind, the capacity for self-care becomes a means of re-establishing human identity and human agency, but this identity or agency crucially extends beyond the physical human body. In this sense, the body becomes an ironic space, for, as Jonathan Cole and Shaun Gallagher have observed, in a similar vein to Canguilhem, "in most healthy, everyday activities, the body-as-subject remains phenomenologically absent," and it is only when we get sick or injured – that is, we become patients – that we "change our conscious attitude towards the body – it becomes more present as an object to be considered" (Cole and Gallagher 2016, 379). Cole and Gallagher go on to state provocatively that "much of medicine is concerned with a breakdown of the absence of the body, or of habitual (and in some sense thoughtless) agency" (379), a claim that reveals humanity's psychological desire to distance itself from its fragilities and temporality. Medicine's intervention, then, can be seen as a means to reinstate, as much as possible, the myth of perpetuity, and it is seen to fail when this myth is not achieved. Moreover, medicine is used in attempts to regain perceived lack of agency, as expressed by Luna Dolezal:

The notion that the body can be changed at will in order to meet the desires and designs of its "owner" is one that has captured the popular imagination and underpins contemporary medical practices such as cosmetic surgery and gender reassignment. In fact, describing the body as "malleable" or "plastic" has entered common parlance and dictates common-sense ideas of how we understand the human body in late-capitalist consumer societies in the wake of commercial biotechnologies that work to modify the body aesthetically or otherwise.

(Dolezal 2016, 310)

Within the impossible desire to maintain authority over bodies that will ultimately fail, the medical humanities are also positioned to help moderate the limitations of medicine, as well as extend the capacities of the individual human to establish the agency that is possible, through the recognition of the aspects of the human that go beyond the physical body.

Exploring what it means to be human

Underlying each section of *Medicine, Health and Being Human* is a recognition of the tension between the human being and the human body, and the consequent understandings of human identity, whether that identity is exerted through individual, communal or sociocultural agency. As in any study, there are limits to what can be covered, necessarily in a volume seeking to contribute to a field as vast as the medical humanities. The most obvious limit here is that, apart from forays into Brazil and South Korea, our study is primarily contained within a West-centric medical and historical tradition. Within this scope, it engages with a variety of forms and concepts that contribute to understandings of humanness, from discussions of the human soul to the human body, human identity and human rights, as well as the lines drawn between the human and animals, monsters, and technology. The three sections follow a narrative path from exploring the integrity of the human soul, through to the perception of the material human body, and then to the limits of medical intervention when that body breaks down. Each section maps an historical trajectory to the present in order to emphasise the entwined development – one might say, entangled development – of medicine and culture. Appropriately, the volume begins with Michelle Pfeffer's "Physicians and the soul," which, in opening the section on "Situating the soul, self, and mind," pinpoints a significant moment of transition in early-modern medical science, where a shift took place from positioning medicine within theological or spiritual responses to health and wellness, to an arguably scientific vision of humanity. Crucially, Pfeffer's work is not focused on physicians providing spiritual or moral support to patients, but rather exploring the way that the relationships and boundaries between spirituality, medicine and health were negotiated in ways that radically affected understandings of "humanness." Bonnie Millar, working within the medieval context, uses the historical examples of Margery Kempe, Julian of Norwich and Hildegard of Bingen, and the way these women describe their communication with the divine through the auditory, to critique the understanding of human relationship to the sensory world. The sensory components that contribute to self-identification have a significant impact on the understanding of others, whether by clinicians or the community, as well as one's understanding of self. The fragility of sensory reception, and its potential to fail – hearing "more" or "less" than is considered within the realm of the rational, for example – strongly controverts the realist agenda of modernity, as does the capacity of the human mind to exceed the present to visit the past and future. However, medical thought has been able to contain extremes of sensory experience through psychiatry. Through the nineteenth and twentieth centuries, rather than seeing figures like Margery Kempe as seers (or hearers) of the divine, medicine sought to contain, as Hazel Morrison's chapter discusses, the human mental life, which "is not always tethered to the here and now."

Patrick Seniuk's chapter brings the discussion of the mind, soul and psychiatry through to the present day, challenging the ways in which the disorder categories of the *Diagnostic and Statistical Manual of Mental Disorders* (DSM) were constructed to classify, manage and contain human identity, while at the same time demarcating the limitations of what is acceptable for human experience in scientific terms. The diagnosis of a psychiatric disorder thus amounts to a medicalised understanding of the human identity. Seniuk's critique brings to the fore the limitations and silences in psychiatry that affect the reliability of conceptualising mental disorder. Medical practitioner turned anthropologist Hannah Lesshafft's chapter bookends Part I by stepping back from the individual human identity to look more ethnographically and anthropologically at the ways in which contemporary medicine has been used to construct more communal boundaries of humanness. Lesshafft draws a comparison between the Westernised, scientific use of randomised controlled trials (RCT) and the ritual healing practices of the Afro-Brazilian Candomblé community to interrogate the role of the placebo effect in healing. This cross-cultural approach crucially questions the ideology of scientific objectivity in evidence-based medicine. In this way, Lesshafft challenges the medical boundaries established through derogatory terms such as "quackery" and "charlatanry," and even more importantly, argues that RCT are not able to cancel out human subjectivity and meaning responses.

Part I's engagement with theology, philosophy, science and psychiatry is centred primarily on the individual's human identity – what can make up that identity physically and mentally, and how those definitions can be contained. Part II, "Socio-Medical Narratives," critiques the ways in which medical science, or the pursuit of scientific knowledge, has been used to justify the dehumanisation of various groups, based on race, ethnicity, and ultimately a perception of an unattainable norm of humanity. Professor of nursing turned philosopher Jennifer Greenwood explores the uses of medical trials, and the ways in which medical research has been used historically to justify marginalisation, discrimination, and even genocide, with examples from Nazi medical experimentation to the Tuskegee syphilis study. M. Renee Benham continues the discussion of medical narratives in the early twentieth century, turning though, to perceptions of nursing and efficiency. The mechanisation of health care, and the loss of emotion on the part of the carer, is figured as a loss of humanity. Benham addresses the tension between efficient and sympathetic care in the attempt to maintain humanity, in the context of the Great War, where one was faced with death and the inability to save lives continually.

Given the potential dangers associated with experimentation and efficiency at the cost of human sympathy, Anna Gasperini's discussion of the figure of the doctor in vampire narratives, as well as the iconic Frankenstein trope, takes on a critical role in the way that medical thought has impacted communal and individual understandings of being human, and the human's position in the world. Gasperini triangulates the concept of "medically improving humanity" through these narratives, the potential for such improvements to lead to "inhumanity," and the agency of the medical scientist to examine the tensions and fears surrounding the material body and the perceived necessity of medicalised improvement of nature as a means of avoiding the boundary between life and death. Corinna Wagner's chapter also contends with the distrust of science, synthesising strands from the history of medicine, literary studies and art history to rethink the nineteenth century's modernist quest for "the real." In particular, Wagner addresses the impact this agenda had in understanding the human being through anatomical and physiological knowledge as means to contain identity, and examines the disillusionment of nineteenth-century artists, like John Ruskin, with the distinction between the impetus to teach art students anatomy, and the actual effects of its practice.

The focus on the physical body in Wagner's essay is a significant departure from the preceding chapters in the section, but it relates to the chapters on scientific experimentation, ethics and empathy by critiquing the ways in which both art and anatomical studies have contributed to human distancing through perceived differences, as well as creating "sympathy" or "common feeling" through recognising similarities. The collapsing of biological, moral and artistic classifications, Wagner argues, fundamentally changed the way the artist – now the "artist-anatomist" – perceives, which holds significant implications for the understanding of humanity and the human figure by redefining what is visually considered "real." The visual narrative at play was as much a redefinition of social narratives as it was applied to medical scholarship. Catherine Jenkins's chapter builds on this critique of the visual, turning to medical technologies such as x-rays, CT scans and MRIs, as means by which diagnostic narratives potentially reshape the patient's understanding of their own humanity. Jenkins questions the privileging of what she refers to as the "disembodied data over the patient voice," and explores the medicalised use of images of the interior human body as a challenge to human identity. This perspective is particularly provocative in relation to the two-dimensional image, a direction that raises questions regarding the limitations of objectivity in diagnosis derived from such images as a literal "flattening" of human identity.

While Part II appears to critique the intrusion of medical narratives on human identity, and the consequent distrust of the medical professions, Part III, "Limits of Medical Intervention," seeks to balance this judgement, acknowledging the limitations of medical science. As much as there is a distrust of doctors, the disillusionment related to it comes from an inability of the patient or the public to accept the humanity of the doctors themselves. This problem of perspective has been addressed by Jane Macnaughton in "Elegant Surgery" (2015), in which she refers to the persistent social narrative of surgeons as "men of action: heroes able to act decisively in moments of crisis, and without the tender sensibility that shunned physical contact with their patients" (Macnaughton 2015, 193). Importantly, Macnaughton addresses the distance of medical practitioners – their "cool intimacy" (175) – as an attitude that is necessary to the retention of the humanity of both the doctor and the patient:

> In modern medical education, surgeons are often the butt of semi-humorous jibes about their lack of communications skills. The word "elegant" is not warm and cuddly; it is standoffish and slightly forbidding, cool in fact. I suspect that for many patients, this is the image they have of their surgeons,

and this is the way that surgeons like to see their work. For patients and for surgeons this emotional distance is necessary. Most patients awaiting the knife do not like to reflect too closely on the nature of the operation, and find it helpful to regard the surgeon as an infallible genius who can deal coolly with any crisis that may arise. Surgeons in turn may themselves find it easier not to be too emotionally aware of the individual with whose flesh they must become intimately, and elegantly, entangled.

(2015, 196)

Yet even within this context, there is an increasing desire to understand proximity, and a quest to find a way to be proximate and human while maintaining professionality on the one hand, and dignity on the other. Both the doctor and the patient, as human beings, have a right to sentient agency; yet in the terms of the doctor-patient relationship, the boundaries of agency are challenged. Carmen Voinea addresses ideas of human agency through her discussion of social narratives of plastic surgery in the South Korean make-over TV show, *Let Me In*. The "before and after" narratives provide individuals with a sense of authority and power over their life narratives, even though this intervention requires the work of the surgeon, and both patient and surgeon borrow terminology from each other's position to negotiate the narratives of physical evaluation and identity. Yet ultimately the relationship is one of the "patient" (or game-show contestant) depending on the surgeons, not just to mend a perceived physical defect, but in doing so, to improve their socio-economic position. In the context of these shows, the doctors, rather than affirming their human limitations, actively assume a social position of god-like power.

Kathryn Bird addresses what she terms "medicine's historical investment in obtaining and anatomising exceptional bodies in its quest to produce a norm of human embodiment." In doing so, however, she brings to light the failure of bodily, human coherence. She explores the ways in which dehumanised forms are "worked" and "sold" through twentieth-century novels by Alasdair Gray and Hilary Mantel. Building on the Frankenstein model, Bird examines the definitions of the human form in the history of medicine, and the compulsion to dissect that which is considered monstrous. April Patrick's chapter draws out this "conflict between medicalised body and the human being," and attempts to reconcile "medical realism" and "humane sympathy" through her readings of literary medical figures. The short stories by Dr John Brown and Katharine Tynan that Patrick examines provide narrative examples of the medical practitioner's recognition of the impact of illness, not just on their patients' bodies, but on their broader lives, dealing specifically with cases of breast cancer. The patient characters not only face their own mortality but also losing their identities as women through the breakdown of the integrity of their body: their "female" form. The doctors retain their humanity, and are written as comforting their patients who are dying, or whose bodies become unalterably fragmented through mastectomies.

Uzo Dibia's chapter provides a crucial intervention at this point, providing a medical doctor's perspective on the role of literary study and narrative in medical practice. As a medical consultant, Dibia engages with the literary works of Chekov, Kafka, Solzhenitsyn and T.S. Eliot, specifically in relation to their doctor figures who grapple with their own humanity, as well as that of their patients. He argues that the literary space enables such exploration and reflection for the "real" medical practitioner, particularly when facing limitations of scientific capacity. Dibia argues that there has been a disconnect from humanity as medical science has progressed technologically; yet one of the most provocative aspects of his chapter is the way in which he positions the physician in relation to end of life moments and the rehabilitation of patients who have nearly evaded death. Dibia uses these literary cases as examples of narratives that can help lead medical practitioners "back to the tenets of empathy, patience and understanding of ourselves" – importantly the physician's understanding of him or herself as likewise human.

Rodríguez-Prat and Escribano appropriately close the volume with a history of the communication between health professionals and patients (in broad terms) that death is unavoidable – not just as a general concept, but for the individual human. While this chapter, as well as Dibia's, can be seen as a departure from the "entanglement" framework, returning to ideas of "humanising" healthcare, it remains an important inclusion because it addresses the ways in which healthcare professionals need to contend with the limits of their capacities once a patient can no longer be helped, or passes away. While the medicalisation of the human figure and the development of technology have sanitised and distanced humanity *for a time* from the reality of death, Rodríguez-Prat and Escribano offer a humanist perspective on the power of language to transcend scientific models of mortality management. The ultimate inability of science to prevent death is a clear demarcation of its limitations; and as a result, the humanities need to step into the breach in an attempt to bring reconciliation to the individual human's "vulnerability, dependency and finitude," the "self that feels fragmented by illness." Rodríguez-Prat and Escribano argue that the dialogue of imminent death is "hampered" by scientific jargon and look to identify the ways in which words can be used therapeutically and palliatively, which is important both for the patient and the medical professional.

The limits of science and the humanities, rather than being in opposition, flow into and through each other towards defining what it means to be human. Within this study's trajectory from the medieval to the contemporary world, and spanning the globe in terms of contributors and locations of case studies, what undergirds the project is the understanding that incremental historical and cultural influences have brought humanity to its current relationship with medicine, in which the medical is ingrained, sometimes consciously, sometimes unconsciously, and usually as a mode of legitimisation. Yet as the borders of medicine's power to provide legitimacy fail, it is important to realise the ways in which medicine itself, rather than being pure, objective science, is influenced and shaped by cultural, economic and social privileging. We engage with questions that Otniel Dror raises about medical knowledge, such as racial and gender assumptions and the "variety of cultural and social forces that define, categorize, and constitute 'disease' and 'health'" (2007, 318), with a desire to forward the project of the critical medical humanities to entangle disciplines from the sciences and humanities towards a clearer understanding of the human being both within the human body and within the human world.

Reference list

Bleakley, Alan. 2015. *Medical Humanities and Medical Education: How the Medical Humanities Can Shape Better Doctors*. London and New York: Routledge.

Bolton, Gillie. 2003. "Medicine, the arts, and the humanities," *The Lancet*, 362: 93–94.

Bowman, Deborah. 2014. "On identity in (the) *Medical Humanities*," *Medical Humanities*, 40.1: 1–2.

Bradby, Hannah. "Medical Migration and the Global Politics of Equality," in *The Edinburgh Companion to the Critical Medical Humanities*, edited by Anne Whitehead and Angela Woods, 491–507. Edinburgh: University of Edinburgh Press.

Brieger, Gert H. 2004. "Bodies and borders: a new cultural history of medicine," *Perspectives in Biology and Medicine*, 47.3: 402–21.

Bronfenbrenner, Urie, ed. 2005. *Making Human Beings Human: Bioecological Perspectives on Human Development*. Thousand Oaks, CA and London: Sage.

Canguilhem, Georges. [1966] 1978. *On the Normal and the Pathological*, translated by Carolyn R. Fawcett. Dordrecht: D. Reidel.

Chiapperino, Luca and Giovanni Boniolo. 2014. "Rethinking medical humanities," *Journal of Medical Humanities*, 35: 377–87.

Cole, Jonathan and Shaun Gallagher. 2016. "Narrative and Clinical Neuroscience: Can Phenomenologically Informed Approaches and Empirical Work Cross-Fertilise?" in *The Edinburgh Companion to the Critical Medical Humanities*, edited by Anne Whitehead and Angela Woods, 377–94. Edinburgh: University of Edinburgh Press.

Dolan, Brian. 2010. "Second opinions: history, medical humanities and medical education," *Social History of Medicine*, 23.2: 393–405.

Dolezal, Luna. 2016. "Morphological Freedom and Medicine: Constructing the Posthuman Body," in *The Edinburgh Companion to the Critical Medical Humanities*, edited by Anne Whitehead and Angela Woods, 310–24. Edinburgh: University of Edinburgh Press.

Dror, Otniel. 2011. "De-medicalizing the medical humanities," *The European Legacy*, 16.3: 317–26.

Fitzgerald, Des and Felicity Callard. 2016. "Entangling the Medical Humanities," in *The Edinburgh Companion to the Critical Medical Humanities*, edited by Anne Whitehead and Angela Woods, 35–49. Edinburgh: University of Edinburgh Press.

Gilman, Sander L. 2015. *Illness and Image: Case Studies in the Medical Humanities*. New Brunswick, NJ: Transaction.

Grant, V.J. 2002. "Making room for medical humanities," *Journal of Medical Ethics*, 28: 45–58.

Hooker, Claire. 2014. "Ethics and the Arts in the Medical Humanities," in *Ethics and the Arts*, edited by Paul MacNeill, 213–24. New York and London: Springer.

Howes, David and Constance Classen. 2014. *Ways of Sensing: Understanding the Senses in Society*. New York and London: Routledge.

Macnaughton, Jane. 2015. "'Elegant' Surgery: The Beauty of Clinical Expertise," in *The Recovery of Beauty: Arts, Culture, Medicine*, edited by Corinne Saunders, Jane Macnaughton and David Fuller, 175–98. Basingstoke: Palgrave Macmillan.

Macnaughton, Jane. 2011. "Medical humanities' challenge to medicine," *Journal of Evaluation in Clinical Practice*, 17: 927–32.

Pickersgill, Martyn. 2015. "Enhancement, ethics and society: towards an empirical research agenda for the medical humanities and social sciences," *Medical Humanities*, 41: 136–42.

Rees, Geoffrey. 2010. "The ethical imperative of medical humanities," *Journal of Medical Humanities*, 31: 267–77.

Saunders, Corinne. 2016. "Voices and Visions: Mind, Body and Affect in Medieval Writing," in *The Edinburgh Companion to the Critical Medical Humanities*, edited by Anne Whitehead and Angela Woods, 411–27. Edinburgh: University of Edinburgh Press.

Schleifer, Ronald and Jerry B. Vanatta. 2013. *The Chief Concern of Medicine: The Integration of the Medical Humanities and Narrative Knowledge into Medical Practices*. Ann Arbor: University of Michigan Press.

Shapiro, Johanna, Jack Coulehan, Delese Wear and Martha Montello. 2009. "Medical humanities and their discontents: definitions, critiques, and implications," *Academic Medicine*, 84.2: 192–98.

Sullivan, Erin. 2008. "The art of medicine: melancholy, medicine, and the arts," *The Lancet*, 372: 884–85.

Viney, William, Felicity Callard and Angela Woods. 2015. "Critical medical humanities: embracing entanglement, taking risks," *Medical Humanities*, 41: 2–7.

Whitehead, Anne and Angela Woods. 2016. "Introduction," in *The Edinburgh Companion to the Critical Medical Humanities*, edited by Anne Whitehead and Angela Woods, 1–34. Edinburgh: Edinburgh University Press.

Winning, Jo. 2016. "Afterword: The Body and the Senses," in *The Edinburgh Companion to the Critical Medical Humanities*, edited by Anne Whitehead and Angela Woods, 325–35. Edinburgh: University of Edinburgh Press.

Woods, Angela. 2011. "The limits of narrative: provocations for the medical humanities," *Medical Humanities*, 37: 73–78.

Part I

Situating the soul, self and mind

1 Physicians and the soul

Medicine and spirituality in seventeenth-century England

Michelle Pfeffer

There has been of late a vigorous interest in combining medical practice and spirituality to facilitate the provision of holistic patient treatment. According to this vision, it is only by considering the whole person – body, mind, soul and spirit – that optimal health can be obtained. What is at stake in these discussions is not only the connection between the "spiritual" and "biological" aspects of a person, but the very existence of a human soul and/or spirit. That is, a certain conception of "humanness" is a basic assumption of all claims for or against a combination of medicine and spirituality. This is important because the conceptual frameworks upon which medicine is practiced guide the ways that people see and define themselves. As Marilyn Schlitz has argued, if medicine plays a role in defining the human, then an "integrated" medical perspective "requires a deep examination of our core assumptions about reality and our place in it" (2011, 151).

The second half of the seventeenth century in England was a time when – like today – the relationship between the body, soul and spirit and the relations between medicine, spirituality and health were under negotiation. A key figure in these discussions was the Anglican and university-trained physician and anatomist Thomas Willis (1621–1675). Like today's supporters of spiritually inclusive medicine, Willis's views about humanity were the basis of his medical theory and practice. In this chapter, I will first examine common seventeenth-century ideas about the nature of the human and the study of the soul, showing how Willis reinforced and subverted different aspects of the mainstream position. From this point, I examine the ways Willis applied his philosophical ideas to his medical practice. His notion that the physician could and should play a role in healing the soul was built upon a complex blend of personal, theological, clinical and anatomical knowledge and experience. Crucially, Willis's work in turn served both to subvert and reaffirm different theological approaches to human nature in the seventeenth century, and the final section of the chapter will explore three religious responses to his widely read work. The fact that we can discern contrasting levels of acceptance of Willis's various findings suggests that medicine does not merely dictate what it means to be human, but instead provides a set of resources with which people can grapple, and accept, reject, or modify according to their pre-existing values and beliefs.

Despite originally intending a career in the church, Willis shifted his sights to medicine while studying at Oxford University and was awarded a Bachelor of Medicine in 1646. While his career began rather slowly in rural Oxfordshire, his rising social status on account of his involvement with prominent natural philosophers and his post as Sedleian Professor of Natural Philosophy from 1660 onwards meant that by the mid-1660s his career had advanced to such an extent that he was earning the large sum of £300 a year (Hawkins 2011). While a keen interest in chemistry in many ways guided his research, Willis soon became fascinated with anatomy and directed his attention to the soul and its relationship with the body. His medico-anatomical texts, *Cerebri anatome* (1664), *Pathologiae Cerebri et Nervosi Generis Specimen* (1667) and *De anima brutorum* (1672) in particular, were immediately influential.[1] In his application of medical and anatomical experience to the question of the soul, Willis was highly apologetic, in the sense that he was seeking a conception of the human that would fit with his clinical practice and his anatomical work as well as his religious beliefs (Bynum 1972). Willis constructed an understanding of the human that would go on to organise his approach to disease and illness. In early modern England, the human soul was typically considered the spiritual and immortal aspect of a person, and while Willis agreed with this vision, he also ensured that the soul was a medical patient.

Body, soul and spirit

In his first letter to the Thessalonians, St Paul wrote: "the very God of peace sanctify you wholly; and I pray God your whole spirit and soul and body be preserved blameless unto the coming of our Lord Jesus Christ" (1 Thessalonians 5:23). For Willis and the prevailing tide of opinion in the seventeenth century, these words were an accurate representation of the composition of a person. Humans possessed a body, a spirit, and an immortal, rational soul. While brute animals also had a body and a sensitive spirit (or sensitive soul), the rational soul was possessed by humans alone. The Bible was the foundational text of early modern English culture and implicated every area of society, so the scriptural support offered to this three-fold framework made it particularly attractive. But, like any text, the Bible could often mean different things to different people, and the same passages could be used to support divergent ideas and agendas. Accordingly, 1 Thessalonians 5:23 was combined with various "biological" understandings of humanity and mobilised in support of competing visions of humanness. For the most part disagreement centred on the spirit/soul that humans had in common with animals. Some, like Henry More, claimed that the sensitive soul of both humans and brutes was immaterial. Others, like René Descartes, believed that the word "spirit" in 1 Thessalonians referred to the "animal spirits," those extremely subtle particles in the nerves that controlled bodily functions like muscle movement, sense perception and the passions. Animal spirits were corporeal, but very "fine," and were therefore considered able to mediate between the physical body and the immaterial soul. Willis, however, like many of his contemporaries, complained that Descartes's distinction between the *res cogitans* and the *res extensa* did not adequately explain how two radically different substances could influence each other. Thus, Willis decided that a mediator was necessary, and his solution was the "corporeal soul," a refined and subtle substance that communicated between the body and soul (Willis 1683, 40–1).

The corporeal soul was composed of two parts: the "vital" spirit in the blood and the "sensitive" spirit in the brain and nerves (Willis 1681a, 95). While for Descartes the animal spirits belonged to "a totally different genus" from the rational soul (Descartes 1649, 131–3), for Willis the boundaries between soul, spirit and body were much more fluid (Bynum 1973, 456–7). Yet, for Willis, the human remained composed of a corporeal sensitive soul, an immaterial rational soul and a physical body, just as St Paul had described.

Whether they held the sensitive part of humans to be an immaterial soul, a corporeal soul or simply part of the body, early moderns saw a divide between the rational and sensitive aspects of humanity. This division implied that while the latter was the proper province of the physician and physiologist, the former was out of the bounds of naturalistic enquiry, knowable instead through metaphysics, theology and spiritual practices. The rational soul not only facilitated a relationship with God, but was responsible for what many saw as the two key aspects of the *imago dei*: thought and will. As an immaterial substance, it was believed to be incorruptible and thus liable only to moral and spiritual decay. The sensitive, corporeal part, meanwhile, responsible for the bodily functions of growth, nutrition and sense, was susceptible to physical disease and decay. Yet because the rational soul, residing in the brain, relied upon the "Images and Impressions" of the corporeal soul in order to exercise reason, judgement and will, its "mental" functions were liable to deteriorate with the sensitive ones (Willis 1683, 32). The health of the rational soul relied on the health of the corporeal soul, and, as we will see, the opposite was also the case.

The sensitive/rational division had a long history spanning back to classical philosophy. According to the principles of Aristotle, whose *oeuvre* had largely directed Western philosophy from the eleventh and twelfth centuries onwards, the soul was the "form" of the body, and manifested at nutritive, sensitive and rational levels. In *De partibus animalium* Aristotle suggested that natural philosophers should study the nutritive and sensitive levels, but *not* the rational level. So which discipline should examine the soul's intellective functions? While nearly all Latin commentators located psychology in natural philosophy, in the Renaissance some speculated that the soul was an *ens medium* – a middle thing – belonging to both, with its nutritive and sensitive parts in natural philosophy and the rational part in metaphysics (Bakker 2007, 151–78). In general, however, the soul *qua* soul was placed in metaphysics, and the soul *qua* animating principle was studied in natural philosophy (Wolfe and van Esveld 2014, 374).

The faculty structure of English universities long reflected this division. Oxford students like Willis would have learned about the nutritive and sensitive souls in natural philosophy and the rational soul in metaphysics (Vidal 2011,

3–4). Outside the pedagogical system, however, the continued collapse of Scholasticism in the seventeenth century altered this Aristotelian divide (Funkenstein 1986, 6). In practice, the soul crossed the borders between physics, metaphysics and theology. The prominent natural philosopher Robert Boyle (1627–1691), for example, argued that theology and natural philosophy should be used alongside each other: in regards to the soul, "much may be deduced from the light of reason … [but] divine revelation teaches it us with more clearness, and with greater authority" (Boyle [1674] 1999–2000, 22). Boyle advised that "the judicious estimates of reason, improved by philosophy, [should then be] enlightened by natural theology" ([1691] 1999–2000, 348). In Charles Wolfe and Michaela van Esveld's phrase, the soul was a "go-between concept;" it was the subject of "shared territory" where various disciplinary perspectives were useful and legitimate (2014, 379). Seventeenth-century writers on the soul purported to use the best information gathered in dialogue with different disciplines. They wanted their practice to be informed by well-rounded, cross-disciplinary truths.

Within this context, the soul in the later seventeenth century tended to be discussed in texts that claimed to use natural philosophical and theological methods simultaneously. But could medicine provide any insights on the soul? Medical students at Oxford were exposed not only to the Aristotelian corpus, but also to Hippocratic practice and Galenic anatomy (Booth 2005, 50). Galen had described the soul as dependent upon bodily temperaments, and there was an influential tradition that emphasised the need to treat the body and soul together (Gowland 2006, 47; Lund 2010, 113). While the soul thus had a long history of being within the purview of medical practitioners, seventeenth-century physicians in particular built for themselves a persona that emphasised the spirituality of their practice. The physician's long-held reputation for immorality and atheism – summed up in the medieval adage *ubi tres medici, duo athei* – was based on both their supposed tendency to treat disease "naturalistically" (Henry 1989, 88; Kocher 1956, 241; Wolfe, 2006) and the common perception that physicians were greedy, untrustworthy and morally suspect (Sumich 2013, 2, 22). In their defence, physicians increasingly emphasised the spiritual facets of their practice. While physicians were sure to "disentangle their intended services from those of the minister" (their priority was the body; the health of the soul was a "by-product") (29), the close connection between soul and body meant that in practice, "the duties and functions of the two professions often overlapped" (Hawkins 1995, 107). This was the case for Willis.

Willis studies the soul

The seventeenth century is often heralded as the period in which the important move from speculative to experimental natural philosophy began to take place (Anstey 2005). In the preface to *Anatomy of the Brain*, Willis discussed how his university position required him to provide some comment on the soul, and while he had "thought of some rational Arguments for that purpose, and from the appearances raised some not unlikely Hypotheses," he nevertheless "seemed to my self, like a Painter, that had delineated the Head of Man ... at the will of a bold Fancy and Pencil, and had followed not that which was most true, but what was most convenient" (1681a, 53). This quotation discloses the generally unstable position of speculative reasoning in the seventeenth century, and Willis's decision to apply himself instead "to the study of Anatomy ... [, that] a firm and stable Basis might be laid" is demonstrative of a physician's attempt to situate himself firmly within the zeitgeist (53). Accordingly, the first treatise of *Two Discourses on the Souls of Brutes* was "Physiological, shewing the Nature, Parts, Powers, and Affections" of the corporeal soul, and Willis's claims in this section emerged from his clinical and anatomical work, but remained rooted in theological presuppositions.

Willis's anatomy revealed that the brains of humans and quadrupeds were similar in form, but the fact that they were so different in function – animals, it was said, could not reason or will like humans – meant that "some immaterial principle in man must be postulated in order to account for the mental differences in men and animals" (Bynum 1973, 447). Willis's anatomical findings, then, inferred the existence of an immaterial, immortal soul.

In an example of the communication between physician and theologian that existed during this period, Willis dedicated *Cerebri Anatome* to the Archbishop of Canterbury. For Willis, religious leaders reside "over all our Temples and Sacred Things," and this includes the temple of the mind – "the living and breathing Chapel of the Deity" (1681a, 51). Willis did not deny the spiritual authority of religious institutions; however, he admitted he was fearful that church authorities would be upset because he was treating a theological subject in a scientific way: "[c]oncerning the Soul, I have enter'd upon a great and difficult thing, and full of hazard; where we may equally fear the Censures of the Church, as the Schools" (51). Willis knew he was touching a matter of great theological importance. Some believed that by declaring the sensitive soul corporeal, there would be no evidence for human immortality or even for God himself. However, Willis was confident that his propositions were in line with Biblical doctrine. He claimed that he was in "a place of Safety, in that the Arguments and Reasons fight on my Side, and that I have got the Suffrages of the ancient Philosophers, and the holy Fathers" (51).

Willis argued that his medical theories adhered to the Biblical doctrine of the spirit/flesh divide – that is, between the fallen, sinful flesh and the immortal, immaterial spirit: "the Corporeal Soul adhering to the Flesh, inclines Man to Sensual Pleasures, whilst in the mean time, the Rational Soul, being help'd by Ethical Rules, or Divine favour, invites it to good Manners, and the works of Piety" (1683, sig. A4^r). This highly theological interpretation of human physiology meant that, as Willis explained, his view was "altogether Orthodox, and appears agreeable to a good Life, and Pious Institution: from hence the Wars and Strivings between our two Appetites, or between Flesh and Spirit, both Morally and Theologically inculcated to us, are also Physically understood" (sig. A4^r). For Willis, medical and anatomical analysis of the corporeal soul meant that "the wonderful things of God are very much made known," so much so that "not only the Face and Members, but also the inward Parts" of animals "shew them to be of a most Elegant and Artificial and plainly Divine Structure" (sig. A4ᵛ). Medical knowledge, then, can help an individual to live piously. Medicine served apologetic and theological purposes, and the soul was thought to be connected to the body on moral, theological and physical grounds. And if the body and soul and medicine and spirituality were so closely connected, the soul could be within the purview of the physician and might be medically treated.

Treating the sickly soul

After writing at length on the nature of the soul, Willis moved to focus on its diseases and treatments. He was explicit in providing not only physiological and theological explanations for this connection, but medical and pathological ones. As Willis wrote

> the Corporeal Soul doth extend its Sicknesses, not only to the Body, but to the Mind or rational Soul, ... and that it often-times involves it with its failings and faults, I think is clear enough in our Pathology or Method of Curing.
>
> (1683, sig. A4ʳ)

This example gives us a glimpse into Willis's rather covert way of medically treating the rational soul. Indeed, while his title clearly designated the corporeal soul as the topic of discussion, Willis spent half of the section on pathology discussing diseases that affect the rational soul. It is in this section that it becomes clear that Willis was using explicitly medical cures to treat parts of the soul that were traditionally reserved for the minister and the moral philosopher. Physicians had long noticed that medical, physical, bodily treatments could cure diseases of the corporeal soul, but it was rare for physicians to extend their medical management explicitly to the rational soul. While many physicians called upon the "physician of the soul" for assistance, or combined medicine with prayer, Willis attempted to treat the rational soul with medical remedies. In this section I will discuss his approach to two "diseases" of the soul: melancholy and stupidity.

In *Two Discourses*, after first addressing the causes and cures of headaches, lethargy, comas, nightmares, vertigo, apoplexy and palsies, conditions which, Willis noted, affect the corporeal soul but leave the rational soul alone so that "the Intellect for the most part remains clear and lively," Willis moved to delirium, phrensie, melancholy, madness and stupidity, distempers in which the rational soul is the sufferer (179). The bond between body and soul made it possible for the rational soul to be troubled and suffer from "deformed, distracted ... and very confused" thoughts if the corporeal soul was "so disturbed, or perverted, that it ... evilly composes ... the species and notions brought from the Sense or Memory" (179). There are "many ways, by which the Imagination, and by consequence the mind and will, and the other powers of the superior soul, are wont to be perverted or depraved," but it is possible to delineate them in the following way: when the rational soul is disturbed for only a short period of time, it is delirium; when for a long period with a "Feavour" it is "phrensie;" or for a long period without a fever but with "raving, sadness, or stupidity," it is either madness, melancholy or foolishness respectively (179). Each disease could be caused by bodily issues – plague, problems with the blood, too much wine, and ingestion of poisonous substances (like night-shades or the roots of wild parsnips) – and could be treated by a range of bizarre Galenic cures. Phrensie, for example, can be treated with "*Emetick*" potions, leeches, cupping-glasses and "*Cataplasms* of Rue, Chamomel, Vervine, Bryony, Roots, red Poppies, with Sope ... or instead of them ... Pigeons or Chickens, cut up and laid warm" over the feet (185). Willis was clear: while this was a case of a physical ailment affecting the rational soul, because the distemper had a corporeal cause – established upon an understanding of tripartite humanness – it was part of his medical purview.

Many of these "diseases" of the rational soul had a history of being treated by physicians, of which melancholy is a principal example. As Jeremy Schmidt has suggested, in antiquity both the moral philosopher and the physician were interested in melancholy, but they divided it "strictly into the disciplinary compartments of body and soul" (2007, 27). Robert Burton's *Anatomy of Melancholy* (1621) was a foundational text: this huge tome is known for its suggestion that melancholy was "a common infirmitie of Body and Soule, and such a one that hath as much need of Spirituall as a Corporall cure" ([1621] 1652, 16). Burton thought that when treating melancholy, "we must first beginne with prayer, and then use Physicke," for "all the Physicke we can use is to no purpose without calling upon God" (222). For Burton, one could be "a Priest & a Physitian at once" – and Christ was the supreme example (15).

Willis worked within this established framework. For Willis, melancholy came in many forms but normally presented with a complaint that the patient was "almost continually busied in thinking" but "comprehend[s] in their mind fewer things than before" (1683, 188). This is clearly an ailment of the rational soul, responsible for thought. The reason for these disordered thoughts was that the corporeal soul, normally transparent, subtle and lucid, had become obscure, thick and dark, "so that [it] represent[ed] the Images of things, as it were in a shadow, or covered with darkness" (189). That is, the rational soul was receiving disturbed sensory information. Yet such perturbations of the corporeal soul were often caused by the rational soul: love, sadness, fear, envy, shame and immoderate study could all cause melancholy (192). Accordingly, as Willis explained, the physician's first step was to discover whether there was an obvious mental cause for a patient's melancholy and if so, the opposite affection should be applied: "to desperate Love ought to be applied ... indignation and hatred; [and] sadness is to be opposed with the flatteries of Pleasure, Musick, a desire of vain glory or also a *pannick* terror" (193–4). The physician should attempt to heal the animal spirits with "pleasant talk, or jesting, singing, Musick, Pictures, Dancing, Hunting, Fishing, and other pleasant Exercises ... [including] *Mathematical* or *Chymical* Studies, also Travelling" (194).

However, many cases of melancholy required strictly medical treatments. If the above remedies did not produce results, the physician could reduce the blood "to a better temper" through phlebotomy, purging, vomiting or certain "Pills, Boluses, Powders, or Syrups"; herbs and minerals, including Extract of Steel and filings of iron in a glass of orange juice, were also useful (194–7). In his Oxford casebook, Willis recorded his treatment of a melancholic patient who was suffering from vertigo, stupor and "aberrations of the mind." Willis prescribed two "scruples of powder of tartar" and one "scruple of resin of jalap," which made the patient pass six stools. The next day, Willis applied leeches to his haemorrhoids, and finally the patient found himself "completely better" (at least until a couple of months later when he complained of heart palpitations) ([1650–1652] 1981, 108).

Importantly, melancholy was closely tied to spiritual health for Willis. "[T]he Stupid *Deliriums* of Melancholicks," he reflected, "have driven some, both from the Communion of Saints, and from the Society of men," and the physician should work to make sure they not only grow physically well, but leave behind their "Errors" and "become Wise" (1681b, sig. C4ᵛ). That physicians should be concerned with their patients' spiritual health becomes clear in Willis's discussion of a type of melancholy which he termed "Superstition, and a despair of *Eternal Salvation,*" which "seem to require the care of a Physician" (1683, 199–200). The illness strikes when salvation is thought to be in danger of being lost. The rational soul impresses its worries onto the corporeal soul, and the corporeal soul, "presently growing hot, moves inordinately the Blood and Spirits." It opposes "spiritual objects," and "endeavours to draw the man to its side." It thus follows that there is "a continual skirmish between the two Souls": the corporeal soul becomes increasingly "Melancholick" and consequently the imagination furnishes the intellect with only "undecent [*sic*] and monstrous notions," leaving it "perverted from the use of right reason" (200). Willis seems to be describing something like a bodily experience of temptation and spiritual doubt. While he provided no direct cures for this ailment, the fact that he described it as a type of melancholy requiring the care of a physician suggests that it was probably responsive to the same behavioural and medical remedies.

In his discussion of "stupidity" and "foolishness," Willis again deployed his theory that the rational soul relied on the corporeal soul to produce reasoned thoughts. The corporeal soul's faculty of imagination, seated in the middle of the brain, was responsible for sharing sensory images with the rational soul, so the health of the corporeal soul, the imagination and the brain were directly in tune with the vigour of the rational soul. Thus, as Willis explained, when the corporeal parts are "defective or hindered, … the eye of the Intellect, as if covered with a veil, is wont to be very much dulled, or wholly darkned [*sic*]" (1683, 209). While Willis claimed that stupidity was often inherited, he warned that it could also come from old age, brain injury, drunkenness, violent passions and brain disease (210–11). While Willis admitted that many types of stupidity were incurable, from time to time stupidity could be corrected by "the work both of a *Physician* and a *Teacher*" (212–13). The teacher's role was to "sharpen" the souls "by perpetual exercise" (213). "[M]edical Remedies," meanwhile, included the purifying of the blood through phlebotomy (which, in "fat folks," should be performed between the shoulders), trepanning, prescribing a better diet and environment, and various pharmaceutical remedies such as "the Spirits of Armoniacum, succinated, or with Amber six drams" and "the fresh leaves of Misletoe [*sic*] of the Apple tree six handfuls" (213).

Was the rational soul itself sick? No: its instruments were. Nevertheless, Willis was happy to define stupidity as a disease that "most chiefly belongs" to the rational soul because it "signifies a defect of the Intellect or Judgment" (209). While not itself sick, the rational soul was nevertheless the sufferer. Willis was quick to remind his readers of the relevance of spirituality to the treatment of these diseases. He suggested that

> the Physitian, however Skillfull he be, ought allways to Implore the help of the Heavenly Power, to be assisting to him, being above all the Strength of Medicines. Therefore … Disease [should] be cured no lesse with prayers and fastings than with Medicines, and therefore [physicians] should desire greatly to call upon the Authority of Holy men, and to be helped by the Power of your Sanctity.
>
> (1681b, sig. B4ʳ)

Notably, like Burton, Willis pointed out that Jesus Christ used "this method," because he knew that "the health of the Soul, should take its beginning from the restored health of the Body" (sig. B4ʳ).

Three religious responses to Willis

While some historians have characterised the medical work of Willis as being open to atheistic interpretations (Henry 1989, 94; Wolfe and van Esveld 2014, 384–92), his strong reliance on theology and his efforts to align his findings with scripture meant that many contemporary theological interpreters of his work were in fact overtly positive about his medical contributions. Indeed, Willis's findings were assimilated not only into natural philosophy, but also into the work of many theologians. This section will discuss three late seventeenth-century religious responses to Willis's work on the soul and brain. The fact that Willis enjoyed a heterogeneous reception demonstrates the ability of his readers to engage in creative responses to his work. Some accepted him wholeheartedly, others accepted very few of his findings, and others again modified his claims somewhat so that they agreed with their own suppositions. Medicine does not simply dictate what it means to be human, but it also provides resources with which people can engage. The way individuals respond to medical claims about the nature of humanity is engendered by the beliefs and values that they bring with them. Thus, divergent ideas about what constituted "true" Christian anthropology and the proper relationship between medicine and religion meant that divergent "Christian" responses to Willis's medical texts are perhaps to be expected.

In 1680, Samuel Haworth published *Anthropologia, or, A Philosophic Discourse concerning Man being the anatomy both of his soul and body*, in which he argued against Willis's positions. While Haworth believed that studying the soul would help one to "know thy self" (sig. A10ʳ), he maintained that knowledge of the soul was "above the reach of Sense" (14). As he went on to explain

> nothing can penetrate into the Bowels of this Golden Mine, or explicate the hidden Mysteries therein contained, but the Soul it self; she who is immaterial her self, can best by a reflex speculation explicate the Nature of a Spirit.
>
> (14)

Knowledge of the soul was acquired "by Profound Contemplation" rather than "Actual and Manual Dissection of Bodies" (74). That is, the immortal, immaterial, rational soul was out of the bounds of medicine and anatomy. For this reason, it is unsurprising that Haworth disagreed with Willis's claims: they both held fundamentally different positions about what disciplines could produce knowledge of the soul. Yet it was also a question of two different understandings of matter: while Willis believed that matter could be active, Haworth contended that matter was fundamentally inactive, and thus, in contradistinction to Willis, *all* sensation and reason must come from an incorporeal soul (35, 44). Willis's position, for Haworth, was a contradiction.

Other theologians were more than happy to fold Willis's medicine and anatomy into their work. In 1695, Matthew Smith contended that the findings of physicians – and he specifically mentioned Willis – were of considerable importance to Christian understandings of the human soul. In his *A Discourse on the Nature of Rational and Irrational Souls*, Smith advised his readers to "subscribe to the universal Judgement of Physicians" when discussing the soul, for it is physicians who understand this matter best. If a physician like Willis demonstrated that the sensitive souls of men and beasts were corporeal, Christians should accept this. Indeed, "[w]hen therefore we assert the Animal Part of Man incorporeal, we at once discard all Physicians in a matter which they should best understand" (1695, 17). Hence, Smith was clear that Willis – in *De anima brutorum* – had written in "vindication" of scriptural anthropology (Smith 1695, 7). In fact, Smith went so far as to suggest that theologians who assert the opposite might actually be assisting atheists: "those Divines help much to confirm them in their Opinion, who assign the office of Sensation to the Rational Soul, and allow Reason to other Animals" (18). Willis's findings, meanwhile, were "truly serviceable to [Christians]," because they "preserve[d] the dignity of Humane Nature, by shewing an essential difference between the Spirit of Man and the Souls of other Animals" (21). While some had misinterpreted Willis, his opinion in fact "helps us … it does not disservice" (24). In his *A Physico-Theological Discourse* (1698), John Turner, vicar of Greenwich, agreed. While the sensitive soul was corporeal, in humans there is something in us, "essentially differing from, distinct and superior to other Animals," and Turner supported his conclusion with several long quotes from the "very sagacious" Willis (83, 92). For Turner, knowledge of the soul – especially its immortality – was "not only credible by Faith or upon Authority Divine, but also demonstrable by Reason, or the Light of Nature" (99). Thus, the findings of "Dr. Willis" were important for theologians to grapple with. Turner urged his readers to contemplate the evidence that "naturally aris[es] from a Philosophical or Physical Enquiry," because this "Evidence ... is impossible to withstand" (103). In any case, as Turner made clear, Willis's medical and "Anatomical Disquisition[s]" had demonstrated the pre-eminence of the rational, immortal soul (104).

As some historians have pointed out, Willis's findings were also modified so that they would support a wholly *materialistic* understanding of human nature (Thompson 2008, 23; Wolfe and van Esveld 2014, 387). His suggestion that the rational soul could be impacted by the unwell body, as well as his contention that a corporeal soul could explain some mental functions, was mobilised in support of an anthropology to which Willis was himself opposed. The lawyer Henry Layton (1622–1704), for example, published several materialist treatises in the late seventeenth and early eighteenth century, where he argued that both the sensitive soul *and* the rational soul of humans were material. When one of his friends gave him Willis's *De anima brutorum*, Layton was surprised to find "all the particulars of my Opinion, fully delivered;" even though Willis "maintain[ed] an Immortal Soul in Man," Layton suggested that Willis had perhaps been wary of publishing his true opinion of the matter (1706, 23). Nevertheless, Layton was confident that Willis's work on brain pathology and the localisation of brain functions was convincing (1703, 11). While later eighteenth-century French writers would combine this extension of Willis with atheism (Wolfe and van Esveld 2014), Layton argued for the material rational soul upon the grounds of "religious reformation" (1692, 82). The immaterial soul, he argued, was not only opposed to medical findings, but was a pagan invention that had been adopted by Catholics to support the lucrative doctrine of purgatory. And, in a strange twist, the fact that the biblical writer St Luke was "a Learned Man, and a *Physician*," and appeared to present a more materialist account of humanity than other gospel writers, was deployed by Layton to argue against the idea that humans possessed an immaterial soul (82).

Despite Layton's admittedly heterodox religious foundations, it was this sort of denial of the immaterial soul that saw Willis often associated with atheism. While they agreed with Willis's positions, Smith and Turner saw their radical potential: "the reason why some Physicians ... have been atheistically enclin'd, is because they are able to demonstrate, that Sen[s]e is made by Matter and Motion, and therefore have carelessly concluded Reason to spring from the same Principle" (Smith 1695, 18; Turner 1698, 85). When the physician William Coward, another materialist interpreter of Willis, responded to Turner, he asked his opponent: "do you think it an infringement of your Prerogative, that a Physician should search into the Grounds of Religion...?" (1704, sigs. A8ʳ–B1ᵛ). Medicine, Coward was clear, could play a role in reforming theological doctrine. This, however, did not stop the clergyman Matthew Hole from directing Coward to Willis's *De Anima Brutorum*: "By which Lights, I hope I have given the Doctor an opportunity to ... rectifie his mistake of [confounding] the *Rational Soul*, for the *Sensitive*" (1702, 66). Medicine, then, was central to theological discussions of the soul.

The soul, medicine and what it means to be human

While some historians have denied the bearing of medicine to early modern theological discussions of the soul (Henry 1989, 93), as Wolfe has argued "it seems patently difficult to separate medical theory, medically nourished philosophical speculation, and metaphysics" (2006, 343–4). When it came to the soul in the seventeenth century, the interrelations between medicine, philosophy and theology were remarkably fluid. When searching for "true" knowledge on the soul, Smith argued that one should make use of the "assistance from Holy Writ" alongside "a strict search into the Nature of Things" (1695, Sig.A2ᵛ). Smith's contention encapsulates the study of the soul in the seventeenth century, a period during which the soul forged strong paths of communication between the early modern disciplines of medicine and theology. The more that functions of the immaterial soul were seen to rely in some way on the body, the more aspects of the soul were placed in the hands of those experienced in pathology and medical treatment. Yet this shift in dominant explanatory power did not imply by necessity a move away from religion; as we have seen, the work of Willis remained steeped in religious aims and implications.

Even today discussions about the physician's ability to provide spiritual care and to contribute to spiritual knowledge arise from underlying assumptions and beliefs about human nature. As John Peteet, Michael Balboni and Michael D'Ambra have written,

> [w]e assume that one cannot engage [in] basic questions regarding the nature of what medicine itself should be like without heavily resting one's argument on philosophical or theological foundations, which are grounded in traditions. There is a need, as the philosopher Alasdair MacIntyre has argued, to personally admit, "I find myself part of a history and ... whether I like it or not, whether I recognize it or not, one of the bearers of a tradition" (1984, 221). Traditions, and the moral communities that embody them, shape the limits, ethics, and goals of medicine ... Consequently, medicine as a practice is shaped by moral, philosophical, and religious traditions and is embodied by practitioners who are inevitably members of the communities that carry these traditions.
>
> (Peteet, Balboni and D'Ambra 2011, 25)

When we talk about spirituality and medicine today, there is a need to acknowledge our unconscious assumptions and conscious beliefs about what it means to be human, and to historicise those beliefs. Yet there is also a need to discuss the ways in which medicine has reaffirmed or at times redirected socio-cultural and religious understandings of humanness, and the means available to individuals to accept, reject or modify the claims of medicine. Ultimately, if medicine plays a role in defining the human, then medical practitioners have a responsibility to examine their assumptions and to be transparent about them, especially in times when, in the seventeenth-century as well as today, the incorporation of spirituality into medicine is under negotiation.

Note

1 The first was translated as *Anatomy of the Brain* (in *Five Treatises*) in 1681, the second as *An Essay of the Pathology of the Brain and Nervous Stock* in 1681, and the third as *Two Discourses on the Souls of Brutes* in 1683.

Reference list

Anstey, Peter R. 2005. "Experimental Versus Speculative Natural Philosophy." In *The Science of Nature in the Seventeenth Century*, edited by Peter R. Anstey and John A. Schuster, 215–42. Dordrecht: Springer.

Bakker, Paul J.J.M. 2007. "Natural Philosophy, Metaphysics, or Something in Between? Agostino Nifo, Pietro Pomponazzi, and Marcantonio Genua on the Nature and Place of the Science of the Soul." In *Mind, Cognition and Representation: The Tradition of Commentaries on Aristotle's* De Anima, edited by Paul J.J.M. Bakker and Johannes M.M.H. Thijssen, 151–78. Aldershot: Ashgate.

Booth, Emily. 2005. *"A Subtle and Mysterious Machine": The Medical World of Walter Charleton (1619–1707)*. Dordrecht: Springer.

Boyle, Robert. [1674] 1999–2000. *The Excellency of Theology compar'd with Natural Philosophy*. In *The Works of Robert Boyle. Electronic Edition*, edited by Michael Hunter and Edward B. Davis, volume 8, 1–99. London: Pickering & Chatto.

Boyle, Robert. [1691] 1999–2000. "Greatness of Mind Promoted by Christianity." In *The Works of Robert Boyle. Electronic Edition*, edited by Michael Hunter and Edward B. Davis, volume 8, 345–67. London: Pickering & Chatto.

Burton, Robert. [1628] 1652. *Anatomy of Melancholy*. London: Hen. Crips & Lodo. Lloyd.

Bynum, William F. 1973. "The Anatomical Method, Natural Theology, and the Functions of the Brain." *ISIS* 64, no. 4: 444–68.

Coward, William. 1704. *Farther Thoughts Concerning Human Soul*. London.

Descartes, Rene. [1649] 1985. "The Passions of the Soul." In *The Philosophical Writings of Descartes*, edited by John Cottingham, volume 1, 325–404. Cambridge: Cambridge University Press.

Dewhurst, Kenneth. 1981. *Willis's Oxford Casebook (1650–52)*. Oxford: Sanford.

Funkenstein, Amos. 1986. *Theology and the Scientific Imagination from the Middle Ages to the Seventeenth Century*. Princeton, NJ: Princeton University Press.

Gowland, Angus. 2006. *The Worlds of Renaissance Melancholy*. Cambridge: Cambridge University Press.

Hawkins, Michael. 1995. *A Most Excellent Antidote: Thomas Willis, the* Diatribae Duae *and the Physician's Duty*. MA Thesis for Edmonton, Alberta.

Hawkins, Michael. 2011. "Piss Profits: Thomas Willis, His *Diatribae Duae* and the Formation of his Professional Identity." *History of Science*, 49: 1–24.

Henry, John. 1989. "The Matter of Souls: Medical Theory and Theology in Seventeenth-Century England." In *The Medical Revolution of the Seventeenth Century*, edited by Roger French and Andrew Wear, 87–103. Cambridge: Cambridge University Press.

Hole, Matthew. 1702. *An Antidote against Infidelity*. London: John Nutt.

Kocher, Paul H. 1969. *Science and Religion in Elizabethan England*. New York: Octagon Books.

Layton, Henry. 1692. *Observations upon a Sermon Intituled, A Confutation of Atheism from the Faculties of the Soul, Alias, Matter and Motion Cannot Think*. London.

Layton, Henry. 1703. *Arguments and Replies*. London.

Layton, Henry. 1706. *A Second Part of Treatise Intituled A Search after Souls*.

Lund, Mary Ann. 2010. *Melancholy, Medicine and Religion in Early Modern England*. Cambridge: Cambridge University Press.

Peteet, John R., Michael J. Balboni and Michael N. D'Ambra. 2011. "Approaching Spirituality in Clinical Practice." In *The Soul of Medicine: Spiritual Perspectives and Clinical Practice*, edited by John R. Peteet and Michael N. D'Ambra, 23–44. Baltimore: The Johns Hopkins University Press.

Schlitz, Marilyn. 2011. "Spirituality and Health: Assessing the Evidence." In *Spiritual Healing: Scientific and Religious Perspectives*, edited by Fraser Watts, 140–52. Cambridge: Cambridge University Press.

Schmidt, Jeremy. 2007. *Melancholy and the Care of the Soul: Religion, Moral Philosophy and Madness in Early Modern England*. Aldershot: Ashgate.

Smith, Matthew. 1695. *A Discourse on the Nature of Rational and Irrational Souls*. London: Richard Baldwin.

Sumich, Christi. 2013. *Divine Doctors and Dreadful Distempers: How Practicing Medicine Became a Respectable Profession*. Amsterdam and New York: Rodopi.

Turner, John. 1698. *A Physico-Theological Discourse upon the Divine Being, or First Cause of all Things*. London: for Timothy Childe.

Vidal, Fernando. 2011. *The Sciences of the Soul: The Early Modern Origins of Psychology*, translated by Saskia Brown. Chicago: University of Chicago Press.

Willis, Thomas. [1644] 1681a. "The Anatomy of the Brain." In *Five Treatises*, translated by S. Pordage. London: Thomas Dring.

Willis, Thomas. [1667] 1681b. *An Essay of the Pathology of the Brain and Nervous Stock: in which Convulsive Diseases are Treated*, translated by S. Pordage. London: J.B. for Thomas Dring.

Willis, Thomas. [1672] 1683. *Two Discourses on the Souls of Brutes*, translated by S. Pordage. London: for Thomas Dring.

Wolfe, Charles T. 2006. "Tres medici, duo athei? The Physician as Atheist and the Medicalization of the Soul." In *Early Modern Medicine and Natural Philosophy*, edited by Peter Distelzweig, Benjamin Goldberg and Evan R. Ragland, 343–66. Dordrecht: Springer.

Wolfe, Charles T. and Michaela van Esvald. 2014. "The Material Soul: Strategies for Naturalising the Soul in an Early Modern Epicurean Context." In *Conjunctions of Mind, Soul and Body from Plato to the Enlightenment*, 371–421. Dordrecht: Springer.

2 Hearing differently

Medical, modern and medieval approaches to sound

Bonnie Millar

Modern approaches to hearing impairments, or non-normative hearing, tend to medicalise the presentations and to favour the prescriptions of pharmaceutical or device interventions to control the manifestations. Many of those who receive hearing aids do not use them or rarely use them, leaving these devices in drawers (Hogan and Phillips 2015, 73). Those who hear voices or noises often take numerous concomitant medications daily for stress, anxiety, depression and sleep, and they may experience the strain of trying to communicate, the social isolation due to difficulties in hearing conversations in noisy situations, the inability to explicate what they hear internally for which there are no external stimuli, and the need to recount the story of their phantom noise or voices. The voices or sounds can be indications of a number of conditions according to contemporary scientific and medical theory. Alternatively, they could be instances of the internal dialogues all people experience. Further possibilities are that they could be emotive, vivid dreams or spiritual instances of divine or magical intervention. Many struggle and do not request acoustic assistance and understanding with these disparate auditory situations as they do not wish to align themselves with what they perceive to be the disabled population.

Auditory models and perceptions of hearing impairment vary across culture and through time, ranging from the positive to the negative. If one considers medieval paradigms, voice or sound-hearing and even deafened states could be viewed very differently from modern medical interpretations. In this chapter, I draw on medieval theological, philosophical, biographical and literary examples in addition to stories collected during modern clinical research. The early Christian theologian and philosopher Augustine's conceptualisation of the human being's relationship to the sensory realm is juxtaposed to modern views, and the medieval ideal of musical harmony is compared to present-day understanding of how healthy bodies sound. Central to the discussion are the accounts of female mystics and nuns from the twelfth to fifteenth centuries and two literary examples from the fourteenth century. By comparing these medieval descriptions with reports from modern research, it is possible to note connections between the medieval instances and contemporary medicine as well as assess the impact of hearing differently on the understanding of being human. Medical science challenges the social/cultural positioning of events/experiences like hallucinations, while the corollary is also evident in that cultural/philosophical/ theological exemplars disrupt the medical.

Contemporary clinical narratives

Researchers, like clinicians and other professional listeners, hear narratives that may not gain the attention of others (Charon 2006, 178). Those suffering ill- nesses or chronic conditions can require more than care pathways; they can seek "recognition" that they have lost "something of value" as they negotiate the pain of their symptoms and the impact on their life (17). Illness is an impetus for stories; it instigates stories. These stories begin in what Frank terms "wreckage," when people flounder on the rocks of affliction, losing their direction (Frank 2013, 54; 73; 75; 164; 197; 220). The narratives are born in dislocation, a dislo- cation which they use as new channel for their life story. The tellers of these tales do not necessarily have the building blocks for their stories, so they draw on the repository of existing narremes and topoi. By moving beyond sequential ordering and working with the fragments of discourse, one could tap into the mediated residue of these illnesses, such as the accounts of tinnitus in question- naires collated during research. These tinnitus histories bear interesting parallels with medieval accounts of sound and voice-hearing and the mixing of interior and exterior sounds.

The accounts collected are ritualised in form, often with no contextual data as to how the participants appeared, conducted themselves, or sounded as they completed these questionnaires. Responses tend to be collated from original formal paper-based formats and input into more uniform electronic records, in standardised rows and columns. Despite this it is possible to uncover the tem- poral scaffolding of the tinnitus narratives, that is, their order, duration, story- time before addressing the lacunae and seeming contradictions. Through such close readings recipients could become more attuned to tinnitus storylines and what these experiences reveal about human identity.

The stories contained in these data sets reveal poignant tales of individuals, including that of a 66-year-old male, who developed tonal tinnitus gradually after having a stroke 12 years previously.[1] He experiences it constantly and finds that it is adversely affected by headaches. He also notes that he finds it pulsates with headaches, though it is not clear from the record whether the pulsating is solely confined to periods of headache. His main source of respite is listening to stories in the kitchen, after conducting choir. For someone with a deep interest in music and music participation it is easy to see how tinnitus would prove annoy- ing 70 per cent of the time. The stories that mask or distract him from his symp- toms could be recounted by family members or be relayed on the radio.

A second example details how a 56-year-old male experiences hissing and ringing (occasionally high-pitched) inside the top of his head, sounds which commenced abruptly for reasons he cannot fathom. He surmises that it may have something to do with it being a stressful period in his life between moving house and having a difficult job. Then again, it may be due to a hard press on the mandible below his left ear during self-defence training. He uses sound maskers and, occasionally, relaxation CDs, but has desisted with his hearing aid, which he used for a mere three months. Environmental and mechanical sounds like hair dryers and kettles used to help, but he finds that he no longer requires them. Sleep problems and stress both exacerbate his tinnitus precept. As this narrative unfolds, it is possible to detect two threads in particular: the exacerbations of stress and the ameliorative effect of sonic media.

A further story furnished by this repository recounts the experiences of a 60-year-old woman who abruptly got tinnitus for two weeks, before it disappeared. Later, it returned on a permanent basis in both ears, though it is worse in the left. In response to the question of causation she lists having labyrinths twice, medical treatment for flu, abscesses and jaw infection. Although her tinnitus is constant, she thinks that it might be louder at certain times. She describes her tinnitus as being like a noisy backdrop with layers of added sounds such as whistling kettles. She finds that radios, principally conversational programmes, mask her noises, though loud sounds, particularly machine-based, have an adverse effect. She thinks she is developing age-related hearing loss, and that pressure is increasing in her ear. Furthermore, she is also prone to headaches. As this tale unfolds it is possible to read it as indicative of indecision with the use of modal verbs like "might." Alternatively, she might be struggling to find a way of expressing her situation. She draws on tangible things she has experienced, medical treatments and everyday objects like kettles to articulate her condition, turning to the familiar for respite: the company of human conversation on the radio.

All three stories could be defined as quest narratives, journeys born in loss, a loss of their inner peace for which they cannot ascribe origins. They try a succession of approaches to mask or distract themselves from their dislocated lives. Significantly, due to the way the stories are recorded, references to human agency are erased. We do not hear of family members or friends assisting. Conversations and choirs are chronicled as disembodied activities. This is in part due to the particularities of this style of recording. Yet despite this ritualisation of the narratives, the individual voices still emerge as they retell their tinnitus stories, seeking recognition and solace. The discourse variables used to record the reverberations reveal hearers' endeavours to articulate and explain perceptions and management of their internal soundscapes. The enterprise of explication can in turn become a painful encounter in which words fail. In other words, articulation, trying to convey something that cannot be fully externally verified, can smart.

The essential difference between contemporary and earlier accounts of voice and sound hearing are the manner in which they are interpreted (Saunders 2016, 423; Sayers 2010, 81–92; Singer 2010, 39–52). The ability to differentiate clearly between interior and exterior incidents, "reality monitoring," plays a fundamental role in hallucinations, both auditory and visual (Fernyhough 2016, 239). Voice-hearing is a form of communication, that is, one hears a voice when one wishes to communicate (230). In these internal auditory experiences, verbal, non-verbal and even non-vocal sounds can mingle (222). "Sensory perception" is immeasurably more than "a physical act" (Rice 2013, 6); it has additional cultural and social dimensions. Indeed, Rice emphasises "the agency of sound to disturb, dissolve and re-configure the boundaries of private and public space" (40). Sound knows no bounds and has the ability to dissolve dichotomies between interiority and exteriority, bodies and minds, well and unwell. In his discussion of auscultation and hospital soundscapes, Rice notes the importance of "acoustic illumination," that is, the "visualization of the bodily interior through sound," and listening to what the body expresses through sound (163, 179). A healthy body is a body which, when heard through modern medical instrumentation, sounds healthy (178), which resonates with the classical and medieval concepts of musical harmony (*musica munda* and *musica humana*). Pythagoras theorised that music ordered the world, with musical harmony the acoustic articulation of numbers (Reilly 2001, 13; see further Crawford *et al.* 2015, 89–95). Harmonious music could soothe the spirit, while its discordant counterpart could trouble the spirit. The teachings of Pythagoras, elaborated upon by Plato and perpetuated in the influential writings of Boethius, dominated musical theory for centuries (Reilly 2001, 14). Conversely, the dislocation of music, its fragmentation, and the jettisoning of tonality, similar to the erasure of "objective moral order," adheres to the premise that there is no "hierarchical and ordered universe" (15).

Medieval voice-hearing

The differences between prevailing views of voice-hearing and alternative assessments become more apparent when one turns to medieval accounts such as those furnished by the fourteenth-century Middle English poem *Sir Orfeo*. Sir Orfeo loses his beloved wife to the king of fairies and, distraught at his loss, he renounces his kingdom and lives in solitude in woods. After a 10-year sojourn in these copses, Orfeo's inscape returns to harmonious balance and he is re-united with his wife. His self-imposed exile is a quest for healing, wholeness and a means of understanding his bereavement. The lay is a story about loss, the disappearance of his beloved, just as the passing of quiet occasions the tinnitus stories. The poem dwells on Orfeo's ability to harp:

> And harped at his owhen wille:
> Into alle þe wode þe soun gan schille,
> Þat alle þe wilde bestes þat þer beþ
> For joie aboutten him þai teþ ...
> (*Sir Orfeo* lines 271–74)

The exterior soundscape of this tale is filled with the reverberations of minstrelsy, hunting, falconry and the court, as well as the woods with all their wildlife.

There is also a more liminal arena of sound and voice interaction. As Orfeo's wife, Heurodis, sleeps under an apple tree one hot May morning, the fairy king and his retinue come to her and take her on a tour of their land, where she is to live come the morrow:

> And made me wiþ him ride
> Opon a palfray bi his side,
> And brouȝt to his palyas
> Wele atird in ich ways,
> And schewed me castels and tours,
> Rivers, forestes, friþ wiþ flours,
> And his riche stedes ichon,
> And seþþen me brouȝt oβain hom
> Into our owhen orchard,
> And said to me þus afterward:
> "Loke, dame, tomorwe þatow be
> Riȝt here under þis ympe-tre,
> And þan þou schalt wiþ ous go ..."
>   (*Sir Orfeo*, lines 155–67)

Yet while this journey and these conversations appear very real to Heurodis, to her companions she seems to be gently sleeping, shaded by apple trees. *Sir Orfeo*'s sonic fabric with its interior, exterior and liminal voices and sounds, framed by references to performance and listening, offers paradigms for the experience of hearing sound and voice, which can both illuminate and be illuminated by contemporary medical and non-medical conceptions. Human beings' relationship to the auditory, as this passage from *Sir Orfeo* amply illustrates, is more than what can be tangibly measured and evidenced.

Hearing differently

The diverse nature of hearing and humans' relationship to sound indicates how restrictive current medical models of hearing and deafened states can be, given their emphasis on interventions. What appears to be called for is a cultural change, an alteration in the paradigm, a holistic person-centred rather than intervention-based model. To tackle this, one needs to look at the social construction of hearing impairments as well as the physicality of the hearing conditions. Hearing differently need not be something one wishes to keep secret. In both medieval self-narratives and fictional stories, hearing and authority can be intrinsically linked. Non-normative hearing patterns and auditory transformations are indicative of virtue and communication with the divine, or of female authority. Teresa de Cartagena, a fifteenth-century nun, in her autobiographical account *Arboleda de los enfermos*, depicts her acquired profound deafness as a virtue, which facilitates her withdrawal from the temptations of worldly vanities and enables her to focus on the path to salvation. Chaucer's Wife of Bath, who becomes partially deafened through a fight with her husband, is freed from listening to male authority and able to voice her own arguments, confronting male Latinate textual authority. Conversely, the sounds and voices heard by Margery Kempe, Julian of Norwich and Hildegard of Bingen, resembling contemporary accounts of tinnitus and auditory verbal hallucinations, were interpreted as evidence of their transition into vehicles of divine communication. The multifarious nature of the sounds Margery Kempe, a fourteenth-century English mystic, hears, "a peyr of belwys, blowing in hir ere," "voys of a dowe," "voys of lityl bryd" are interpreted by contemporary audiences as spelling out God's instructions. The sensory components of these women's visions have spawned a number of alternative retrospective modern medical diagnoses ranging from migraine attacks, neurosis and bipolar disorder, to temporal lobe epilepsy and Tourette's syndrome. However, through auditory transformations, the nun, three mystics, together with the fictional model of the Wife of Bath, are translated into authoritative figures in their narratives.

In the medieval period, there was an established tradition of advising sovereigns and sovereigns in waiting, with many texts written with the intention of encouraging self-reflection in princes. Advising those in power was fraught with difficulty and proffering counsel in a deferential manner was necessary. Queenly intercession was a particularly effective way of guiding a monarch as the wise words came from a non-threatening source (Schieberle 2014). Indeed, Gower and Chaucer aligned themselves in the *Confessio Amantis*, *The Tale of Melibee* and *The Legend of Good Women* with female counsellors and were thereby able to offer guidance in a deferential manner to those in power.

Chaucer's Wife of Bath is a vibrant personality from *The Canterbury Tales* who has been married five times and is not wont to follow the instructions of others. After an argument with her husband Jankin she loses some of her hearing:

> But afterward repented me ful sore.
> He nolde suffer nothing of my list
> By God, he smoot me ones on the lyst,
> For that I rente out of his book a leef,
> That of the strook mine ere wax all deef.
> Stibourne I was as is a leonesse,
> And of my tonge a verray jangleresse,
> And walke I wolde, as I had doon biforn,
> From hous to hous, although he had it sworn.
> (*Wife of Bath's Prologue*, lines 632–40)

This deafness does not impede her in any way other than to render her free from hearing of the teachings of patristic authorities. This facilitates her being able to use her own lived experience as her text and the authority behind her words.

Similar to the fictional wife, Margery Kempe uses her life experiences rooted in the world of guilds, merchants and townlife in her narrative. After having 14 children, she took a vow of chastity and travelled extensively on pilgrimages. She expressed her faith through the gift of crying, driven to weeping by the beauty of the divine. Toward the end of her life she dictated an account of her life's journey, reputedly the first autobiography in English. Following the difficult birth of her first child she experienced an unsoundness of mind and while thus incapacitated she had her first vision of Christ. Through time, Margery disengages from typical female roles such as those of housekeeper and wife, pursuing her own path of devotion, guided by the sounds, music and voices to which only she is privy.

Written probably in the late 1430s, *The Book of Margery Kempe* is framed by two prefaces written by the scribe who supposedly recorded Margery's oral account of her memories, which situate the narrative within the conventions of female sacred biography:

> Sometimes she heard with her bodily ears such sounds and melodies that she could not hear what anyone said to her at that time unless he spoke louder. These sounds and melodies she had heard nearly every day for twenty-five years when this book was written, and especially when she was in devout prayer, also many times while she was at Rome, and in England too.
>
> (*The Book of Margery Kempe*, 124)

Margery Kempe mentions going to Norwich to speak with Julian of Norwich, an important Christian mystic, in around 1414. The details of Julian of Norwich's life are sketchy, but she was an anchoress attached to the Church of St Julian in Norwich. Her narrative indicates that she was probably born around 1342 and died around 1416, and she may have been from a privileged family residing in or near Norwich. Her *Revelations of Divine Love*, written around 1395, is the first book in the English language known to have been written by a woman. Julian was also acclaimed as a spiritual authority within her community, where she served as a counsellor and advisor.

When she was 30 and living at home, Julian succumbed to a life-threatening illness and received the last rites of the Catholic Church on 8 May 1373. As part of the ritual, the priest held a crucifix aloft and, despite her failing sight and feeling physically numb, she saw the figure of Jesus begin to bleed as she gazed upon the object. Over the next several hours, she had a series of 16 visions of Jesus Christ during the five days or so that she was severely ill, which she documented thereafter in a version of the *Revelations of Divine Love* now known as The Short Text. Many years later, Julian rewrote this account with a theological gloss and commentary teasing out the meaning of the visions, known as The Long Text, which appears to have been revised many times before it was finished, perhaps in the 1410s or even the 1420s:

> And after this, ere God shewed any words, He suffered me for a convenient time to give heed unto Him and all that I had seen, and all intellect that was

therein, as the simplicity of the soul might take it. Then He, without voice and opening of lips, formed in my soul these words: *Herewith is the Fiend overcome*. These words said our Lord, meaning His blessed Passion as He shewed it afore.

(Revelations of Divine Love, The Fifth Revelation, 49)

Here Julian describes how in her weakened state she hears God speak to her internally, with no external stimuli. It is an affirmative experience that transforms her life and provides her with food for thought throughout the rest of her life, which she feels is valuable to communicate to others.

The Norwich nun was preceded in her mystical experiences by Hildegard of Bingen, a German Benedictine abbess, writer, composer, philosopher, Christian mystic, visionary and polymath, who was considered by many to be the founder of scientific natural history in Germany. Hildegard was elected *magistra* by her fellow nuns in 1136 and went on to found the monasteries of Rupertsberg in 1150 and Eibingen in 1165. She wrote theological, botanical and medicinal texts, as well as letters, liturgical songs, drama and poems, and invented her own language, the *Lingua Ignota*.

Hildegard experienced poor health and visions from a tender age. According to her own accounts she first saw the "Living Light" at the age of three, and by the age of five she realised that she was experiencing visions that could prove unfathomable to others. Her visions were multi-sensory experiences involving all five senses: sight, hearing, taste, smell and touch. Within her extensive *oeuvre*, her most significant works are her three volumes of visionary theology: *Scivias* ("Know the Ways"); *Liber Vitae Meritorum* ("Book of Life's Merits"); and *Liber Divinorum Operum* ("Book of Divine Works"). These volumes record her visions and their multi-sensory nature, together with a theological explanation. The first work, *Scivias*, was inspired by hearing an instruction from God to "write down what you see and hear":

When I was forty-two years and seven months old, a burning light of tremendous brightness coming from heaven poured into my entire mind. Like a flame that does not burn but enkindles, it enflamed my whole heart and breast, just like the sun that warms an object with its rays ... A voice from heaven was saying, O weak person, you who are ash of ash and decaying of decaying, speak and write what you see and hear. Since you are timid about speaking, and simple in your explanation, and unskilled in writing about these things, speak and write ... as one who hears and understands the words of a teacher and explains them in his own way.

(Scivias, 60–61)

Scivias comprises three sections which delineate the nature of creation, redemption and salvation. As if these literary and theological accomplishments were not enough, she also preached publicly, addressing a variety of clerical and lay audiences.

There is a tension between embracing this ability to hear differently, alternative auditory states, and the desire to alleviate auditory otherness. Hildegard's medicinal and scientific writings have been interpreted as thematically complementary to many of her ideas in her visionary works. Similarly, they are the result of Divine communication, although her experience helping in and then leading the monastery's herbal garden and infirmary and reading played their parts. The practical skills she developed over many years in diagnosis, prognosis and treatment of physical illnesses she combined in a whole-person approach dealing with the emotional and spiritual aspects of the diseases. During her lifetime she became renowned for her ability to cure the ill and for her herbal remedies. Hildegard catalogued both her theory and practice in two encyclopaedic works, the *Physica*, which details the scientific and medicinal properties of various plants, stones, fish, reptiles and animals, and the *Causae et Curae*, which explores the physicality of the human body and its place in the natural order, together with the causes and cures of diverse ailments. Among the many cures Hildegard records is the following recipe to alleviate deafness and tinnitus:

> If some disease or bad humors fall upon one's ears, so that he becomes as if deaf and his ears ring, he should take the forenamed gum [of the cherry tree] and dissolve it in a small dish over the fire. He should pour it, thus warmed, over crumbs of rye bread and place this in the openings of his ears at night. He should cover his ears and temples with these crumbs smeared with the gum and tie a linen cloth over them. If he does this often, the disease, bad humors, and ringing will be chased away, and he will be cured.
>
> (*Physica* Book 3 Trees, Chapter VI Cherry Tree, 111)

Hildegard perceived plants and natural elements of the garden to be directly linked to the maladies, humors and elements of the human body. Interestingly, although Hildegard privileges her ability to hear differently, she still invests considerable time and effort, both physical and intellectual, in working out medicinal recipes to ensure others did not have a non-normative relationship with the auditory. This distinction between the aural sensory experience of the religious and that of those beyond the convent walls perhaps parallels the difference in religiosity evident in the life of a nun, and that of a devout layperson who pursues a more worldly path.

A final example of a woman who contended with auditory otherness, Teresa de Cartagena, was a Spanish author and nun who fell deaf between 1453 and 1459. This experience influenced her two known works, *Arboleda de los enfermos* ("Grove of the Infirm") and *Admiración operum Dey* ("Wonder at the Works of God"). The latter work represents what many critics consider as the first feminist tract written by a Spanish woman. Before losing her hearing, Teresa entered the Franciscan Monasterio de Santa Clara in Burgos around 1440 and nine years later moved to the Cistercian Monasterio de Las Huelgas in Burgos. She wrote her first work *Arboleda de los enfermos* upon embracing her new-found deafened state. Approximately one to two years later, she turned pen to paper once more, resulting in the *Admiración operum Dey*, an explanation of how a woman could and did write the former text. Both of her writings have survived in a single manuscript completed by the copyist Pero López del Trigo in 1481. Her deafness permits her to zone out the noise of the tangible external world and to focus on the delivery of the delicious sounds of the divine:

> Silence has already been imposed on me by the hand of God, who commands me to be quiet, and my foolish persistence has been checked with that finger that I now understand, showing me openly that it behoves me to be totally silent, to cut myself off completely from worldly chatter and desires; for it would be of little profit to separate myself from these worldly things if my desire and care were still involved with them. For my involvement would produce so much noise that I could not understand the voices; in order to hear them, I am commanded to maintain such an extreme silence.
>
> (*Grove of the Infirm [Arboleda de los enfermos]*, 28)

For all these figures, the propensity to hear differently ultimately proves an impetus to write, or compose, to distil their experiences in order to guide and counsel others. These capacities arise from illness or mishap and lead them to eschew traditional female roles and pursue more independent pathways. By embracing their auditory transformations they forge new authoritative positions for themselves, women and humanity. They interpret their sensory experiences positively and value the benefits they perceive to have gained from them.

Beyond the sensory

In medieval theological and philosophical traditions there is a premium laid upon being able to move beyond the world of the senses, beyond the tangible to the world of reason and intellect, to a place where the essence of human beings meets the divine. Augustine, especially in his earlier works, distinguishes between the intelligible and the sensible, asking his readers to forgo the world of the senses and concentrate on the intellect (*De Libero Arbitrio* II.7). What we perceive through our senses is ephemeral while what we learn through our intellect is eternal (*De Libero Arbitrio* II.6; *Confessions* XI.xxxix.39; *Confessions* IV.xii.18). It is only by loosening the chains that bind us to the world of the senses, and turning to intellectual paradise with God at the centre, that we can be released from care. The intelligible realm, with God as its source, promises the only lasting relief from the anxiety prompted by the transitory nature of the sensible realm.

The human soul, as Augustine conceives it, can understand its relationship to the sensory world and channel this connection so that it perceives what lies above (*Confessions* VII.x.16 and VII.xvii.23). Thus, in the Augustine schema, human beings begin with sense perception and move upward to reason. Even among the five senses there is a hierarchy to be unravelled with taste and smell being private, hearing and sight public, and touch occupying a median position.

Co-ordinating the senses is what Augustine terms the "inner sense" (*De Libero Arbitrio* II.3), and it is this faculty that is unique to humans, setting us apart from animals.

Interactions with sound

The human relationship to sound is more complex than just the facility to hear and interpret auditory stimuli. Moreover, if one surveys some of the discussion in modern popular culture, one can find the ongoing controversy, for example, about the ethics of implantation of cochlear implants in young children, and how the Deaf community has had to change its attitude towards implantation as cochlear implants have been more widely adopted by deaf persons. Great debate has been waged about the bioethical issues raised by the conflict between parents' desires to raise children in their own culture, the best interest of the child and the interests of Deaf Culture, the long-term survival of which might well be threatened by routine cochlear implantation in deaf children. The extensive literature on this topic can be amply illustrated by the following sources (Balkany 1996; Bognar 2015; Christiansen and Leigh 2006; Crouch 1997; Edelist 2016; Edwards 2005; Jones and Saladi 2014; Lane and Bahan 1998; Lane and Grodin 1997; Lee 2012; Levy 2002a, 2002b, 2007; Mauldin 2012, 2014, 2016; Sparrow 2005, 2010).

Those who are deafened, suffer hearing loss or hear internal voices or sounds are more attuned to difference as they are accustomed to trying to listen and not catching everything: they hear differently. So, what does the relationship between individuals and auditory worlds reveal about what it means to be human? First, it underlines how the sense of hearing is more than just a means of collecting external stimuli; it is also an internal process of sound gathering and interpretation. Some will have had no direct experience of auditory input. Internal soundscapes, be they silent or filled with noises and voices, are fundamental to the human condition and to well-being. The sensory world of sound encompasses a cornucopia of human subject positions where agency can lie with persons or with the resonances. These auditory associations are constantly evolving on both an individual and a social level and the modern medical model of hearing as something which functions or needs a cure does not reflect the richness of this human sensory experience. By hearing and listening differently, individuals can be transformed or transform themselves, they can become isolated or gain incredible authority and influence. The auditory realm constitutes a microcosm of the potential and the limitation of the human.

Note

1 These three stories come from the Tinnitus Data Repository, a collection of material from studies conducted at a UK research unit.

Reference list

Augustine. 1955. *De Libero Arbitrio*, trans. Dom Mark Pontifex. Westminster: Newman Press.

Augustine. 1991. *Confessiones (Confessions)*, trans. Henry Chadwick. Oxford: Oxford University Press.

Balkany, T.J., A.V. Hodges and K.W. Goodman. 1996. "Ethics of cochlear implantation in young children," *Otolaryngology – Head and Neck Surgery*, 114: 748–55.

Bliss, A.J., ed. [1954] 1966. *Sir Orfeo*, 2nd edn, Oxford: Clarendon Press.

Bognar, Greg. 2015. "Is disability mere difference?" *Journal of Medical Ethics*. doi: 10.1136/medethics-2015-102911.

Burrow, J.A. and Thorlac Turville-Petre. 1992, 1996, 2005. *A Book of Middle English*, 3rd edn. Oxford: Blackwell.

Charon, Rita. 2006. *Narrative Medicine: Honoring the Stories of Illness*. Oxford: Oxford University Press.

Chaucer, Geoffrey. 1996. *The Wife of Bath*, edited by Peter G. Beidler. Boston and New York: Bedford Books.

Christiansen, J.B. and I.W. Leigh. 2006. "The Dilemma of Paediatric Cochlear Implants," in *The Deaf Way II Reader*, edited by H. Goodstein, 363–69. Washington, DC: Gallaudet University Press.

Crawford, Paul, Brian Brown, Charley Baker, Victoria Tischler and Brian Adams. 2015. *Health Humanities*. Houndsmill, Basingstoke and New York: Palgrave Macmillan.

Crouch, R.A. 1997. "Letting the deaf be deaf: reconsidering the use of cochlear implants in prelingually deaf children," *Hastings Center Report*, 27.4: 14–21.

Edelist, Tracey. 2016. "Capitalising on cultural dichotomies: making the 'right choice' regarding cochlear implants," *Social Theory & Health*, 14.3: 293–311.

Edwards, R.A.R. 2005. "Sound and fury; or, much ado about nothing? Cochlear implants in historical perspective," *The Journal of American History*, 92: 892–920.

Fernyhough, Charles. 2016. *The Voices Within: The History of How We Talk to Ourselves*. London: Profile Books, in association with Wellcome Collection.

Frank, Arthur W. [1995] 2013. *The Wounded Storyteller: Body, Illness and Ethics*, 2nd edn. Chicago and London: University of Chicago Press.

Hildegard of Bingen. 1990. *Scivias*, trans. Columba Hart and Jane Bishop, Introduction by Barbara J. Newman, Preface by Caroline Walker Bynum. New York: Paulist Press.

Hildegard of Bingen. 1998. *Physica*, trans. Priscilla Throop. Rochester, VT: Healing Arts Press.

Hildegard of Bingen. [2006] 2008. *Causes and Cures of Hildegard of Bingen*, trans. Priscilla Throop. Charlotte, VT: MedievalMS.

Hogan, Anthony and Rebecca Phillips. 2015. *Hearing Impairment and Hearing Disability: Towards a Paradigm Change in Hearing Services*. Farnham: Ashgate.

Jones, Cynthia M. and Shawn P. Saladi. 2014. "Fixing deafness," *The Journal of Philosophy, Science & Law*, 14.3: 16–32.

Julian of Norwich. 2013. *Revelations of Divine Love*, edited by Grace Warrack. Milton Keynes: Digireads.com Book.

Kempe, Margery. [1985] 1994. *The Book of Margery Kempe*, trans. B.A. Windeatt. London: Penguin.

Lane, H. and B. Bahan. 1998. "Ethics of cochlear implantation in young children: a review and reply from a deaf-world perspective," *Otolaryngology – Head and Neck Surgery*, 119: 297–308.

Lane, H. and M. Grodin. 1997. "Ethical issues in cochlear implant surgery: an exploration into disease, disability, and the best interests of the child," *Kennedy Institute of Ethics Journal*, 7: 231–51.

Lee, Chongmin. 2012. "Deafness and cochlear implants: a deaf scholar's perspective," *Journal of Child Neurology*, 27.6: 821–23.

Levy, N. 2002a. "Reconsidering cochlear implants: the lessons of Martha's Vineyard," *Bioethics*, 16: 134–53.

Levy, N. 2002b. "Deafness, culture, and choice," *Journal of Medical Ethics*, 28: 284–85.

Levy, N. 2007. "Must publicly funded research be culturally neutral?" *Virtual Mentor*, 9.2: 140–42.

Mauldin, Laura. 2012. "Parents of deaf children with cochlear implants: a study of technology and community," *Sociology of Health & Illness*, 34.4: 529–43.

Mauldin, Laura. 2014. "Precarious plasticity: neuropolitics, cochlear implants, and the redefinition of deafness," *Science, Technology, & Human Values*, 39.1: 130–53.

Mauldin, Laura. 2016. *Made to Hear: Cochlear Implants and Raising Deaf Children.* Minneapolis, MN: University of Minnesota Press.

Padden, Carol and Tom Humphries. 2005. *Inside Deaf Culture.* Cambridge, MA and London: Harvard University Press.

Reilly, Robert R. 2001. "The music of the spheres, or the metaphysics of music," *The Intercollegiate Review*, Fall: 12–21.

Rice, Tom. 2013. *Hearing and the Hospital: Sound, Listening, Knowledge and Experience.* Canon Pyon: Sean Kingston.

Sacks, Oliver. [1989] 1990. *Seeing Voices: A Journey into the World of the Deaf.* New York and London: Picador.

Saunders, Corinne 2016. "Voices and Visions: Mind, Body and Affect in Medieval Writing," in *The Edinburgh Companion to the Critical Medical Humanities*, edited by Anne Whitehead and Angela Woods, 411–27. Edinburgh: Edinburgh University Press.

Sayers, Edna Edith. 2010. "Experience, Authority, and the Mediation of Deafness: Chaucer's Wife of Bath," in *Disability in the Middle Ages: Reconsiderations and Reverberations*, edited by Joshua R. Eyler, 81–92. Farnham: Ashgate.

Schieberle, Misty. 2014. *Feminized Counsel and the Literature of Advice in England, 1380–1500*, Disputatio 26. Turnhout, Belgium: Brepols Publishing.

Singer, Julie. 2010. "Playing by Ear: Compensation, Reclamation, and Prosthesis in Fourteenth-Century Song," in *Disability in the Middle Ages: Reconsiderations and Reverberations*, edited by Joshua R. Eyler, 39–52. Farnham: Ashgate.

Sparrow, Robert. 2005. "Defending deaf culture: the case of cochlear implants," *Journal of Political Philosophy*, 13.2: 135–52.

Sparrow, Robert. 2010. "Implants and ethnocide: learning from the cochlear implant controversy," *Disability & Society*, 25.4: 455–66.

Taylor, George and Anne Darby, eds. 2003. *Deaf Identities*. Coleford: Douglas McLean.

Teresa de Cartagena. 1988. *The Writings of Teresa de Cartagena*, trans. Dayle Seidenspinner-Núñez. Rochester, NY and Woodbridge, Suffolk: Boydell and Brewer.

Tucker, B.P. 1998. "Deaf culture, cochlear implants, and elective disability," *Hastings Center Report*, 28.4: 6–14.

3 Sensing the self in the wandering mind

Hazel Morrison

"Nothing": says Meisters "so well illustrates the nature of our thinking faculties as to consider them in different conditions of waking and sleeping, and in that intermediate state between sleeping and waking, where the external senses are in a more perfect state of quiet and rest ... when the active inner sense is cut off from the external world."

(Boismont 1859, 29)

Human mental life, write psychologists Smallwood and Schooler (2015), is not always tethered to the here and now; rather, consciousness ebbs and flows. Attention shifts between the immediacy of our external environment to thoughts and feelings internally generated. Notions of an interiority, to which our attentions shift, have long been based on philosophical distinction between "inside" and "outside." This distinction, argues Sawday (1995), lies at the heart of Western accounts of the self. Yet the language of the self and its interiority has historical character (Grosz 1994, vii; Kristeva 1990, 14; Smith 1997, 49). Conspicuously, it shifts, as experimental investigations into "intermediate" states of consciousness, such as daydream, reverie, mind wandering and hallucination, have generated multiple, often conflicting insights into this notion of a human interiority.

The potential value of such studies to our understanding of the human has recently been brought to light through exchanges between philosophers of the mind, psychologists and others working in the cognitive sciences. An "enduring and intimate" relationship is recognised to exist between mental activity that occurs when the mind is "at rest" and the "neural architecture" of the self, which has significant ramifications for various clinical studies (Callard and Margulies 2011). Rest, as conceptualised within the cognitive sciences, facilitates perceptual disengagement from ongoing external events. Rest enables one's immersion in thoughts and feelings, which hold little or no immediate relation to the goings on of the world around us. Clinical studies of attention deficit hyperactivity disorder (Seli *et al.* 2015), obsessive compulsive disorder (Seli *et al.* 2016) and schizophrenia (Shin *et al.* 2015) – commonly construed as "self-related reflective thought disorders" (Allen and Williams, 2011, 8) – have each engaged with this emergent area of research, which is seen as having the potential to re-orient concepts of self within academic and wider cultural and medical spheres (Gallagher 2000; Callard and Margulies 2011). Foregrounding this research is enquiry into the phenomenology of variously classified resting states, namely daydream, self-generated thought and mind wandering. It is through examination of these ordinary, everyday perambulations between intrinsic and extrinsic sources of perception that philosophies of the self intersect with medical theory and practice.

The role of this chapter is to provoke critical reflection, and historical enquiry, on the longstanding role of experimental investigation into "resting states" in shaping conceptualisations of the self. The wager is that across nineteenth- and twentieth-century Western societies, studies of mental phenomena that disconnect us from our immediate physical and social environments, such as reverie, daydream and mind wandering, have historically, mutually, interacted with notions of the "self," as explored through medical, literary, philosophical, psychological and theological paradigms. To review these literatures is to reveal a history of transience, in which successive incarnations of this notion of the self are framed in relation to spatial and semantic dualisms. Inner and outer, mind and body, reason and sensation, imagination and perception, these dualisms predominate (Grosz 1994; Sawday 1995). Significantly, this history reveals the productive potentiality of past experimental investigation into daydream, reverie and mind wandering to challenge the legitimacy of such bifurcations.

Beginning with an investigation of Cartesian mind-body dualism, a well-worn subject in studies of the human, this chapter acknowledges the role of the wandering mind in destabilising Descartes' classical philosophy of the self. Investigation then moves towards the reception of Cartesian paradigms of the self within nineteenth-century French medical, literary and philosophical circles. Here, experimental descents into states of reverie, daydream and, in extremity, hallucination, are shown to have instigated radical re-appraisals of the notion of self. Moving then to turn-of-the-century Britain and North America, this chapter looks to psychological investigation of daydream and reverie in relation to the adolescent self and associated mental pathologies. To conclude, this history is brought into conversation with modern day investigation into daydream and mind wandering. Charting a history of the self, ranging from Cartesian notions of its unity to pragmatist notions of its fragmentation, from psychological through to psychiatric investigation of its pathologies, this longitudinal history is shown through its entangled relationship to states, variously categorised under the umbrella term of the wandering mind.

This paper, this fire, the first experiment

The history of modern philosophy is often traced to the Renaissance writings of René Descartes (1596–1650), to the overarching concern of his life's work – the philosophy of truth and certainty. Embedded in his seventeenth-century writings is a concept of selfhood that is analogous to the Christian soul. Defined as a

"thinking substance" and an indivisible unity, the Cartesian self is conceptualised as existing apart from, and being independent of, the "extended substance"
of the human body (Grosz 1994, 8). The significance of Descartes to Western
conceptualisations of the self indelibly lies with this ontological separation of
mind and body; for the carving of an interiority, considered non-spatial, spiritual
and separate from mankind's corporeal existence, that from Descartes on is
increasingly seen as constituting human identity (Burkitt 1994, 8; Kristeva 1990,
14; Strozier 2002, 210). Yet, as Kim Atkins relates, his is a history both "fascinating and deservedly famous" for the various "ambiguities he continually
uncovers [while] he attempts, unsuccessfully to delineate the mental from the
physical in the context of the human body" (Atkins 2008, 7). By engaging with
one of Descartes' most famous thought experiments, as expressed in *Meditations
on First Philosophy* (1641), this section draws attention to Descartes' carving of
an ambiguous and un-reconciled set of relations, between mind and body, interiority and exteriority, in which the functioning of the self becomes problematic.
Such relations Descartes recognises to occupy the liminal territories between
waking and dreaming, in which the mind is recognised to "wander":

> How many times has it occurred that the quiet of the night made me dream
> of my usual habits: that I was here, clothed in a dressing gown, and sitting
> by the fire, although I was in fact lying undressed in bed!
>
> (Descartes 1960, 18)

Seated by the fireside, holding a piece of paper and wrapped in his dressing
gown, Descartes, in this now well-worn scene of thought experimentation,
reports that he knows not how to distinguish this experience, this body, this
paper, from perception experienced during dreams. The mind, he states, is "a
vagabond who likes to wander" beyond "the strict bounds of truth" and therefore
he must doubt the reliability of sensory-based perception (Descartes 1960,
28–29).

Perception, as Grosz attests, "is the psychical registration of the impingement
of external and internal stimuli on the body's sensory receptors" (1994, 28). It is
a concept that "exists in the breach between mind and body," and therefore
posed significant epistemological questions for Descartes' theory of mind-body
dualism (28). As Descartes defines the self as an entity separate to the body and
its senses, the only certainty voiced by Descartes is that he is conscious of his
capacity for thought, that is, *cogito ergo sum*, usually translated into English as
"I think therefore I am." This, he writes, is indisputable evidence of his self-
existence. So how, asks Descartes, can the certainty of self-consciousness be
used to perceive reality from illusion? "I now recognise that our memory can
never bind together and join our dreams one with another and with the whole
sequence of our life as ... is accustomed ... when we are awake" (Descartes,
quoted in James 1995, 3). As the work of Tony James (1995) demonstrates, Descartes found his answer by establishing a division between the self during
waking states, and the self during dreams. During waking hours Descartes

defines himself as possessed of self-awareness, conferred by a sense of temporal and psychological continuity as constituted by memory. The self when experienced in dreams, observes Descartes, lacks such psychological continuity, indeed may even lack conscious awareness of its own capacity for thought. Descartes' *cogito*, that is, the "certitude of consciousness" being conterminous with the certainty of the self, makes divisible the self of waking hours from the self experienced during dreams (Berrios 1996, 230). Dreams, he observes, do not reproduce the kind of sequential linear consciousness experienced in waking life. Dreams have neither the coherence nor the stability of waking perception. To experience elements of both waking and dreaming *simultaneously* was for Descartes considered as "anomalous," even pathological, threatening to disrupt the unity of the conscious self (James 1995, 6; Descartes 1960, 18).

It is within this liminal space carved by Descartes, between sleep and waking, that the wandering mind is conceptualised as having space to roam. Here lurks this second, unverified self that threatens the stability of its waking counterpart. For perception to breach the boundaries between waking and sleeping, was equated by Descartes with insanity (Descartes 1960, 18), and for thinkers emerging from the Renaissance, the wandering imagination is often described as a principal source of human error (Redpath 1998, 69). How then, does the wandering mind become an experimental apparatus in the proceeding centuries, and what impact has this had on Western scientific and humanistic accounts of the self?

A space to roam

The relationship between "vision, consciousness and memory" (Pick 1997, 189), was a subject of longstanding debate by the time of the late nineteenth century, deliberated within medicine, art and philosophy, while questions raised by Descartes, as to the role of perception, memory and consciousness in anchoring mankind's sense of identity permeate the intellectual culture (Pick 1997; Taylor 1997). The desire to "regulate and control" these relations ran counter to the desire to explore the "hidden depths of the mind" that so absorbed the Romantics, and it is through this frisson between the sciences and humanities – between medicine, art, literature and philosophy – that the wandering mind becomes an experimental and conceptual device through which to explore emergent notions of selfhood (Marx 2008, 316; Taylor 1997).

Jennifer Ford and Shane McCorristine's work on the Romantic poet Samuel Taylor Coleridge demonstrates how this relation between selfhood, waking and dreaming perception is experimentally explored through the prism of the wandering mind. Like Descartes, Coleridge regarded dreams as a period in which critical judgement and will are in suspense; where the loss of will indicates "disturbances in the very concept of the self" (Ford 1998, 35). However, it is the stance taken by Coleridge to studies of self in relation to the wandering mind – to those "half-waking" states between sleep and waking – that medical and philosophical insights meld and invite new understandings of self. In parallel with a medical model of hallucination that was emerging on the continent, Coleridge identifies a state, below full waking consciousness, where visions and imaginings may take on the appearance of extrinsically oriented perception. In both published and private works, this semi-conscious state is identified as a space in which poetic creativity germinates; where the partial loss of the "Will," and suspense of the "Ich," brings to ascendance flights of "Fancy" (McCorristine 2010, 37–39). In France, where authors such as Victor Hugo and Honoré de Balzac directly use the word *hallucination* to denote such half-waking states, this emerging concept is used to signify a "break in the continuity" of characters' "sense of self" (James 1995, 75–76). Their novels demonstrate conceptual slippages between this emergent medical paradigm, and a sense of self imagined to exist within a semi-conscious realm.

Maintaining a geographical orientation towards France, the following section looks to the publications of the French physician, Alaxandre-Jacques-François Brierre de Boismont (1797–1881) a noted authority on the subject of hallucination, and the French psychologist, historian and literary critic, Hippolyte Taine, noted for his studies on the human subject. Through both their works, the state of reverie is used to refigure notions of the self in regards to the physiology and psychology of perception and insanity. Notably it is through their engagement with the arts and humanities, with poets, artists and dramatists, that these authors may ultimately use studies of daydream, reverie and hallucination to question what it means to be human.

Hallucination and hashish

> When I arrived I found, amongst the persons who were present, M.M. Esquirol, Ferrus and others well-known in science, literature, and art … Three persons had taken the liquor … At one time [B., a painter and musician] … exhibited the singular phenomenon of the *Double man*, … he heard, he said, music with one ear, and what was spoken with the other.
>
> (Boismont 1859, 329–31)

The term *hallucination*, a derivative of the Latin *allucinor*, had since the sixteenth century denoted only that of a wandering mind (Sacks 2012, ix; Leudar and Thomas 2000, 8). Yet as it enters the medical lexicon at the turn of the nineteenth century, hallucination is brought into equation with mental pathology. First given medical definition in France in 1817 by the proto-psychiatrist Jean-Étienne Esquirol (1772–1840), hallucination came to be defined as an "inward conviction of a presently perceived sensation … when no external object [is] capable of arousing this sensation." For Esquirol, hallucination came to represent a breach in the paradigm of sleep and waking; "visionaries and ecstatics are hallucinatiors" writes Esquirol in 1832, "are dreamers who are wide awake" (Esquirol 2000, 263). For psychiatrists such as Moreau de Tours, a pupil of Esquirol, this rift, if penetrated, offered the possibility to "descend within ourselves." Removed from Descartes' philosophical concern with truth and certainty, hallucination promised for Moreau de Tours opportunity to observe the "mind … taking on … a quite new, independent existence" (James 1995, 107).

The above experiment concerning the unidentified liquor was reported on by Brierre de Boismont, a member of Esquirol's inner circle of "aliénistes" (Goldstein 2001, 262). In Boismont's widely translated text *Des Hallucinations* (1845) he reports how, in 1840, he attended a medical inquiry, in which the state of hallucination was induced through the intake of hashish. "Esquirel, Ferrus and others well-known in science, literature, and art" were the subjects of enquiry. Their heightened artistic abilities seen to enable a more detailed description of the fantastical sensory and perceptual experiences that unfolded before and within them (Boismont 1859, 329–31). To understand how such experiments, and their insights into hallucination, shape nineteenth-century paradigms of the self, this section looks to Brierre de Boismont's studies of mental pathology through the lens of reverie and drug-induced hallucination. An assessment of the impact this makes upon prevalent philosophical models of self will extend into the proceeding section on Taine. The following section establishes how, in such cases, the proto-psychiatric profession took on an increased degree of ownership of the concept of the self, as psychiatry breached Cartesian boundaries between the study of mind and matter.

Philosophers, rather than physicians? The material reproduction of an idea

> A vast abyss, it is said, separates philosophical questions from those of practical and experimental medicine; the understanding, the mind, the soul, must be left where this principle should rest. The physician who would be useful and practical, must only study the organs, their functions … in short, there is no advantage to introducing spiritualism to medicine.
>
> (Boismont 1859, vi)

In the 1850s, Brierre de Boismont is writing at a time of debate as to whether diseases of the mind might better be treated by philosophers rather than physicians (Kendell 2001). Within the persistent Cartesian mind-body dualism in the medical discourse of this period, a prevailing, if contentious view (expressed above with what is assumed to be a large dose of sarcasm) was that medicine was to administer to "organs and their functions," leaving philosophy to administer to the mind. Hallucination, defined by Esquirol as a disturbance of "memory … without the intervention of the senses," is deprived of an organic aetiology *if* read within the Cartesian dualist tradition. To claim hallucination a matter of medical concern Brierre de Boismont needed to establish physiological causation: "The branch of medicine that disrupts this dualist assumption is that of mental disease … [they push the physician to] resort to the most difficult of metaphysical problems" (Boismont 1853, vi).

As demonstrated above, the disruptive potentiality of Brierre de Boismont's work to the Cartesian dualist paradigm of the self is well recognised in *Des*

Hallucinations, and in 1855, as the French Société Médico-Psychologique met to debate the emergent diagnosis of hallucination, there arose a second reason for Brierre de Boismont's need to claim hallucination as a matter of medical concern. Should, asked contributors to the 1855 debates, seeing, hearing and otherwise sensing that which is not externally present, as proposed by Alfred Maury, be considered fundamentally pathological? And if so, were "great thinkers" of the past, such as Socrates, Luther and Joan of Arc, guided not by visions but by the products of their own insanity? (Haggerty 2003, 9). For Breirre de Boismont, a Roman Catholic doctor present during these debates, to align hallucination to the loss of reason was to deny the reality of the visions and apparitions of some of the most revered religious figures and philosophical thinkers. To oppose such views, it was necessary to retain the possibility that hallucination may be consonant with reason. The first step in *Des Hallucinations* is to turn to the study of states of mind not considered pathological, but those which nonetheless blur such body-brain boundaries. "The state of reverie has been experienced by everyone," writes Boismont, and "shows how easily hallucination may be produced" (1859, 28): "Carried away by these day-dreams, these castles in the air, ... our thoughts expand, chimeras become realities, and all the objects of our wishes present themselves before us in visible forms" (30). Identifying reverie as a state in which consciousness is in suspense yet not altogether absent, where the coherent boundaries of the rational self are "fissured" but do not permanently "brake" (Bullen 1997, 147), Boismont uses the common experience of reverie to demonstrate hallucination co-existing with reason. To do this he offers two lines of argument, which offer points of departure from Descartes' conceptualisation of the self. First, he defines a class of hallucination which he terms "physiological." These he defines as cases that demonstrate "derangement" having "not exceeded the sphere of the sensorial faculties" (Boismont 1859, 71). Second, he argues that hallucination may be the product of voluntary evocation, a theme later taken up by Taine. To sustain his arguments, Boismont first portrays hallucination in relation to the experience of reverie, identifying environments in which external stimulation of the senses are quieted, where the internal functioning of sensory faculties come into their own: "This condition usually proceeds or follows that of sleep, ... especially when we are placed amidst the silence of nature, in the recesses of a forest, or are surrounded by the darkness of the night" (Boismont 1859, 29). Then, wanting to demonstrate these faculties with greater intensity and precision, he extends his study to visions and auditory hallucinations as related by artists, musicians, literary authors and religious followers whose sensory faculties, he argues, are more extensively developed. In such cases, he aims to demonstrate that those of heightened creative and intellectual abilities may experience hallucination yet maintain an intact sense of self:

> The person under the influence of haschish had a maniacal exaltation; his ideas were unconnected, and succeeded each other with great rapidity; they were in a state of excitement, which placed them beyond the influence of

the will. The mind was under the dominion of hallucinations ... Things of the past could be recalled, and revived, as though they were actually present ... In the midst of this disordered career of ideas, ... the feeling of personality was preserved.

(Boismont 1859, 29)

Influenced by Esquirol, Boismont embeds his argument in contemporary theories of human anatomy, proposing that "repetition of the same mental operations" may carve actual physical channels along the nerves of the brain (Taylor 2014, 143). His reasoning reflects contemporary principles of association psychology, allowing him to suggest the repetition of ideas, sensations and memories such as in periods of intense study or devout contemplation, may result in hallucinations that possess the same intensity, the same perceptual integrity, as when those impressions were first made upon the mind, and yet may occur with the retention of reason (Boismont 1859, 310). Such a theory allows Brierre de Boismont to go beyond the binary division between body and mind, as established by Descartes. Hallucination, by Boismont's logic, binds man's spiritual and physical faculties through this form of altered perception:

Considering its duality we think that an idea is, like man, composed of two parts – the one spiritual, the other material; and hallucination, considered in its characteristic phenomena, is the material reproduction of an idea. It is the highest degree of tension of which the deep thinker is capable – a real ecstasy.

(Boismont 1853, 21)

An elusive unconscious, it may be said, is emerging in this period, albeit more akin to notions of automatic cerebral functions than later psychoanalytic notions of an interior psychic space (Taylor 2014). Yet it reflects a growing instability of Descartes' notion of a unified, divisible self that equates only to consciousness. As reverie, daydream and hallucination are states of mind that shift between, blur and blend intrinsic and extrinsic sources of perception, they bring notions of reality and fantasy into dialogue with philosophical, medical and literary configurations of embodied selfhood. Perhaps most significantly, these mental states magnify the uneasy delineation of the mental from the physical in Cartesian philosophic tradition, and in turn, foreground new theoretical configurations of mind-body relations.

Returning to Brierre de Boismont's 1840 experiments with hashish, this attempt to intensify and physiologically induce hallucination represents the growing ability of literary, artistic and medical men to adjudicate over a new set of relations from which to understand the self. However, in distinguishing pathological from non-pathological hallucination, it is notable that Boismont does not openly challenge the Cartesian notion of the *unity* of the self; of its spiritual, incorporeal and innermost dimensions. His fashioning of the hallucination diagnosis ultimately works *within* the murky recesses of the Cartesian model of self to the extent that insanity proper is still considered a disease of the mind/soul and not of the material body. It was for others, taking up Boismont's research, that the metaphysical notion of the unity of the self is undermined, as experimental descents into states of reverie further his insights into the relations between perception, consciousness, memory and selfhood.

"When alone and in silence," Hippolyte Taine and the illusion of the self's unity

The notion of a multiplicity of possible selves, reacting and adapting to mental simulations during daydream and reverie, may be traced to the development of positivist psychology in the nineteenth century, as critical thinkers such as Hippolyte Taine (1828–1893) and William James (1842–1910) rejected Cartesian philosophies of the "unity of the self" that had persistend into the nineteenth century (James 1995, 154; 220). Taine, a French critic, historian and psychologist, published *De l'intelligence* (1870), in which he experimentally engages with mental states such as daydream, reverie and hallucination. By rejecting the notion of self as somehow "unique, persistent" and a "substance" unto itself, Taine redefines the self as made up of a series of "events," comprising "sensations, images, recollections, ideas and resolutions" (1889, 204; 209). By experimentally inducing unto himself a state of reverie, Taine uses "events" such as this to magnify, and show in its constituent parts, the formation of perception, which he argues constitutes the edifice of human knowledge. "When alone and in silence," writes Taine, and "reclining in a chair I abandon myself to reverie, and when by the obliteration of ordinary sensations, the internal phantasmagoria becomes intense, and if sleep draws on, my precise images end by exciting actual hallucinations" (209). Sitting back, closing his eyes, and entering into a state of reverie, Taine charts a continuum between "perception, memory, reverie, dreaming and hallucination" (James 1995, 154). Allowing "simulacra," or mental images, to fill his mind, the transition from extrinsic to intrinsic sites of perception is the pivotal subject of exploration: "At this moment a slight touch arouses me, the images become undone; the imaginary sounds lose their tone and sharpness; the colors fade; ... they ... lose their solidity and consistence" (Taine 1889, 242). It is, however, in analogy to the composition of selfhood that Taine's anatomisation of perception offers his most powerful attack on Cartesian based philosophies of the self. By theorising how mental representations are formed, Taine perceives the human nervous system as possessing two antagonistically functioning parts, one which predominates as sleep draws on, the other taking control upon waking. These, he postulates, regulate our perception of exteriority and interiority: "the waking state, as it draws to a close, confers the ascendency on images by taking it from sensations, and that the close of sleep deprives images of their ascendency by restoring it to sensations" (Taine 1889, 243). Rather than employ the Cartesian argument that the certitude of a conscious, unified self forms the basis from which to distinguish true from false perception, Taine flips this argument on its head. Using the state of reverie to shine a lens on the functioning of the human nervous system when the two modes of perception function at their most antagonistic, Taine poses the study of perception as analogous to the study of the unity of the self. Both, he argues, are products of an illusion: "Take the case of a table," he writes, "I see it, touch it, perceive it." Yet this perception of the table as a unified object is a mere "phantom," an "illusion," as the mind reduces its many characteristics to form the abstract idea of an object (Taine 1889, 227). This reductive process is seen as analogous by Taine to the constitution of the Cartesian self. The unified "Self" or "Ego," writes Taine, "is but a verbal entity and a metaphysical phantom," its unity "seen to vanish," as does the unity of the table, when the mechanisms of its perception are examined more closely. No longer "[is it] a question of knowing how an unextended substance, termed soul, can dwell in an extended substance, termed body;" rather, Taine declares the self to be made up of events comprising "sensations, images, recollections, ideas and resolutions," themselves considered aggregate functions of a wider web of "nervous functions." Bringing into consideration both physiological and psychological bases of conscious and unconsciously operating "events," Taine declares it is "these [which] ... constitute our being, our self has no other elements" (Taine 1889, 214).

A "sharply defined and securely discernible visual field" was giving way during this period to "a more ambiguous inner space" (Pick 1997, 190). The confidence in clear seeing, as outlined by Descartes through relations of consciousness, memory and the certainty of *cogito*, is undermined, as Taine argues all perception, even that during our most consciously experienced states of wakefulness, a form of hallucination. Taine, an avid reader of Brierre de Boismont and the 1855 debates, (James 1995, 162), feeds his ideas with medical publications on hallucination such as produced by Maury. L.F. Alfred (1848) and Baillarger (1846). Re-entering the 1855 debates, Taine argues that individuals predisposed to visual hallucination, such as during illness or periods of intense artistic, musical and literary creativity, demonstrate in extremity the "the internal event" – that is, the production of images in distinction to the reception of sensation – shown in a state of a "colored, intense, precise and localised semblance" (Taine 1889, 226). Ordinary conscious perception, as in the exemplar case of the table, is understood by Taine as hallucination, modulated by the sensory centres of the nervous system. Turning contemporary definitions of hallucination on its head, Taine declares "external perception" to be but "an internal dream which proves to be in harmony with external things." "[I]nstead of calling hallucination a false external perception," concludes Taine, "we must call external perception a true hallucination" (Taine 1889, 226).

For Taine, the unusual capacities of both the insane and the artist showed in extremity the functioning of perception. To gain a deeper understanding of perception in relation to one's personal sense of self, he, like Brierre de Boismont, turns to culture and literature to understand this intrinsic component of human experiential life. As James's research has unveiled (1995, 154), Taine took influence from his connections in literary circles to differentiate creative hallucination from the hallucination of madness. The literary author Gustave Flaubert wrote to Taine in 1888 that "[A]rtistic intuition ... actually resembles hypna-gogic hallucination: it flits before your eyes, and that is where you must grasp it, avidly" (Flaubert 1982, 97). Where the difference lies between the artist and the "man genuinely hallucinating," writes Flaubert, is in the joy felt by the poet, in contrast to the terror of "feel[ing] your personality slipping away from you" (James 1995, 167). This perspective reflects the argument made by contemporar-ies Buchez, Peisse, Moreau de Tours and Brierre de Boismont, who state that the line between pathological and artistic hallucination is drawn, not in terms of the presence of hallucination, but in terms of control. In the physiological hallucina-tions of artists and musicians, argues Buchez, the internal visions and auditory images are prepared and voluntary, but in cases of pathology they are spon-taneous and involuntary (Leudar and Thomas 2000, 9). Moreau de Tours wrote in 1855 that "Dreams begin where the freedom to direct our thoughts ceases," and further that when "notions from the outside are confused with those [whose] origin is the very organ if thought," abnormality arises in the waking state, con-current with this loss of freedom" (James 1995, 107; 109). To lose control over one's interior and exterior boundaries; to confuse imagination with reality: this was consonant with the loss of reason and therefore the loss of self (Leudar and Thomas 2000, 9).

In establishing a relationship between the wandering mind, experiment and re-conceptualisations of self within philosophy, medicine and literature, the final section of this chapter looks to the turn of the twentieth century, to a period in which studies of daydream and reverie are drawn into narrative, and increasingly psychoanalytically oriented studies of character. These studies each engage with, as well as mould, notions of the unconscious self during the period of adoles-cence. The focus is on British and North American psychiatric and psychological studies of mental pathology during adolescence; adolescence being a period of life described by the pioneering North American psychologist and educator Granville Stanley Hall (1844–1924) as a time of "dreamery and reverie" (Hall 1904, 351). Alighting on the examples of Stanley Hall, as well as the British psychiatrist James Crichton-Browne (1840–1938), and psychologist Cyril Burt (1883–1971), these cases are demonstrative of a shift in the early twentieth century away from studies of perception, and towards narrativity, case-taking and storytelling. The wandering mind, while formerly experimentalised through investigation of perception, moves now into the sphere of discourse analysis, through which new paradigms of the self begin to emerge.

"To see stars or sea phosphorescence in sunshine": daydreams and adolescence

The normal soul always soon comes back to the world of reality, perhaps wakes with a start, or may slowly ebb back, and is as powerless to revisit this subthalmic realm at will as it is to see stars or phosphorescence in sun-shine ... Adolescence is the golden age of this kind of dreamery and reverie which supplants reality ... It is a state from which some of the bad, but far more of the good qualities of life and mind arise. These are the noble lies of poetry, art, and idealism.

(Hall 1904, 312; 351)

Collapse of a sense of self; disorientation as to one's connection to the world; doubt as to the boundaries between dreaming and waking – these are the threads linking Cartesian, Romantic, proto-psychiatric and positivist psychologies of the self during periods of daydream, reverie and mind wandering, to the psychoanalytically invested studies of adolescence in the early twentieth-century:

> As Browne has well shown, if this efflorescence of meditativeness or introspection has been too rank, prolonged, or frequent, the subject may fall to thinking ... As Blood did on emerging from the influence of drugs ... that nothing is real but thought, feeling and sensation ... he may lose even a sense of his personal identity.

(Hall 1904, 312)

For Hall, the legacy of his forebears who experimentally explored drug-induced hallucination and descents into reverie informs his two-volume text, *Adolescence; its Psychology and its relations to physiology, anthropology, sociology, sex, crime, religion and education* (1904). Here, he charts the dangers of prolonged introspection during states of daydream and reverie to the health and stability of adolescent self-development. Notably, this is in causal relation to sexuality, criminality, morality and intelligence. The longstanding significance of Hall to the study of self are the insights that he offers to the study of adolescent mental pathology, in which he invokes methods of childhood education and upbringing aimed to increase mankind's virility, health and power (Bederman 2008, 78). Yet Hall's work is also influential in the wider field of understanding man's humanity. It is in relation to the notion of an unconscious, as elaborated by Sigmund Freud – as a driving force in the production of "poetry, art and idealism" – that Hall's widely read works explore the creative and elucidating potentiality of adolescent descents into daydream and reverie. "Indeed in the reverie and day dreaming common at this age," writes Hall of adolescence, "when the soul transcends its individual limitations and expatiates over the whole field of humanity, past, present, or future," the "soul" or self comes into contact with "unconscious cerebration" (Hall 1904, 312). Here, in Hall's text, the unconscious is envisaged as something separate from, and a space that distorts the functioning of, the conscious self, and yet to enter this unconscious realm through daydream and reverie was to be freed of the constraints of time, memory and consciousness, that are so central to Cartesian models of self and self-knowledge. Hall stresses a fundamental relationship between these dreamy mental states and the highest achievements of humanity. Achievement in art, poetry and idealism are accounted for by an individual's transcendence of the boundaries between reality and illusion; for entering into states of daydream and reverie where the senses are heightened, where a firm sense of individuality recedes. Such transcendence was deemed characteristic of the age of adolescence.

While Hall's psychology of adolescence is influenced by Freud, he is similarly indebted to the work of his British contemporary, James Crichton-Browne. In Britain, studies of adolescence in relation to daydream and reverie conducted by Crichton-Browne – the famed specialist in the nervous diseases of children – are published in his 1895 "Cavendish Lecture on Dreamy Mental States." Taking influence from the literary evocations of dreams, daydream and reverie penned by Coleridge, William Wordsworth and Thomas Hardy, his lecture focuses on the popular 1889 monograph of John Addington Symonds, *Sleep and Dreams*, through which to demonstrate the phenomenology of dreamy mental states. Like Hall, Crichton-Browne defines the wandering mind as a window into the unconscious: such states are "rents in conscious life through which glimpses of the supra-conscious may be obtained" (Crichton-Browne 1895, 74). Yet, unlike Hall, they are considered ultimately morbid, a cause of neurological deterioration and disintegration of a sense of self that hark back to Descartes:

> Symonds ... suffered from dreamy mental states which left on him discernible traces. "Suddenly in church or in company" he said, "when I was reading, and always, I think, when my muscles were at rest, I felt the approach of the mood. Irresistibly it took possession of my mind and will, lasted what seemed an eternity.... It consisted in a gradual but swiftly progressing obliteration of space, time, sensation, and the multitudinous factors of experience, which seem to qualify what we are pleased to call ourself."
>
> (Crichton-Browne 1895, 74)

The case to which this section turns its final attentions is that of Cyril Burt, whose publication, "The Dreams and Day-Dreams of a Delinquent Girl" (1921), exemplifies a period in which psychoanalytic theories and practices are precipitating a new metaphysics of *character* to emerge during early twentieth-century Britain. Alongside Sigmund Freud's *The Interpretation of Dreams* (1899), "Creative Writers and Day-Dreaming" (1908) and Dr J. Varendonck's *The Psychology of Day-Dreams* (1921) having reached a British readership, Burt's investigations offer British educationalists, psychologists and criminologists alike an understanding of self that is constituted through biology and heredity, as well as factors of environment, education and affluence. For Burt, the study of self is the study of biography – the study of character – as constituted through a "precipitate of fantasies, desires, and dreads," of past and present experiences, that overlay, exaggerate or modify mankind's more primitive impulses, reactions, intellect and emotions (Marcus 2014, 11; Burt 1925). Far from an understanding of self as something separate from, and independent of, the "extended substance" of body and environment, Burt regards these elements as integral to the self's formation (Burt 1921, (I) 3). Burt's psychoanalytically informed study of the dreams and daydreams of adolescents labelled as delinquent employs an iterative investigative process, by which daydreams are recovered and recited through interview. Featuring the choice case of a young domestic servant, Nellie Malone, his publication uses the resulting co-constructed narrative to support an emergent body of psychiatrists and psychologists who challenged the then dominant medical and legal classification of mental delinquency (Burt 1923; Shrubsall 1926; Tredgold 1926). In taking a life history that pivoted around the "delinquent['s]" recital of dreams and daydreams, Burt rejected the notion of mental delinquency as a form of criminal and antisocial behaviour to which an individual is hereditarily pre-disposed. In doing so, Burt investigated the plot lines and narrative tropes that bound Nellie's inner, psychic life to the external social, familial, educational and economic environment. Here Burt investigates the role of the social in the fashioning of the self, while the daydream becomes an avenue to intervene in the formation of character:

> [Nellie's] thoughts were fixed far more upon the fictitious world of fantasy which she had created for herself than upon the actual world of fact. When tidying her mistress' bedroom, she had one day found, and worn before the looking-glass, [a] chain necklace with a heart-shaped locket. This instantly appealed to her as being such a gift as the princely stranger might present, in token of his lasting affection.... She related, I think with unfeigned shame at her own childishness, the shock with which a call from her mistress startled her out of her musing before the mirror.... The day-dream was resumed the same night in her own room; and there seemed always something quasi-hypnotic in the ease with which she could throw herself into a state of trance-like fantasy by simply gazing at her image in the glass.... One evening ... she crept to the bedroom and stole the jewellery.... The easiest way to escape a troublesome conscience was always to return to her fantasies and self-told stories.
>
> (Burt 1921, 72)

Conclusion

Today, mental activity known variously as daydream, fantasy, self-generated thought and mind wandering, are recognised to occur within regions of the brain that increase in activation during periods of rest (Callard and Margulies 2011). These investigations are bound to the identification of a "default mode network" (DMN) of the brain, identified as such because within experimental fMRI scans, participants, when not engaged in cognitively demanding tasks and asked simply to rest in the scanner, consistently display *heightened* rates of metabolic activity in specific regions of the brain (Fox *et al.* 2013, 2). Mind wandering is understood to occur when the DMN is active, and it is here, tangibly situated within these networks of the brain, that conceptualisations of the self are again being revised.

When contemporary experimental investigations into the wandering mind are read with foreknowledge of a historical trajectory, such as that described in this chapter, it suggests that the shifting of the boundaries of the self have, in significant ways, been shaped by mind wandering investigation. Looking to contemporary studies, the self is now taking on new neurological boundaries, with human interiority no longer predominantly considered incorporeal, but rather as ostensibly situated within the body and the brain. Within laboratory environments perception of the self may now, in part, be conducted through fMRI scans that look beneath our outer surface. Of course, this is only partially to perceive what truly makes us human. At bedrock, studies of the self through the daydreaming, wandering, revelling mind are directed by the introspective individual, who alone has the most immediate and arguably authentic access to whatever constitutes our subjective interiority (Singer 1966, 6). Early psychological investigations, in addition to those focused upon in this study, such as Mary Learoyd's "The 'Continued Story'" (1895), Theodore L. Smith's "The Psychology of Day Dreams" (1904), Anna Freud's "The Relation of Beating Fantasies to a Day-Dream" (1923) through to Jerome L. Singer's substantial twentieth-century reports on *The Inner World of Daydreaming* (1966), compile tens, hundreds, even thousands of first-person reports on the phenomenology of the self and its interiority during mind-wandering states, have steered philosophical and medical theory and practise.

Beyond these formative studies, new formations of the concept of self are burgeoning in the twenty-first century through studies of the wandering mind (see for example Gallagher 2000; Smallwood *et al.* 2011; Allen and Friston 2016). Of most significance may be the observation that such studies have and continue to engender interdisciplinary working practices that link the insights of medicine and science to the arts and humanities in our endeavours to understand the human.

Reference list

Allen, Micah and Karl J. Friston. 2016. "From Cognitivism to Autopoiesis: Towards a Computational Framework for the Embodied Mind." *Synthese*, 1–24.

Allen, Micah and Gary Williams. 2011. "Consciousness, Plasticity, and Connectomics: The Role of Intersubjectivity in Human Cognition." *Frontiers in Psychology*, 2: 20.

Atkins, K. 2005. "Commentary on Descartes." In *Self and Subjectivity*, edited by Kim Atkins. Blackwell Readings in Continental Philosophy. Oxford: Wiley.

Bederman, G. 2008. *Manliness and Civilization: A Cultural History of Gender and Race in the United States, 1880–1917*. Women in Culture and Society. Chicago, IL: University of Chicago Press.

Berrios, German E. 1996. *The History of Mental Symptoms: Descriptive Psychopathology since the Nineteenth Century*. Cambridge: Cambridge University Press.

Boismont, A. Brierre de. 1853. *Hallucinations, Or, The Rational History of Apparitions, Visions, Dreams, Ecstasy, Magnetism, and Somnambulism*. Second Tr. Philadelphia: Lindsay and Blakiston.

Boismont, A. Brierre de. 1859. *On Hallucinations: A History of Explanation of Apparitions, Visions, Dreams, Ecstasy, Magnetism, and Somnambulism*, edited by Robert T. Hulme. London: Henry Renshaw.

Bullen, J.B. 1997. *Writing and Victorianism*. Crosscurrents Series. London: Taylor & Francis.

Burkitt, Ian. 1994. "The Shifting Concept of the Self." *History of the Human Sciences*, 7 (2): 7–28.

Burt, Cyril. 1921. "The Dreams and Day-Dreams of a Delinquent Girl." *Journal of Experimental Pedagogy and Training College Record*, 6: 66–77.

Burt, Cyril. 1923. "Delinquency and Mental Defect (II)." *British Journal of Medical Psychology*, 3 (3): 168–78.

Callard, Felicity and Daniel S. Margulies. 2011. "The Subject at Rest: Novel Conceptualizations of Self and Brain from Cognitive Neuroscience's Study of the 'Resting State.'" *Subjectivity*, 4 (3): 227–57.

Crichton-Browne, James. 1895. "The Cavendish Lecture: On Dreamy Mental States. Delivered before the West London Medico-Chirurgical Society, on Thursday, June 20, 1895." London: Baillière, Tindall and Cox.

Descartes, Rene. 1960. *Meditations of First Philosophy* (1641), translated by Laurence J. Lafleur. New York: The Bobbs Merrill Company.

Evans, Martyn. 2001. "Philosophy and the Medical Humanities." In *Medical Humanities*, edited by Martyn Evans and Illora G. Finlay, 250–63. London: BMJ Books.

Fitzgerald, Des and Felicity Callard. 2016. "Entangling the Medical Humanities." In *The Edinburgh Companion to the Critical Medical Humanities*, edited by Angela Woods and Anne Whitehead, 35–49. Edinburgh: Edinburgh University Press.

Flaubert, Gustave. 1980. *The Letters of Gustave Flaubert, 1857–1880*, edited by Francis Steegmuller. Cambridge, MA: Harvard University Press.

Flint, Kate, 2000. *The Victorians and the Visual Imagination*, Cambridge: Cambridge University Press, quoting Esquirol, J.E.D. "Sur Les Illusions de Sens Chez Les Alienes (1832)."

Ford, J. 1998. *Coleridge on Dreaming: Romanticism, Dreams and the Medical Imagination*. Cambridge Studies in Romanticism. Cambridge: Cambridge University Press.

Freud, Anna. 1974 [1923]. "The Relation of Beating-Phantasies to Day-Dream." *Introduction to Psychoanalysis: Lectures for Child Analysts and Teachers, 1922–1935*. London: Hogarth Press and the Institute of Psychoanalysis.

Freud, Sigmund. 1908. "Creative Writers and Day-Dreaming." In *The Standard Edition of the Complete Psychological Works of Sigmund Freud*, edited by James Strachey, 1953–74. London: Hogarth Press.

Freud, Sigmund. 2010. *The Interpretation of Dreams: The Complete and Definitive Text*, translated by J. Strachey. New York: Basic Books. https://books.google.co.uk/books?id=XWrZDaHlRz4C.

Gallagher, Shaun. 2000. "Philosophical Conceptions of the Self: Implications for Cognitive Science." *Trends in Cognitive Sciences*, 4: 14–21.

Goldstein, J.E. 2001. *Console and Classify: The French Psychiatric Profession in the Nineteenth Century*. Studies in Contemporary Linguistics Series. Chicago, IL: University of Chicago Press.

Grosz, Elizabeth. 1994. *Volatile Bodies: Towards a Corporeal Feminism*. Bloomington, IN: Indiana University Press.

Haggerty, John J. 2003. "Voices of Reason, Voices of Insanity: Studies of Verbal Hallucinations." *Psychiatric Services*, 54 (3): 409–10.

Hall, Stanley G. 1904. *Adolescence; Its Psychology and Its Relations to Physiology, Anthropology, Sociology, Sex, Crime, Religion and Education*. New York: D. Appleton and Co.

Harth, Erich. 1999. "The Emergence of Art and Language in the Human Brain." *Journal of Consciousness Studies*, 6: 6–7.

James, Tony. 1995. *Dream, Creativity, and Madness in Nineteenth-Century France.* Oxford: Clarendon Press.

Kendell, R.E. 2001. "The Distinction between Mental and Physical Illness." *The British Journal of Psychiatry,* 178 (6): 490–93.

Kristeva, Julia. 1990. "The Adolescent Novel." In *Abjection, Melancholia, and Love: The Work of Julia Kristeva,* edited by J. Fletcher and A.E. Benjamin. Warwick Studies in Philosophy and Literature. London: Routledge.

Learoyd, Mabel. 1895. "The 'Continued Story.'" *The American Journal of Psychology,* 7: 86–90.

Leudar, Ivan and Philip Thomas. 2000. *Voices of Reason, Voices of Insanity: Studies of Verbal Hallucinations.* London and Philadelphia: Routledge.

Marcus, L. 2014. *Dreams of Modernity: Psychoanalysis, Literature, Cinema.* Cambridge: Cambridge University Press.

Marx, Otto M. 2008. "German Romantic Psychiatry." In *History of Psychiatry and Medical Psychology,* edited by Edwin R. Wallace and John Gach, 313–33. New York: Springer.

McCorristine, S. 2010. *Spectres of the Self: Thinking about Ghosts and Ghost-Seeing in England, 1750–1920.* Cambridge: Cambridge University Press.

Pick, Daniel. 1997. "Stories of the Eye." In *Rewriting the Self: Histories from the Renaissance to the Present,* edited by Roy Porter, 186–99. London: Routledge.

Redpath, Peter. A. 1998. *Masquerade of the Dream Walkers: Prophetic Theology from the Cartesians to Hegel.* Amsterdam: Atlantic.

Sacks, Oliver. 2012. *Hallucination.* London: Picador.

Seli, Paul, Evan F. Risko, Christine Purdon and Daniel Smilek. 2016. "Intrusive Thoughts: Linking Spontaneous Mind Wandering and OCD Symptomatology." *Psychological Research.* doi: 10.1007/s00426-016-0756-3.

Seli, Paul, Jonathan Smallwood, James Allan Cheyne and Daniel Smilek. 2015. "On the Relation of Mind Wandering and ADHD Symptomatology." *Psychonomic Bulletin & Review,* 22 (3): 629–36.

Shin, Da Jung, Tae Young Lee, Wi Hoon Jung, Sung Nyun Kim, Joon Hwan Jang and Jun Soo Kwon. 2015. "Away from Home: The Brain of the Wandering Mind as a Model for Schizophrenia." *Schizophrenia Research,* 165 (1): 83–89.

Shrubsall, F.C. 1926. "The Definition and Diagnosis of Moral Imbecility (V)." *The British Journal of Medical Psychology,* 6: 70–83.

Shulman, Harry Manuel. 1951. "Intelligence and Delinquency." *Journal of Criminal Law & Criminology,* 41 (6): 763–81.

Singer, Jerome L. 1966. *The Inner World of Daydreaming.* London: Harper and Row.

Smallwood, Jonathan and Jonathan W. Schooler. 2015. "The Science of Mind Wandering: Empirically Navigating the Stream of Consciousness." *Annual Review of Psychology,* 66: 487–518.

Smallwood, Jonathan, Jonathan W. Schooler, David J. Turk, Sheila J. Cunningham, Phebe Burns and C. Neil Macrae. 2011. "Self-Reflection and the Temporal Focus of the Wandering Mind." *Consciousness and Cognition,* 20 (4): 1120–26.

Smith, Roger. 1997. "Self-Reflection and the Self." In *Rewriting the Self, Histories from the Renaissance to the Present,* edited by Roy Porter. London: Routledge.

Smith, Theodate L. 1904. "The Psychology of Day Dreams." *The American Journal of Psychology,* 15 (4): 465–88.

Strozier, R.M. 2002. *Foucault, Subjectivity, and Identity: Historical Constructions of Subject and Self.* Detroit, MI: Wayne State University Press.

Sullivan, Jeremiah J. 1973. "Henry James and Hippolyte Taine: The Historical and Scientific Method in Literature." *Comparative Literature Studies*, 10 (1): 25–50.

Taine, Hippolyte. 1889. *On Intelligence*, edited by T.D. Haye. New York: Henry Holt.

Taylor, Jenny Bourne. 1997. "Obscure Recesses: Locating the Victorian Unconscious." In *Writing and Victorianism*, edited by J.B. Bullen. Oxon: Taylor & Francis.

Tredgold, A.F. 1926. "The Definition and Diagnosis of Moral Imbecility (I)." *British Journal of Medical Psychology*, 6 (1): 1–9.

Varendonck, J. 1921. *The Psychology of Daydreams*. London and New York: Macmillan.

4 Soul searching

Psychiatry's influence on selfhood

Patrick Seniuk

The notion of "well-being" is dependent on a breadth of variables, such as material circumstances and social values of a particular historical epoch. Consistent with any notion of human well-being is the tight connection to self-understanding or what we might call first-person perspective. Arguably, any sense of well-being presupposes some sense of what is good for oneself. Hence, at some level, medicine is implicated in the way humans understand themselves. This should not be construed to mean that medicine defines human beings. However, the relationship between medical practice and well-being is such that it cannot help but involve existential concerns, particularly in the face of suffering, life, death and chronic illness.

The proliferation of diagnostic medical technologies has undoubtedly redefined not only how we *see* disease and illness, but also the way we understand the relationship between nature and soul, mind and body. In both medicine and philosophy, the external material world and the private internal world have traditionally been sharply opposed. Given that philosopher and doctor were, at one time, one and the same (for example, Hippocrates), the history of medicine is equally a philosophical narrative about the relationship between body (physical) and soul (mind). "One might argue," writes Rose, "that the most durable philosophies of the human have always had a very close relation to contemporary medical and scientific practices" (2016, 159). With respect to modern psychiatric medicine, if we consider the intersection of the "sciences of the soul" (neuroscience, cognitive science and psychology), there is little doubt that psychiatry has influenced the way humans understand selfhood.

In this chapter, I examine the way contemporary psychiatry has shaped how humans understand selfhood. More specifically, I consider the extent to which psychiatric nosology – via the *Diagnostic and Statistical Manual* (DSM) – has constrained our understanding of what it means to be human in Western culture. A crucial feature in the development of clinical psychiatry has been the appropriation of the categorical diagnostic paradigm used in biomedicine. Despite the kinship of biomedicine and psychiatry, categorical diagnosis is not easily transposed onto clinical psychiatry. One of the enduring issues for psychiatry is not so much medical as it is philosophical: what does it mean to be disordered? Put another way, with psychiatric diagnosis we find a discursive distinction between *being* and *having*: "I am disordered" versus "I have a disorder." And while this distinction may appear to be a mere matter of semantics, there are several philosophical consequences that emerge apropos of this dichotomy, including the status of moral responsibility, and even the nature of reality. In the first half of the chapter I will briefly discuss the influence of Descartes' substance dualism in medicine, as well as a brief history of the DSM published by the American Psychiatric Association. The second half of the chapter addresses selfhood using insights from phenomenological philosophy and concludes by introducing positive possibilities of a dimensional diagnostic model as an alternative to the current categorical model.

Challenging medicine and psychiatry to a "dual"

The most influential and enduring philosophical concept in psychiatric medicine is undoubtedly Descartes' substance dualism. Colloquially, this idea is often referred to as the "mind-body problem." Even though Descartes' famous metaphysical treaty *Meditations on First Philosophy* is over 300 years old, the consequences of his work for psychiatry should not be understated. The Cartesian metaphysical legacy is subtly interwoven not just into psychiatric medicine, but Western culture itself.

The famous claim made by Descartes is that two types of substances exist: one is extended in space (*res extensa*), while the other does not exist in space (*res cogitans*); one substance is material matter, while the other is non-material matter (for example, thoughts). For Descartes, mind or spirit (*res cogitans*) exists on a plane that is wholly distinct from physical objects, which, it should be emphasised, includes the body. The material world in this account is describable in mechanistic terms, as "stuff" subjected to the laws of nature. That a material object is extended is crucial for Descartes, because only extended things may be plotted *in* geometric space. Mind, on the other hand, cannot be described spatially. According to Descartes, our thoughts (or consciousness) do not "exist in space" the way a table extends across space from a fixed point. As a consequence, thoughts or mind do not adhere to external laws of nature. The Cartesian doctrine permeates idiomatic, everyday language, found in phrases such as "mind over matter" or "body and soul."

The mind-matter distinction is logically predicated on what is proper to the mind and what is proper to the body. Reason, will, rationality and faculties of the intellect have historically been viewed as the source of self, this source of self characterised as belonging to the domain of the mind. Affects (or passions), by contrast, are bodily experiences that belong to the passive domain of sensation; they happen to or impress upon the body. Accordingly, desires, feelings and emotions have long been viewed as encumbrances to self-control. For this reason, self is commonly allied with choice, which, broadly speaking, means that self is not heteronomous, or driven by so-called irrational impulses or passions.

While it is clear that the legacy of Cartesian dualism has punctuated many medical concepts, because psychiatry specialises in "the soul," it is unsurprising that this dualism bears a particular conceptual affinity for this branch of medicine. Because the distinction between mind and body is metaphysical, it makes sense that the influence of substance dualism is embedded within broader, commonplace, conceptual schemas. In fact, Cartesianism is arguably interwoven with medicine, psychiatry and psychology in such a way that our intuitive understanding of the nature of human existence (and consciousness) seems unthinkable in any other way.

Let us consider, for instance, how illness and disease are conceptualised in Western medicine. Disease and illness are generally assumed to be something external to the self (subject), something beyond one's control. Even with respect to diseases that are correlated with lifestyle choices (smoking and cancer, diet and hypertension, etc.), the causal mechanisms for such diseases do not always obey universally predictable pathways. For instance, despite the close correlation between smoking and lung cancer, it does not necessarily follow that smoking is the efficient cause of lung cancer. To conclude otherwise would be rather unpalatable to categorically claim the patient *caused* his or her cancer by smoking. It may well be the case that smoking elicited conditions to bring about a disease, but it is equally the case that many cancers have genetic components, and many are idiopathic. Equally, persons who smoke or have poor dietary habits do not necessarily become diseased. The overarching point, then, is that if a person's body becomes diseased or sick, he or she is not responsible for causing the illness. A cancer diagnosis is often simply attributed to chance or bad genetic luck; it is a physiological state beyond one's control. Hence, to *have* a disease implies that a person ordinarily does not invite the disease upon his or her self, and it transcends the realm of personal autonomy.

By contrast, one of the definitive features of *being* a self (a human) is a capacity for, or power to assert, autonomous action. Character, dispositions, thoughts, and so on, are commonly attributed to the realm of the mind – or at least subsumed under something like a mind. It is in the realm of thinking or reasoning that, for Descartes and many following him, we are free from the constraint of natural laws and possess the power of autonomous choice. Consequently, our freedom, or capacity for self-determination, is indivisible from the responsibility that follows from what we choose or choose not to do. In other words, we can say that an autonomous agent's decision to do X has an obverse relation to responsibility; choice X entails responsibility for having chosen X. When we act, our action is underpinned by justificatory reasons for that action, regardless of whether or not the reasons are made explicit. The traditional relationship between choice and responsibility leads us to conclude that we are at some level accountable for who we are and what we do.

For our purpose here, the crucial point I want to highlight about responsibility does not concern the metaphysics of free will. Enough ink has been spilled on that topic over the last 2,000 years without any satisfactory conclusions. The relevance of responsibility in the context of medical psychiatry is that, depending on the way we conceptualise the relationship between mind and body, we also commit ourselves to tacit conclusions concerning the nature of psychiatric disorders. If we hold that bodily states are determined strictly by physiological and biological processes, then it (rightly) seems counterintuitive that we would hold a person responsible for his or her diseased state. In contrast, if the mind is understood to be under explicit control of an agent, then one might contend that certain affective states, dispositions, or inappropriate behaviours are things that one can freely choose, which therefore makes one responsible for choosing this or that action. With respect to the latter, for example, I could choose not to hit my friend in anger; it was – in principle – not beyond my control to act otherwise. Consequently, the self is something to which we have direct and unimpeded access.

The inexorable rise of the DSM

In order to understand the relationship between dualism and psychiatry, it is important to establish a basic outline of psychiatric diagnosis and its history. The Cartesian worldview that mind and body are distinct modes of existence has fallen into disrepute with most philosophical circles over the last half-century.[1] Despite no longer being philosophically *de rigueur*, as I have already suggested, dualist ontology continues to pervade everyday discourse. More importantly, it remains characteristic of the language used in the natural sciences (Husserl [1954] 1970). In some respects, the scientifically inspired development of the DSM's diagnostic categories reflects psychiatry's attempt to resolve the issue of mind and body, disorder and responsibility. A significant consequence of the publication of the DSM is that patients are absolved from responsibility for being disordered. In other words, the depressed person needed medical care because her depression was a physiological pathology beyond her control. As such, the application of a DSM diagnosis means that it was inappropriate to characterise a person's condition as a moral failure or lack of self-control. Instead, mental disorder becomes characterised no differently than any "naturally" occurring somatic disease.

It is now almost unthinkable to mention the DSM without stipulating that it is the near ubiquitous reference manual for diagnosing mental disorder in psychiatry. Before the American Psychiatric Association's publication rose to prominence, the World Health Organization's *International Classification of Disease* (ICD) also served as a clinical guide for psychiatric disorder. Prior to the DSM's inaugural publication in 1952, there had been no definitive psychiatric classification system. At the beginning of the twentieth century, psychiatrists in the United States remained relatively uninterested in mental illness data since there was no reliable method for diagnoses. As of 1840, demographic data collected by the American census bureau was fit into imprecise categories of mental disorder (Grob 1991), offering two vague options: "insanity and idiocy" (Beutler and Malik 2002, 4). Moving forward to the mid-twentieth century, war indirectly proved to be a turning point for psychiatric care. During peacetime, mentally ill persons were treated by removing them from their so-called "noxious environments" (Decker 2013, 7) and placed in asylums. War presented a challenge to this paradigm, since in-patient treatment was most obviously not an option. The nascent influence of psycho-analysis matured into the dominant theory in psychiatry, establishing a foothold by providing treatment to soldiers at the front lines in the form of talk therapy. The result was that a significant number of patients often recovered well enough to return to duty. This therapeutic practice initiated the eventual shift of psychiatric treatment from hospital care to a community setting.

The publication of DSM-I through DSM-III was accordingly imbued with psychoanalytic theory. However, the psychoanalytic approach had little use for diagnosing disorders since psychic disturbances were viewed as internal con-flicts at the unconscious level, and through clinical analysis, the aim was to bring the unconscious conflict to the conscious level, thereby resolving the neurotic behaviour. Unfortunately, this would prove unsatisfactory, as emerging psycho-pathologies failed to fit into the basic categories or could not be captured with nomenclature available to military psychiatrists. The soldier-patients presented symptom clusters that could not be adequately accounted for (Grob 1991, 428). Psychodynamic labels like "neurosis" did not square with the psychosomatic disorders psychiatrists were faced with. Both the Army and Navy were com-pelled to create their own classification system, which eventually inspired the APA to publish the DSM-I in 1952.

The third revision of the DSM (DSM-III) signified a decisive conceptual and clinical shift in American psychiatry. One notable reason for the shift that occurred in the classification of mental disorder was anxiety over diagnostic validity, a problem that undermined psychiatry's categorisation as a medical science. Without distinct conceptual boundaries for categories of disorder, evid-ence that a diagnosis actually pointed out a "real" disorder was scant. As a result, psychiatry was portrayed unfavourably by some as arbitrary and unscientific.[2] Doubt was cast on psychiatry's claim to scientific rigor because of the inconsist-encies in diagnoses between different clinicians as well as the over-theorised influence of psychoanalysis. The overarching problem was psychiatry's inability to achieve successful communication among clinicians, not to mention research-ers. It became clear that enhancing communication among psychiatrists would not only enhance professional integrity (for example, shared diagnosis across multiple psychiatrists), it would also make it possible for researchers to work from well-delineated categories, that would develop empirical data on causation and ultimately vindicate psychiatry's scientific status by validating disorders.

This transition essentially committed psychiatry to jettison a nominalist meta-physical view of the human person, that is, a view in which the person is viewed as a wholly unique phenomenon whose psychic disturbance is solely related to their specific life situation, for a realist view, which re-envisaged psychic distur-bance in terms of common human experience. The result was that while persons by definition remained "individuals," the disordered experience became seen as something common to many individuals. Because of this commonality, it was understood that a real disorder entity existed as a separate factor and could be readily picked out across a larger population. The result was that the inner work-ings of the self were not unique to the individual but were universally vulnerable to dysfunction. Even though disordered self-experience remains *mine*, the reason for disordered experience could be the same for other selves. Hence, one conclusion is that the self could be characterised as normal or abnormal; the absence of the real entity X meant that psychic processes functioned normally. The presence of X meant it was possible to show objectively that self-experience was abnormal.

Thus, there are two distinct ways psychiatric nosology became relevant for the way we understand selfhood. One the one hand, the psychoanalytic tradition (predating categorical diagnosis) viewed self-control and self-understanding as a chimera. What one desires, how one behaves, is partially the result of unconscious forces beyond conscious control, making it clear that the self was a divided self. For psychoanalysis, the self or experiencer was an assemblage of conscious, unconscious and biological interactions, which, metaphorically speaking, suggested that conscious life (ego) was comparable to a bus steered by an invisible (unconscious) driver. Self was an elusive and unbound phenomenon.

The introduction of categorical diagnostics, on the other hand, engendered a static notion of self; distance was placed between self and mental disorder. The intransigent and capricious psychic economy of psychoanalysis became reified in psychiatric medicine; self-experience or subjectivity could be cleaved from medically definable dysfunction independent of the person *qua* person. No longer did one suffer a "malady of the soul," but rather of the physical body. One consequence of psychiatric nosology is a polarity of self-understanding, a shift from unseen forces in the inner depths of self to something concrete and distinct, existing independently of the external forces exerted on the body. Psychiatric disorder becomes localisable; it may be present or absent, a foreign invader that is something *other* than myself.

The ontology of category

The brief historical overview of psychiatric nosology serves to illustrate why categorical diagnosis is a salient issue for conceptualising selfhood. Matters are complicated, however, when we focus on *what* is being categorised by the DSM. It is, perhaps, taken for granted that mental disorders remain without clear etiological explanation.[3] The DSM categories are not supposed to make reference to the cause of a disorder since current science is only able to establish correlations. The category of X is merely intended to describe the signs and symptoms that point to the underlying presence of X. To take a simple example, if a car is emitting black smoke from its exhaust and making a clunking sound, a mechanic would take these to be signs or symptoms of some underlying problem. Reciprocally, when experiencing a headache, the resultant pain and sensitivity to noise have no causal connection to the headache as such. For the clinician, these positive descriptions point to something beyond the symptoms of pain and sensitivity.

Likewise, psychiatrists do not have the diagnostic tools similar to those of the general physician. The psychiatrist cannot issue a requisition for a test in the way a general physician is able to perform a throat swab to detect *streptococcus*.

Thus, one of the underlying – but overlooked – tensions in contemporary psychiatry is the ontology of disorder. Despite the fact that psychiatry is modelled on biomedicine, psychiatric disorders are much more elusive. It must be taken for granted that beneath the signs and symptoms there is an underlying pathology, even if that pathology remains inchoate for current science. A clinician meets with a patient because it is assumed there is something (unseen) that is clinically significant. In turn, the intention is to identify what is wrong in order to return to a state of normality. Unfortunately, this view bifurcates the self into negative and positive poles; normal selfhood lacks nothing, or has no deficiency, while abnormal selfhood is a state in which the deviation is measured against the relatively static self in normalcy. The problem with this view is well documented by Georges Canguilhem, who notably contends that the difference between normal and abnormal cannot be determined by reference to the normal state. He insists that in pathology, what we witness is the formation of new phenomena, new bodily and self-norms that do not efface previous benchmarks, and further, that it is not possible to return to the same state of self after serious illness (Canguilhem 1989). Alternatively, we can say that it would be a mischaracterisation by the clinician to view the patient as someone who needs to return to a previous normality. Self-experience in mental disorder evokes an entirely new phenomenon; a return to the so-called normal self requires a static or concrete point of reference, something that serves as a reference point for any deviation. This subsequently evokes a question regarding the nature of somatic medicine and psychiatric medicine: if a broken hand restored to full function remains the same hand, does a person who is no longer suffering from major depression return to the state of self?

Do psychiatrists identify discrete and locatable entities? The brief of somatic medicine is typically to assess whether or not a disease or dysfunction is present in a patient. An orthopaedic surgeon investigates whether a person has broken a bone using a variety of assessments, including x-ray imaging. A radiograph is intended to confirm or deny the presence of a suspected fracture. In the case of a positive diagnosis, one may say that a fracture is present; the patient *has* a fracture. Similarly, a variety of tests make it possible for an oncologist to confirm that a person *has* cancer. The physician is tasked with making a categorical claim that one either has or does not have X.[4] By contrast, psychiatrists cannot confirm the presence or absence of a mental disorder by locating a concrete entity. The signs and symptoms presented by the patient are taken to be indicative of disorder, but the disorder cannot be confirmed simply by looking "inside" the patient.

Psychiatric diagnostics is distinguished from other medical sciences primarily by the fact that the symptoms affect what we often refer to as the subjective aspect of experience. The symptoms of mental disorder are inextricable from the patient's self-experience. Then again, the purpose of categorical diagnosis in psychiatry is somewhat in opposition to what is given to self-experience. The diagnostic ideal is to parse signs and symptoms from the experiencer. Of course, in practice, good clinical practice ought to address the particulars of the patient's life (stressors, for example) in order to distinguish disorder from non-disorder. But the diagnostic intention, nevertheless, remains tied to identifying specific criteria. With this in mind, exploring the quality of a symptom only inhibits identification of the symptom.

The proliferation of neuroscience has emboldened some to believe that it is only a matter of time before brain imaging will allow us to confirm the presence of disorder using images that represent the internal working of the brain. Such aspirations would, in principle, allow the clinician to bypass the self-experiential of the patient by relying on a diagnostic test. However, in doing so, such a test is built upon an assumption that mental disorders are restricted entirely to the brain. The overarching implication is that an image or diagnostic test will point to disorder X: there is depression! Yet, when we reflect upon the nature of mental disorders such as depression, we must tread lightly if we assert that it is a discrete, localisable, physiological state. The experience of depression is not localised in the way one experiences a broken bone. The experience of having a broken leg is phenomenologically unique from having depression. Depression by definition permeates every aspect of a person's life; it evokes a change to the way one acts in the world. And it is here that we must consider the not so insignificant question that often arises for patients with mental disorders: *am* I X or do I *have* X? Am I depressed or do I have depression?

The *prima facie* distinction between being something and having something may seem like a pseudo-problem, that what we are presented with is an issue of semantics rather than ontology. On the one hand, to have any malady will undoubtedly change the way in which we engage with the world. Everyday situations that are otherwise experienced as familiar and habitual may become obstacle-like or problematic. A broken leg will transform the way one approaches basic situations such as crossing the street at a traffic light. On the other hand, with respect to mental disorder, while it may well be the case that the world appears obstacle-like, there is, in addition, a distinct change to the affective dimension of experience: "the patient is ill; this means that *his world is ill*, literally that *his objects are ill*, however unusual this may sound" (van den Berg 1972, 46 emphasis original).

Let's find our-self: phenomenology, psychiatry and self

The vast number of available theoretical accounts of human selfhood has been gestured towards in other chapters in this volume. Therefore, rather than summarising them, I will assume that there is *something* we call a human self, with the qualification that it is neither a metaphysical entity, nor a locatable kernel within a subject. Regardless of the metaphysical status philosophers accord to self, one of the intriguing aspects of psychiatry is that it provides us with concrete cases from which it seems evident that mental disorders, even in the most minimal way, always implicate an experiential sense of self.

Phenomenology is an indispensable framework for both clinician and theorist alike. The redeeming feature of the phenomenological approach is that psychiatry can succeed even if it fails to begin with concrete existence; that is, phenomenology recognises that the patient's subjective experience is always, first and foremost, self-experience, which ultimately means that mental disorder is equally a disorder of self (Ratcliffe 2015; Svenaeus 2014). While no one individual can be credited with phenomenology's rise in psychiatry, the appeal of phenomenology is broadly attributable to the challenge it poses to the scientific ideal of objectivity.[5] More specifically, phenomenologists argue that overreliance on third-person observation of the object (patient) is remiss, insofar as third-person approaches must abstract the object of focus from its lived-world context. Phenomenological philosophers of the twentieth century astutely noted that "objective" or scientific thought was guilty of taking for granted the very existence of the world. Our experience of the world is so obvious that we fail to recognise its significance, namely that it is the ground upon which all experience is made possible. The strong claim levelled by the phenomenologist is that any attempt to understand a patient (or person in general) without addressing his or her relationship with the world is destined to fail. And if not an outright failure, then the nature of self-experience is effaced by a (mere) descriptive account experience.

What phenomenology offers contemporary psychiatry is a different way of seeing mental disorder. There is no doubt that phenomenologically inspired psychiatrists and philosophers challenge the conceptual basis of psychiatric nosology, which also includes the validity of various categories used by the DSM. More importantly though, phenomenology, as Merleau-Ponty says, "places essences back within existence and thinks that the only way to understand man and the world is by beginning from their facticity" (Merleau-Ponty [1945] 2012, xx). Phenomenologically inspired psychiatry approaches a patient not as someone with a discrete disorder or disease, but rather as someone whose entire way of relating to the world has become transformed.

Is it me or is it in me?

Do we have good reason to think that the distinction between being disordered and having a disorder is legitimate? Regardless of whether or not such an ontological distinction in fact exists, it is clear that mind-body dualism permeates the discursive development of psychiatric medicine and the way we understand ourselves as human beings. From the phenomenological perspective, it needs to be asked how disorder can be distinguished from the very way one relates to the world. Third-person (clinical) observation ultimately seeks a pathological physiological process independent of the patient *qua* patient. The phenomenological attitude, on the other hand, holds that it is impossible to imagine that a disordered patient's experience could be anything less than an entire way of being-in-the-world.

Taking depression as an example, the categorical diagnostic approach in psychiatry tacitly commits one to an essentialist view of self. Expressed differently, depression is something that I either have or do not have and, accordingly, it is not an essential constitutive component of *who I am*. In principle, if the underlying dysfunction is assuaged, a person can return to a non-disordered (or non-pathological) state. To be depressed means that a person undergoes an "uninvited" intrusion by something external to that person. There is no doubt an intuitive appeal in making a categorical distinction, particularly in light of the fact that one does not choose to become depressed. This intuition mirrors attitudes in somatic medicine, insofar as conditions such as influenza do not respect the boundaries of an autonomous agent's desire to be free of illness. On this account, depression is something *in* me, something foreign or alien to the self.

Because categorical classification of mental disorders characterises mental pathology medically, significant inroads have been made in reducing the stigma often associated with being mentally ill. And yet, with the medicalisation of mental disorder, we equally risk distorting the nature of mental disorder. From the phenomenological perspective, characterising mental disorder as a discrete entity or dysfunction fails to appreciate that this can only occur through abstraction, and as a consequence, precludes consideration for the way disorder is manifested in lived experience. It is not just that a person is disordered or ill; the very structure of conscious experience itself is modified, which in turn affects the phenomenal appearance of the world. Hence, despite the ostensive benefits of a medicalised approach to mental disorder, when we look closer, it becomes clear that we are left with a lacuna.

Staying with the example of depression, the DSM depression category does not investigate the self-experience of a patient in the phenomenological sense. The category does not make room for the fact that there is "a disturbance of something that is fundamental to our lives, something that goes unnoticed when intact. What is eroded or lost is a 'sense' or 'feeling' of being comfortably immersed in the world" (Ratcliffe 2015, 15). I suggested earlier that a categorical approach to mental disorder makes it possible to characterise depression in the same way as influenza, something foreign or unwanted, the upshot of which allows us to absolve the patient of any responsibility for her condition. However, if we adopt a phenomenological perspective, although influenza and depression do have a significant phenomenological overlap with respect to bodily experience, the comparison is not as straightforward as it seems. In fact, the two conditions are experienced in considerably distinct senses. It may be the case that

> depression is often interpreted by the sufferer in a way that differs from how somatic illnesses are generally conceived of. Influenza is a foreign invader that inflicts symptoms on the person from the outside, whereas many depression narratives construe depression as integral to the self.
>
> (96)

A consequence of identifying mental disorder categorically – having or not having a mental disorder – is that it becomes difficult, if not impossible, to establish what properly belongs to the patient. If the disorder is distinct from who I am or how I am, then there must exist some relatively stable index according to which it is possible to discern between "me" and "not me."

As I have noted, the categorical approach to diagnosing mental disorders offers us an unsatisfactory bifurcation: either disorder is present, or it is not. It is equally unsatisfactory to maintain a distinction between being disordered and having a disorder, with respect to the implications for personal responsibility. While it is conceptually compelling to characterise the schizophrenic patient or depressed patient as "being schizophrenic" or "being depressed," it becomes tempting to conclude that mental disorder does not properly belong to the realm of medicine. If, indeed, the self is disturbed in mental disorder, how might we make room for the possibility of understanding mental disorder such that something is wrong with my self, yet nevertheless beyond my control?

There are at minimum two ways to collapse the apparent gap between being disordered and having a disorder. The first and most uncontentious approach is to eschew mind-body dualism. Even in medicine, it has become rather unfashionable to explicitly retain this dichotomy. The rise of person-centred medicine and the bio-psychosocial model are but two examples of the move away from dualism. With respect to mental disorder, the unity of mind and body makes it possible to understand disorders as indivisible from the physiological processes of the body, which importantly includes functions of the brain and the corollary psychological processes. Furthermore, there are extremely compelling arguments to be found in both neuroscience (Damasio 2009) and philosophy (Merleau-Ponty 2012), which illustrate that, not only are mind and body one phenomenon, the very possibility of having an experience of self is only possible by virtue of being embodied. The latter undermines the deeply entrenched view that the psyche (or mind) is the sole constitutive domain of the self.

Having said that, the indivisibility of mind and body has led some to conclude that all subjective experience is explainable by underlying neurobiological processes. The theory of mind known as eliminative materialism (Churchland 2013; Clark 2006) is one model that attempts to do just that. Eliminative materialists hold that the ways we talk about subjective experience, such as emotions, feelings, beliefs and so on, are ultimately (poor) metaphors used as proxies for underlying neurological processes. In other words, emotions feelings and dispositions exist only insofar as they can be reduced to neurophysiological terms. The risk of any reductionist approach to human behaviour is that, with respect to mental disorder, the impetus is to (incorrectly) delimit dysfunction using physiological explanation. In the case of the latter, psychological, sociological and personal dimensions are secondary levels that must concede to the explanation at the primary causal level.

Yet causal explanations, despite their intuitive appeal, exclude considerations for the phenomenal life of self-experience. That is, causal explanations attempt to explain the behaviour of humans without reference to their context. Paradoxically, an attempt to explain the human condition stripped from "being-in-the-world" is a project *by* humans in a very specific, lived-context. But what is perhaps even more significant is that our biological workings are, in part at least, those of persons: the ways in which we pursue even our animal desires, or express even our basic emotions, are conditioned by the human and social context in which we pursue them.

(Matthews 2007, 103)

Thus, we have reasons for doing X or Y that fall outside the purview of the underlying physiology that makes experience possible in the first place. While it is entirely possible to neurologically explain a person's phobia of open spaces (the *how*), such an explanation cannot discern why open spaces are a source of fear for her. The meaning of agoraphobia, or of any phobia, will not coincide with the underlying neurological state, such that the latter cannot itself distinguish between fear of spiders or fear of open spaces. The reduced explanation cannot account for the significations that allow for the possibility of a fearful experience. The causal explanation in this instance is not amenable to predictability: "the biochemistry of fear is the same whatever the intentional object may be" (Matthews 2007, 140). The reason one is fearful of one object or another cannot be determined using a causal explanation.

Just because some theorists have a proclivity for reductive approaches does not mean we must give up on a monist understanding of mind and body. A second possibility to reconfigure how we understand mental disorder involves changing the approach to psychiatric diagnosis, all the while retaining the view that mind and body are one. At the moment, this is the most fruitful of possible resolutions to the current limitations founding categorical diagnosis. The most recent DSM revision (DSM-V) in 2013 has attracted considerable support for the adoption of a new approach to psychiatric diagnosis. Contra the categorical model, a dimensional diagnostic model has been proposed as a significant improvement upon standard practices (Whooley 2014; Regier 2007). For instance, "dimensions may allow clinicians and researchers to better identify more specific diagnostic thresholds and address the nuances of psychiatric disorders, such as individual differences in symptomology, onset course, severity, and treatment response – as well as co-morbid conditions" (Reiner *et al.* 2012, 555). One of the most appealing features of the dimensional model is the inclusion of symptom severity, which is starkly opposed the criteriological approach used in clinical practice "where the realities of patient care confirm that diagnoses are not neatly compartmentalised into hierarchies or categories" (555). On a dimensional diagnostic model, the patient's affliction is not classified categorically. A depression diagnosis is not determined as either present or absent; one is not either strictly depressed or not depressed. Rather, the dimensional model is capacious enough to view disorder as an of-self (belonging to or arising within the self) situated in and by an *Umwelt*, the context within which the world is perceived. Dimensionality is sensitive to the fact that the way one relates to the world is changed, which will be clinically significant, to lesser or greater degrees based on a person's experiential descriptions. The dimensional model introduces a severity spectrum that encourages nuanced diagnosis. A depression diagnosis may range from very mild disturbances up to and including the most sever catatonic manifestations of depression. It also presents us with the idea that normal and abnormal cannot be strictly delimited. Who one is cuts across various dimensions, all of which are more or less dilated at a given point in one's life and are subject to flux.

A revised diagnostic framework enables clinical practitioners to discern gradations of "disorder" within a specific category. A patient who does not present prototypical depression or does not meet the necessary threshold of five out of nine diagnostic criteria could still warrant a diagnosis of depression. In the dimensional framework, the patient may be depressed below the standard diagnostic threshold, or equally, symptom severity may exceed typical clinical presentations. A distinctive feature of the dimensional framework is that it discloses the heterogeneity associated with most mental disorders, which by necessity, was effaced with the categorical approach in order to "facilitate communication between professionals" (Kelly *et al.* 2017, 1), thereby securing inter-rater reliability within the psychiatric profession.

Conclusion

Dimensionality allows for fidelity to the patient's lived-experience of suffering. Not only does it permit degrees of disorder, a dimensional approach is sensitive to the patient as someone whose illness cannot be cleaved from his or her self. The disorder affects the person on a global plane, meaning that it pervades all aspects of life, including self-interpretation and sense-making that always occurs on the tacit background of the world. One should not, however, overstate the virtues of the dimensional approach, since no one change alone will ever resolve all the tensions in psychiatric nosology. Nonetheless, the inclusion of the dimensional approach is a positive movement in diagnosis, if only for the reason that it better reflects the way selfhood is implicated in mental disorder, ways that are less readily apparent in traditional somatic medicine.

Psychiatric medicine has profoundly influenced the way we understand what it means to be human. At best, the history of psychiatric medicine is one of ambivalence: we find both the good and the bad. The use of categorical diagnosis in psychiatry has advanced human well-being, but it has also complicated the very way we understand well-being. However, the introduction of the dimensional approach to diagnosis is a significant step towards resolving some of the vexing conceptual issues associated with nosology. Incorporating dimensionality with categorical diagnosis, I have argued, will make it possible for psychiatry to *see* in a new way.

Notes

1 Notable critics of Descartes are found in both the analytic and continental traditions, and include phenomenologists such as Husserl, Heidegger and Merleau-Ponty, as well as philosophers of mind like Ryle, Sellars and McDowell.

2 Many of these claims emerged from the anti-psychiatry movement, with notable figures who included Szasz, Foucault and Laing.
3 The exception being dementia-related disorders, which, nevertheless, are only identifiable posthumously.
4 There are exceptions to the categorical diagnosis in somatic medicine. Hypertension is one example where a physiological state is assessed according to a continuum, upon which a threshold is used to discern between pathology and non-pathology.
5 This should not be mistaken for rejection of science as such. The criticism rests in the way scientific methods or scientists themselves understand the nature of reality.

Reference list

Beutler, Larry E. and Mary L. Malik. 2002. "The Emergence of Dissatisfaction with the DSM." In *Rethinking the DSM: A Psychological Perspective*, edited by Larry E. Beutler and Mary L. Malik, 3–16. Washington, DC: American Psychological Association.

Canguilhem, Georges. 1989. *The Normal and the Pathological*. New York: Zone Books.

Churchland, Paul M. 2013. *Matter and Consciousness*, 3rd edn. Cambridge, MA: MIT Press.

Clark, Andy. 2006. "I Am John's Brain." In *Theories of Mind: An Introductory Reader*, edited by Maureen Eckert. Lanham, MD: Rowman & Littlefield.

Damasio, Antonio. 2008. *Descartes' Error: Emotion, Reason and the Human Brain*. London: Random House.

Decker, Hannah. 2013. *The Making of DSM-IIIR: A Diagnostic Manual's Conquest of American Psychiatry*. Oxford: Oxford University Press.

Grob, Gerald N. 1991. "Origins of DSM-I: A Study in Appearance and Reality." *The American Journal of Psychiatry*, 148.44: 421–31.

Husserl, Edmund. 1970. *The Crisis of European Sciences and Transcendental Phenomenology: An Introduction to Phenomenological Philosophy*. Translated by David Carr. Evanston, IL: Northwestern University Press.

Kelly, J.R., G. Clarke, J.F. Cryan and T.G. Dinan. 2017. "Dimensional Thinking in Psychiatry in the Era of the Research Domain Criteria (RDoC)." *Irish Journal of Psychological Medicine*, 4.5: 1–6.

Kirk, Stuart A. and Herb Kutchins. 1992. *The Selling of DSM: The Rhetoric of Science in Psychiatry*. New York: A. de Gruyter.

Matthews, Eric. 2007. *Body-Subjects and Disordered Minds: Treating the Whole Person in Psychiatry*. Oxford: Oxford University Press.

Merleau-Ponty, Maurice. [1945] 2012. *Phenomenology of Perception*. Edited and translated by Donald A. Landes. London: Routledge.

Pérez-Álvarez, Marino, Louis. A. Sass and José M. García-Montes. 2009. "More Aristotle, Less DSM: The Ontology of Mental Disorders in Constructivist Perspective." *Philosophy, Psychiatry, & Psychology*, 15.3: 211–25.

Ratcliffe, Matthew. 2015. *Experiences in Depression: A Phenomenological Study*. Oxford: Oxford University Press.

Regier, Darrel A. 2007. "Dimensional Approaches to Psychiatric Classification: Refining the Research Agenda for DSM-V: An Introduction." *International Journal of Methods in Psychiatric Research*, 16: S1–S5.

Reiner, D.A., E.A. Kuhl, W.E. Narrow and D.J. Kupfer. 2012. "Research Planning for the Future of Psychiatric Diagnosis." *European Psychiatry*, 27: 553–56.

Rose, Nikolas. 2016. "Reading the Human Brain: How the Mind Became Intelligible." *Body and Society*, 22.2: 140–77.

Svenaeus, Fredrik. 2014. "Depression and the Self: Bodily Resonance and Attuned Being-in-the-World." In *Depression, Emotion and the Self*, edited by Matthew Ratcliffe and Achim Stephan, 2–21. Exeter: Imprint Academic.

Van den Berg, J.H. 1972. *A Different Existence: Principles of Phenomenological Psychopathology*. Pittsburgh, PA: Duquesne University Press.

Whooley, Owen. 2014. "Nosological Reflections: The Failure of DSM-5, the Emergence of RDoC, and the Decontextualization of Mental Distress." *Society and Mental Health*, 4.2: 92–110.

Zachar, Peter. 2000. "Psychiatric Disorders Are Not Natural Kinds." *Philosophy, Psychiatry and Psychology*, 7.3: 167–82.

5 Faith in healing

Evidence-based medicine, the placebo effect and Afro-Brazilian healing rituals[1]

Hannah Lesshafft

The healing effects of faith have been noted in medicine, with more or less resistance, for a long time (Levin 2009; Seligman 2002). In his 1910 paper, "The Faith that Heals," Oxford Professor of Medicine Sir William Osler wrote: "Intangible as the ether, ineluctable as gravitation, the radium of the moral and mental spheres, mysterious, indefinable, known only by its effects, faith pours out an unfailing stream of energy while abating no jot nor tittle of its potency" (Osler 1910, 1470). Since then, researchers of psychoneuroimmunology and the placebo effect have tried to come to terms with the effects of faith in medicine (see George *et al.* 2000; Khansari *et al.* 1990; Levin 2009), and medical anthropologists have provided many detailed descriptions of healing rituals in cultures around the world (Csordas and Lewton 1998). But while traditional, complementary and alternative healing practices often directly engage with rituals, faith healing, and the subjectivity of human experiences of health and illness, in biomedicine such practices are often ridiculed and rejected as *humbug* or quackery. This chapter argues that biomedicine could become more effective – and even more scientific – if it paid more attention to the importance of human imagination, subjectivity and the role of faith in therapeutic processes.

Opponents of complementary and alternative medicine (CAM) criticise its practices for putting patient safety at risk, and even present CAM practitioners as "enemies of reason" (Dawkins and Barnes 2007). MacArtney and Wahlberg (2014) explain that scientific rationalists often depict the users of CAM as "duped, irrational, ignorant, or immoral" people, who need to be educated about the superiority of scientific medical evidence. Without doubt, patients need to be made aware of and protected from harmful and exploitative practices. But MacArtney and Wahlberg (2014) argue that the portrayal of CAM treatment as ignorant, as put forward by popular authors like Ben Goldacre (2008) and Singh and Ernst (2009), fail to help us understand *how* people choose to take care of their health, and what their reasons for this are. Such medical positivist approaches to health do not consider that healing – even in biomedicine – is more than the objective analysis and manipulation of passive bodies. In practice, treating patients cannot be separated from human subjectivity, as it intertwines with complex social relations, symbolic meaning-making, hopes and fears, and the performative creation of faith. Paradoxically, scientific medicine in its own way employs its principles of objectivity and rationalism to perform medical rituals and create faith in its practice.

Evidence-based medicine (EBM) relies on randomised controlled trials (RCT), which are designed to produce objective and universally valid scientific data. But RCTs are, unavoidably, based on human participants – subjective, complex and context-bound as they are. To control for the human "bias," RCTs distinguish between "placebo effects" caused by the patients' imagination and "real effects" of biochemical substances or clinical procedures. In this way, the placebo effect serves as the methodological bedrock of RCTs to measure efficacy – but it is also their stumbling block, as it exposes EBM's innermost contradiction; it is an important reminder that human experience, sociality and the creation of faith are part and parcel of healing processes and wellbeing. This chapter, from a medical anthropology viewpoint, problematises the tendency of EBM to reduce patients from subjective, imaginative and inherently social human beings to standardised bodies in need of repair. It therefore questions the objectivity of medical knowledge production by highlighting the importance of performativity, faith and social interaction in therapeutic encounters.

My chapter consists of two parts. The first discusses the history and practice of EBM and shows how scientific methods have served to distinguish official medicine from competing healing traditions in Europe. Even long before RCTs were established, deception, fake, quackery and charlatanry have been positioned as opposites of more scientific medicine. But despite all scientific rigor, modern RCTs are not able to cancel out human subjectivity and meaning responses. Drawing on my own experience as a medical doctor, I argue that authoritative statements and symbols of scientific objectivity themselves are used to create faith in medicine. They form part of ritual performances in medical practice and research, and in turn even *contribute* to the placebo effect, instead of controlling for it.

The second part provides a contrast to EBM and its inherent difficulty in coming to terms with human subjectivity, by presenting healing practices in the Afro-Brazilian religion Candomblé, based on my ethnographic research with a Candomblé community in Northeast Brazil. In contrast to EBM, Brazilian Candomblé faith (*fé*) is generated through bodily experience by way of dancing, drumming and elaborate ritual performances, as well as through building kinship networks and reflective identity work. While EBM devalues the "placebo effect" as unreal and even deceitful, in Candomblé social relations and "meaning responses" are actively cultivated to trigger healing self-transformation and improve individual and collective well-being. Moreover, their religious practices respond to motifs of social and historical injustice in Brazil and display a surprisingly pragmatic approach to the creation of faith. By way of confronting EBM with Candomblé rituals, this chapter elucidates key aspects of relational and performative healing practices. Considering practices of cultivating faith in different therapeutic encounters brings social interaction and human experience to the fore and, in consequence, reveals the limitations of scientific objectivity in EBM.

Evidence-based medicine and the placebo effect: origins and development of biomedicine

In medieval Europe, medical practices such as Hippocratic humoral therapy, often exerted by monks and clerics, prevailed alongside local pagan healing methods including magic and herbal medicine. Academic medicine evolved in the twelfth and thirteenth centuries. As Roy Porter (2002) explains, the hegemonic ideal image of a physician of the time became that of an honourable and God-fearing man with a university degree in science and philosophy (34). However, common people were rarely treated by academic doctors. Throughout the Middle Ages and Renaissance, they largely relied on folk remedies, pilgrimages, religious sacrifice and magical healing methods. Examples for the latter are attempts to cure a painful hordeolum (sty) with the touch of a black cat's tail, and treating meningitis by cutting open a living chicken and placing it on top of the sufferer's head (Porter 1997, 283). Unlicensed healers and travelling drug sellers excelled in the art of performance and advertisement:

> [G]audily dressed and flanked by a zany and a monkey, they would erect their stage in the market place, drawing first some teeth, both to the accompaniment of drums and trumpets, giving out gratis a few bottles of julep or cordial, selling a few dozen more, and then riding out of town.
>
> (Porter 1997, 284–85)

The medical elite fiercely refuted such performances and emphasised the value of their academic rational knowledge in destabilising people's belief in non-medical practitioners. Establishing their own authority in the therapeutic landscape of the time, physicians deprecated unlicensed healers as "money-grabbing pretenders" and "swindling quacks" (Porter 2002, 34), and in many parts of Europe laws were implemented to prevent charlatanry. The enlightenment was an important era for the transformation of medicine and the understanding of human bodies. But while the eighteenth century in Western societies has been described as a "time of increased medicalization" (Spray 2011, 82), it also became known as the "golden age of quackery" (Porter 1997, 284). The competitive tension between licensed medical practitioners and unlicensed folk healers became central to the further development of academic medicine, which has since been based on the rejection of magic, miracles and healing spectacles as fraud and deception. Ironically, in this process medical doctors created their own performances to enact and stabilise their authority and superiority, like wearing costumes such as black robes and staging public corpse dissections of criminals in fittingly called "anatomy theatres" (Turner 1995, 32).

According to Foucault in *The Birth of the Clinic* ([1963] 2003), the ascendancy of scientific medicine was part of a modernisation project of society based on control, rational order and discipline. Disease became organised in a system of classifications and hierarchies, and the defined categories were articulated through the patient's pathology and recognised by the doctor "gazing" at the exposed body (Foucault 2003). To confirm diagnoses, tissue and blood samples are sent to laboratories for analysis. Correspondingly, the physician's black robe was replaced by the white lab coat that symbolised scientific accuracy, objectivity, and cleanliness (Jones 1999). According to Foucault, the patient's suffering became seen as little more than an external fact to the natural, rational order of their disease (2003, 7–8). New technologies like microscopy and X-ray made human bodies even more transparent and open to scientific analysis. The objectifying "medical gaze" examined humans not as subjective people with their faith, fears and symbolisms, but instead as measurable bodies or sets of (dys)functional organs.

In distinction to what is considered as "quack medicine," modern biomedicine legitimises its practices by yielding reliable, reproducible studies. RCTs have been described as "the most powerful tool in modern clinical research" (Nystrom *et al.* 1993) because the process of randomly allocating patients into groups who receive (a) an intervention, or (b) a placebo,[2] ensures that all other confounding factors are equally distributed. Therefore, any significant differences between the outcomes of the two groups are attributed to the intervention (Stolberg, Norman and Trob 2004). Without doubt, the achievements of modern biomedicine have contributed overwhelmingly to improving healing methods on a global scale. Notwithstanding, scientific EBM is entangled in some major contradictions, in research as well as in practice. These contradictions become most apparent in the phenomenon of the placebo effect. A placebo is generally understood as a simulated treatment; for example, a pill that lacks medical efficacy. In other words, it is seen as a "fake" intervention intended to deceive the patient (Moerman 2002, 127ff; Peters 2001, xi). But although placebo treatment is set up as a *simulated* treatment, human subjectivity and faith in the procedure have such a strong bodily impact that the placebo effect is a *real* effect, and its relevance is shown precisely where medical evidence is produced: in randomised controlled trials.

The placebo effect: stumbling block of evidence-based medicine

Already the definition of placebo is contradictory. The Oxford Dictionary (2012) describes placebo as "a substance that has no therapeutic effect, used as a control in testing new drugs." But if placebo has no effect, then this turns the placebo effect into an oxymoron: the "no-effect effect." The puzzlement about the placebo effect leads to a question raised by Macedo: "Should it be considered that the placebo effect is not the effect of a placebo?" (Macedo, Farré and Baños 2003, 338). Indeed, it is not the placebo as such that produces the placebo effect, but rather the person responding to meaningful action (Moerman and Jonas 2002); for example, a patient receiving a prescription from his trusted doctor, buying the pills from the pharmacy and taking one every morning before breakfast. Consequently, Moerman and Jonas call this effect the "meaning response" (2002). Nevertheless, I retain the use of the word "placebo" because this is the term commonly employed in EBM. What I want to highlight is that applying a placebo treatment – be it a pill, an injection, or words – is in fact an intervention. This becomes clear when attention is paid to the response process of the patient rather than to the "inert content of a placebo or sham procedure" (Finniss *et al.* 2010, 687). The perceptivity, faith and sociality of patients intervene in medical trials as an important reminder of what it means to be human, and hence undermine their reduction of humans to bodies that mechanically respond to chemical, physical or other treatment.

Paradoxically, RCTs simultaneously acknowledge, use and deny the importance of the placebo effect. They acknowledge the placebo effect as a potent bias; therefore clinical interventional trials are only considered reliable when the "verum group" receiving the "real" treatment is compared with a "placebo group" receiving "fake" treatment. Furthermore, in RCTs both patients and doctors are "blinded" so they do not know who receives what kind of treatment. Only when the effect in the verum group is significantly higher than in the placebo group is the effect seen as a "real effect" and not as a "fake effect." Without doubt, for the patient who gets better, the "fake effect" of the placebo treatment is very real, but that is of no value for the medical trial. Instead, the placebo group is used as a comparative to measure the "true effect." Responses to treatment are thus categorised as "true" only when they are caused by mechanisms that are accepted in biomedical research, like direct chemical drug effects or mechanical surgical intervention. They are labelled as "fake" when they are responses to expectations, hope and meaningful interaction with the practitioner. Therefore, in the attempt to reduce bias, EBM turns a blind eye to effects that do not comply with its positivist approach. This reveals the biomedical tendency to reduce active, social, and imaginative humans to passive bodies (see also Taussig 1980). Biomedicine's difficulty in dealing with the potency of the placebo effect demonstrates that EBM does not comply with its own standards of objectively making sense of empirical evidence.

The significance of the placebo effect has been demonstrated in many studies. For example, a systematic review on the influence of a pill's colour on the outcome showed that blue and green pills in general caused tranquillising effects while red, yellow and orange pills were associated with stimulation (de Craen *et al.* 1996). Not only the colour, but also the application form affects the outcome. Four pills per day work better than two pills per day, as Moerman (2000) showed when comparing data from placebo control groups of different studies about gastric ulcers. Capsules have been described as more effective than pills (Hussain and Ahad 1970), and injections as more powerful placebos than capsules. Furthermore, a placebo pill is not simply a placebo pill. Evans showed that morphine placebos are more powerful than aspirin placebos, although the administered sugar pills are identical (Evans *et al.* 1974). Apart from the application method itself, the performance aspect of the placebo is important, even when the practitioner is not aware that he or she is performing anything. For example, Kaptchuk and Croucher (1986) present a study in which sugar pills were given to patients with bleeding gastric ulcers. In the first group, the pills were administered by a senior doctor who enthusiastically related to them as potent drugs, while in the second group the pills were handed out by a nurse who indifferently stated the treatment may help or it may not. In the first group, 70 per cent of the patients recovered from their gastric ulcers, while in the second the recovery rate was only 25 per cent. The interaction with the doctor and nurse in this study strongly interfered with the patient's faith in the treatment and with the outcome, and hence questions the setup of scientific evidence-making.

To better understand the performative aspects of different healing encounters, Kaptchuk and Croucher compared the dramatic performance of a surgical intervention with a healing ritual of the Native American Navaho (1986, 105ff.). In the Navaho tradition, a patient with repeated episodes of chest pain might first try to get relief by using herbal medicine. When this is unhelpful, they would seek help from a specialised "chanter" or "Navaho surgeon" (105–06). This healer then performs a long and intense ceremony, involving purifying dances, vomit therapy and cleansing procedures with fragrant herbs. Accompanied by drums and rattles, songs are sung and acted out. The chanter tells a story of a hero called Rain Boy, who innocently gets smashed into pieces by a jealous god. But as the song continues, his body is ritually reassembled with the help of different spiritual entities, and his forces are restored. According to Kaptchuk and Croucher, a similarly strong ritual element is present in modern medicine:

> The effect of the smells of strange gases and antiseptics is like incense; the sounds of whirring motors are like drums; the monotonous voice over the intercom is like chants; the gowns and masks are like tribal costumes. The Navaho firmly believes that the chanter knows what he is doing, just as the angina patient has complete confidence in the art and science of surgical procedures.
>
> (Kaptchuk and Croucher 1986, 109)

In biomedical research, the physical responses to such rituals are deemed unreal, because they are seen as "only" a result of the imagination. But it should be noted that, according to the Thomas theorem, "if men define situations as real, they are real in their consequences" (Thomas and Thomas 1928, 571). Hence, if a patient's condition improves after placebo treatment or a healing ritual, this must be acknowledged as a real response to a real treatment. As obvious and straightforward as this approach may be, it does not comply with a reductivist dualistic approach common to biomedical science that separates the sphere of reality, bodies and natural science from the sphere of human experience, imagination and culture.

Considering the social and emotional dimensions of healing, RCTs are ultimately incapable of objectively mirroring how a specific treatment affects a patient. In fact, the setup of clinical trials systematically undermines the participants' (and clinician's) faith in the treatment that is to be tested. When a drug is tested in an RCT, study participants are left with a *double uncertainty*: Have they received the real drug or the placebo? And does the drug to be tested work at all?

In contrast, in a clinical setting, patients take the medicine in the *double certainty* that their doctors administer a "real" drug which has been scientifically proven to be effective. But despite this difference, the results from the study are treated as if they depicted what actually happens in clinical practice. Therefore, not only does the placebo effect interfere with the study results; the study design also interferes with the placebo effect. RCTs are thus ultimately unable to standardise patient-doctor interaction and therefore have no real control over the placebo effect.

Having outlined biomedicine's limitations in coming to terms with the important role of faith, performance and human subjectivity for health and healing, the second part of this chapter will turn to the contrasting example of healing practices in Candomblé; an Afro-Brazilian religion that foregrounds the cultivation of faith through ritual performance and subjective experience as key to improving health and wellbeing. Considering how Candomblé practitioners purposefully cultivate faith through performative practice, and how people perceive their faith as a healing force, can contribute to a more holistic understanding of health and ultimately help biomedicine recognise and overcome its own contradictions.

Candomblé healing practices in Brazil: origins and development of the Brazilian Candomblé religion

Before describing Candomblé healing practices, I will briefly introduce the religion, its origins and the main power conflicts that underlie its development and adaptation processes. This is important as it allows us to understand not only how healing is performed and what traditions it refers to, but also what is being healed. Candomblé historically was a religion of African slaves in Brazil, and the collective memory engraved in its rituals, as well as the continuity of racist oppression and humiliation in contemporary Brazil need to be apprehended to recognise Candomblé as an empowering performance of resistance and dignity, or even, as Merrell puts it, as a "means of survival" (Merrell 2005, 104).

After brutal deportation from their African home countries, the slaves who had survived the transatlantic passage arrived on Brazilian shores with no material goods; but they had brought with them their deities (*orixás*), legends, songs, dances and their mysterious "life force" (*axé*) for much needed protection and healing. On arrival, most slaves were brought to the market in Salvador de Bahia, the so-called "Black Rome" of Brazil (Matory 2005, 40). There, they were often separated from their countrymen by slave owners who, following the motto "divide and rule," chose Africans from different regions to impede fraternisation and resistance (Johnson 2002, 104). Through ethnic mixing, forced Christianisation and contact with indigenous people, over the centuries Candomblé emerged as a diverse, syncretic religion that combined African traditions with Catholic and indigenous elements (Capone 2010; Matory 2005; Voeks 1997).

Central to healing in Candomblé is the cultivation of the mysterious *axé*. *Axé* has been described as life force, energy, and the principle that is essential for the existence of the world as a whole (Prandi 2005), and Robert Thompson calls it the "power-to-make-things-happen" (1983, 5). *Axé* also indicates authority, power, and wisdom (Matory 2005, 123). In Candomblé everything revolves around *axé*, and the community members are constantly engaged in ritual work to strengthen their personal *axé*, as well as the *axé* of the group. *Axé* itself cannot be grasped in words, it can only be experienced and, similar to the Polynesian *mana* (Boyer 1986, 52), it escapes attempts to define it in academic terms.

During my fieldwork with a Candomblé community in Bahia, Northeast Brazil, I learned that while I would never be able to fully understand *axé*, I could observe how *axé* was created through paying respect and providing food to the *orixá* deities, and acts of care for the group members as well as the sacred space of the *terreiro* (temple), for example by keeping the ceremony hall clean and providing fresh flowers and ritual objects for the shrines. The Candomblé priest-ess of the community explained to me that the "Law of Candomblé" consisted of three elements: paying respect; following the rules; and keeping the secrets. By obeying this law, she said, people contributed to the *axé* and flourishing of the community and over time developed faith (*fé*).

The development of faith was a key aspect of healing in the Candomblé com-munity. The members of the Candomblé group mostly used faith not in the sense of "a religious faith," but as having faith that good things were about to happen. Faith in this context is a general attitude towards life: a perspective of hope, trust and confidence in a positive outcome, despite the social insecurity and risk of violence present in everyday life in Brazil. Importantly, in this context faith is more than a mere belief in something. Instead, it is employed as a powerful force that *does* something: it effectively changes reality and provides wellbeing. Like the placebo effect in clinical trials, Candomblé faith turns the anticipation of wellbeing into the physical experience of health. To provide an example of how faith and *axé* are strengthened and experienced I will now describe the "leaf bath" (*banho*), a very important sacred ritual in the Candomblé community that was performed on a daily basis.

Upon arrival in the Candomblé temple, the members, one by one, went down to the small waterfall in the forest to take their *banho* (pronounced: bun-yo). The *banho* serves, first, to spiritually cleanse them by cooling down the "hot" street energy from outside and to make them feel calm; and second, to "close the body" (*fechar o corpo*) to negative influences. A "closed body" (*corpo fechado*) is defined as being immune to injury, be it of a spiritual, emotional or physical nature, while an "open body" (*corpo aberto*) is vulnerable and can easily be attacked (see also Sansi 2011, 274). The "closed body" is a protected, strengthened body.

To close the body to danger, the Candomblé followers used a solution of leaves soaked in water that they fetched from a container by the house. First, they cleaned their bodies in the small waterfall by the lagoon, amidst tropical flowers and lush vegetation. Standing naked on the wet stones, they then poured the leaf solution over themselves to impregnate their body with *axé*. The leaf solution had to run over the whole body and was not to be rubbed off with a towel, meaning people stepped into the sacred white clothes with tiny leftover leaf pieces sticking to their still dripping wet skin. Interestingly, the *axé* that one feels (or is expected to feel) in the *banho* is not simply an effect of the leaves on the body; it is supposed to increase with the faith that one acquires over time. "The more faith you have, the more effective the leaf bath will be," the Candomblé priestess said. A person's faith strengthens the *axé* of the leaf bath. In contrast to EBM, which attempts to delete or at least control the effects of faith and expectations (or the placebo effect), faith in Candomblé is actively created and recognised as a powerful force that protects and facilitates healing.

Human subjectivity is central to the cultivation of faith and healing in Candomblé. Taking the leaf bath as protection against negative influences was directly linked with the sensual experience of standing in the dizzyingly beautiful tropical forest, feeling the cooling plant juice running down one's naked body. Several members of the group told me how much they enjoyed this moment when their stress and worries were washed away and they felt strong, fresh and full of *axé*. In his book *Sacred Leaves of Candomblé*, Robert Voeks writes that the leaf bath could have a "profound psychological impact" and that an initiated person could go into trance just from its smell (Voeks 1997, 95). The visceral expectation of something good to come, this faith, is not only a side aspect of their religious life; it is a central outcome of their ritual practice, and a significant resource for healing.

Notably, faith as an experiential, dynamic human force was more important than belief as a cognitive capacity. As the Candomblé priestess explained, a person would arrive at a Candomblé house with hope (*esperança*), but not with faith, and she added: "one arrives searching, and faith is what one acquires." Providing a personal example, she told me that when she entered Candomblé, she believed in the leader of the Candomblé house, but she had no faith in him. Over time, however, he gradually taught her to have faith by "showing, conversing, [and] exploring" (*mostrando, conversando, explorando*). After having entered Candomblé, she felt that her life became easier, and things started to work out for her. It was through this practical experience that she "learned to have faith." Illustrating the supremacy of experiential faith over cognitive belief, the anthropologist Paul Christopher Johnson (2002) recounts that he told the Candomblé priestess of the house in Rio de Janeiro where he was initiated, that he did not actually believe in the *orixás*. Her reply was pragmatic: "The question is whether you perform the rituals, not whether you believe in them" (Johnson 2002, 13). Hinting at a similar supremacy of acting over believing in medicine, Kaptchuk *et al.* (2010) argue that placebo treatment can be successful even when the patient knows that the administered pills they take contain nothing but sugar. In other words: the *practice* of a therapeutic procedure (for example, performing Candomblé rituals or taking a sugar pill) seems more important than the cognitive *belief* in gods or medical substances.

Social acts, rituals and references can indeed be very effective, even if an individual does not rationally believe in the underlying explanations. Ethnographic examples for the effects of magic and witchcraft on outsider anthropologists can be found in Jeanne Favret-Saada's *Deadly Words* (1980) and Paul Stoller's and Cheryl Olke's *In Sorcery's Shadow* (1987). Favret-Saada (1980) demonstrates that when she learned about witchcraft in a French village, she got more and more "caught up" in it herself because the whole village related to her in terms of witchcraft. Similarly, Stoller, who became a sorcerer's apprentice among the Songhay in Niger (Stoller and Olkes 1987, 148), states that Songhay magic worked for him, not because he believed in it, but because he was integrated in the narrative and social reality of magic. This entanglement went so far that he experienced leg paralysis caused by a sorcerer's attack, which he eventually managed to reverse by using protective charms (Stoller and Olkes 1987). While medical practice uses its own charms and symbols, such as the stethoscope dangling around the doctor's neck, medical authority is based in strictly rational evidence-making. The human experience of health and bodily symptoms, however, does not follow the same rational logic but is shaped by the imagination, suggestion, and social practices.

In contrast to EBM with its aim to establish objective truth, Candomblé healing was very pragmatic and allowed for a surprising amount of relativism. Accordingly, other religions were not seen as wrong, but as different ways to create faith and spiritual protection. This respect towards other religions as other ways to cultivate faith is best expressed in an interview with Lucas, a young member of the Candomblé house. As a recent initiate of Candomblé, he was wearing his white ritual clothes, a turban and colourful religious necklaces around his neck. One afternoon, after all the housework had been done, we were sitting by the lagoon in the afternoon sun as he reflected on the similarities between different religious narratives and practices:

LUCAS: If we look at other stories, at other religions, you will see that they all converge.
ME: So, is there not one true religion?
LUCAS: No, no, no, no, no. I cannot say that Catholicism is wrong, that the Catholic's faith is wrong. There are problems in Catholicism, but there are also problems in Candomblé. In the end, we are humans. The religions are made by people, by humans, with their differences, similarities, their agonies, their histories, their fears.... I don't believe that my religion is better than any Evangelical, or any Catholic. I don't think it is. Buddhists, Islam. But I think that my faith is my faith. That is enough for me.

Lucas' explanation presents Candomblé as a pragmatic religion, made *by humans for humans*, considering "their agonies, their histories, their fears" in the cultivation of faith. Such religious pragmatism has previously been described by Max Bondi (2009, 6) and Marcio Goldman (2003), who characterise Candomblé as a "praxeological" religion, that is not built on ideas of an ultimate truth, but on the faith in the efficacy of their rituals. In this sense, in Candomblé the creation of faith appears not as a side product, but as a main purpose of religious activity. While biomedical trials try to delete the effects of the unwanted bias of patients' faith and subjectivity from their study results, Candomblé is an example of a healing practice that recognises the value of faith for healing and systematically uses rituals to cultivate it as a central and effective source of wellbeing.

Conclusion

Both biomedicine and Candomblé are imbued with meaning, symbols and the hope to get better, and both are concerned with the role of faith in their respective healing practices. The authority of the medical doctor, justified by long years of study and often self-sacrificial work attitudes, is displayed in titles, certificates and symbols like the stethoscope around the neck and the white coat. Likewise, the Candomblé priestess has earned her authority in a seven-year long initiation process, which is embodied in her ritual clothes and necklaces. The doctor and the Candomblé priestess both aim to improve the wellbeing of their patients or clients, who (at least ideally) have faith in their abilities and knowledge and in the respective treatment or ritual to help them.

A crucial difference between the two healing systems, however, is that biomedicine creates evidence by *subtracting* the effect of the patients' hope, their faith in the practitioner and the ritual effects of medicine (the placebo effect or meaning response), while the healing rituals in Candomblé systematically aim at *cultivating* faith as an effective healing resource in itself. When an RCT shows that the treatment that is to be tested works no better than the placebo in the control group, then it will be evaluated as ineffective. In Candomblé, however, a protective leaf bath is prepared, handled and taken with the greatest care to follow the rules and show respect for the *orixás* as to strengthen and experience their divine power, the mysterious *axé*. While in medicine, scientific objectivity is the base of creating trustworthy data, in Candomblé subjectivity is key to creating faith. The leaf bath in the waterfall, the long chants and rituals, the intense smells, repetitive drumming and communal excitement all contribute to an experiential, embodied feeling of being strengthened and protected. And over time this feeling is to grow stronger: and the Candomblé priestess stated, "The more faith you have, the more effective the leaf bath will be."

Another important difference is that biomedicine is highly regarded in Candomblé, and the priestess would often send her patients to see a medical doctor in addition to coming to the Candomblé house. Conversely, medicine as a discipline generally rejects healing practices that do not conform with its scientific standards (although individual practitioners might hold different positions), and mockery of complementary and alternative medicine is commonplace. Here, I need to point out again that dangerous practices or those that delay medical interventions must be prevented to protect the patient. But measuring non-medical healing practices with scientific standards of objectivity misses the point, when the strength of the rituals lies not in their objective reproducibility and rigor (and the control of the placebo effect), but in the subjective experiences that generate an attitude of faith in healing. Indeed, when the proven effects of the "placebo effect" are treated as unwanted bias in medical trials, medicine derives itself from a huge and little understood resource to support and enhance patient well-being. As Jeremy Laurance writes in *The Lancet*: "The placebo effect may be one of the most underused weapons in the medical arsenal. We should find ways to exploit it" (2010, 885). A respectful consideration of often-mocked healing practices in other cultures and religions, like Candomblé, may shed light on underexposed ritual aspects in medical treatment and the value of faith and subjective experiences for human health. Medical anthropology provides rich ethnographic research that can help EBM to move from a positivist science of standardised human bodies towards a more holistic and deeper understanding of our shared yet diverse humanity.

Notes

1 I would like to thank Prof. Ian Harper, Dr. Maya Mayblin and Prof. Alexander Edmonds for their support and input during my research. I gratefully received funding from the DAAD (Deutscher Akademischer Austauschdienst, German Academic Exchange Service), and the University of Edinburgh (Principal's Career Development Scheme).
2 For ethical reasons, the control group in many clinical studies receives the current standard treatment against which a new drug is tested. However, in this text I focus on placebo-controlled studies in order to carve out the biomedical difficulty of handling the placebo effect.

Reference list

Bondi, M. 2009. "Things of Africa – Rethinking Candomblé in Brazil." Working paper no. 02/2009. London: UCL. www.scribd.com/doc/53615307/Things-of-Africa-Rethinking-Candomble-in-Brazil-Bondi (accessed 14 August 2017).

Boyer, P. 1986. "The 'empty' concepts of traditional thinking: A semantic and pragmatic description." *MAN: Journal of the Royal Anthropological Institute*, 21.1: 50–64.

Capone, S. 2010. *Searching for Africa in Brazil: Power and Tradition in Candomblé*, Durham, NC: Duke University Press.

Csordas, T.J. and Lewton, E. 1998. "Practice, performance, and experience in ritual healing." *Transcultural Psychiatry*, 35.4: 435–512.

Dawkins, R. and Barnes, R. 2007. "The irrational health service." [Television series, episode 1]. In A. Clements (Producer), *Enemies of Reason*. London: IWC Media.

De Craen, A.J., Roos, P.J., De Vries, A.L. and Kleijnen, J. 1996. "Effect of colour of drugs: Systematic review of perceived effect of drugs and of their effectiveness." *British Medical Journal*, 313.7072: 1624–26.

Evans, F.J. 1974. "The placebo response in pain reduction." In J.J. Bonica (ed.) *Advances in Neurology, Vol. 4: Pain*, 289–96. New York: Raven.

Favret-Saada, J. 1980. *Deadly Words: Witchcraft in the Bocage*. Cambridge: Cambridge University Press.

Finniss, D.G., Kaptchuk, T., Miller, F. and Benedetti, F. 2010. "Placebo effects: Biological, clinical and ethical advances." *The Lancet*, 375.9715: 686–95.

Foucault, M. 2003 [1963]. *The Birth of the Clinic*. London: Routledge.

George, L., Larson, D., Koenig, H. and McCullough, M. 2000. "Spirituality and health: What we know, what we need to know." *Journal of Social and Clinical Psychology*, 19.1: 102–16.

Goldacre, B. 2008. *Bad Science*. London: Fourth Estate.

Goldman, M. 2003. "Observações sobre o 'sincretismo Afro-Brasileiro.'" *Kàwé Pesquisa. Revista Anual do Núcleo de Estudos Afro-Baianos Regionais da UESC*, 1.1: 132–37.

Hussain, M.Z. and Ahad, A. 1970. "Tablet colour in anxiety states." *British Medical Journal*, 3.5720: 466.

Johnson, P.C. 2002. *Secrets, Gossip and Gods. The Transformation of Brazilian Candomblé*. Oxford: Oxford University Press.

Jones, V.A. 1999. "The white coat – Why not follow suit?" *Journal of the American Medical Association*, 281.5: 478.

Kaptchuk, T.J. and Croucher, M. 1986. *Healing Arts: A Journey Through the Faces of Medicine*. London: British Broadcasting Corporation.

Khansari, D.N., Murgo, A.J. and Faith, R.E. 1990. "Effects of stress on the immune system." *Immunology Today*, 11.5: 170–75.

Laurance, J. 2010. "Magic is acceptable." *The Lancet*, 375.9718: 885.

Levin, J. 2009. "How faith heals: A theoretical model." *EXPLORE: The Journal of Science and Healing*, 5.2: 77–96.

MacArtney, J. and Wahlberg, A. 2014. "The problem of complementary and alternative medicine use today: Eyes half closed?" *Qualitative Health Research*, 24: 114–23.

Macedo, A., Farré, M. and Baños, J.E. 2003. "Placebo effect and placebos: What are we talking about? Some conceptual and historical considerations." *European Journal of Clinical Pharmacology*, 59: 337–42.

Matory, J.L. 2005. *Black Atlantic Religion: Tradition, Transnationalism, and Matriarchy in the Afro-Brazilian Candomblé*. Princeton: Princeton University Press.

Merrell, F. 2005. *Capoeira and Candomblé: Conformity and Resistance through Afro-Brazilian Experience*. New York: Markus Wiener.

Moerman, D.E. 2000. "Cultural variations in the placebo effect: Ulcers, anxiety, and blood pressure." *Medical Anthropology Quarterly*, 14.1: 51–72.

Moerman, D.E. and Jonas, W.B. 2002. "Deconstructing the placebo effect and finding the meaning response." *Annals of Internal Medicine*, 136.6: 471–76.

Nystrom, L., Rutqvist, L.E., Wall, S., Lindgren, A., Lindquist, M. and Rydén, S. 1993. "Breast cancer screening with mammography: Overview of Swedish randomised trials." *The Lancet*, 341.8851: 973–78.

Osler, W. 1910. "The faith that heals." *British Medical Journal*, 1.2581: 1470.

Peters, D. 2001. *Understanding the Placebo Effect in Complementary Medicine*. Edinburgh: Churchill Livingstone.

Porter, R. 1997. *The Greatest Benefit to Mankind: A Medical History of Humanity from Antiquity to the Present*. London: Harper Collins.

Porter, R. 2002. *Blood and Guts: A Short History of Medicine*. London: Penguin.

Póvoas, R.D.C. 2011. *Da Porteira para fora: Mundo de preto em terra de branco*, Ilhéus: Editus.

Prandi, R. 2005. *Segredos guardados: Orixás na alma brasileira*, São Paulo: Companhia das Letras.

Sansi, R. 2011. "Shrines, substances, and miracles in Afro-Brazilian Candomblé." *Anthropology and Medicine*, 18.2: 271–83.

Seligman, M.E. 2002. "Positive psychology, positive prevention, and positive therapy." *Handbook of Positive Psychology*, 2: 3–12.

Singh, S. and Ernst, E. . 2009. *Trick or Treatment? Alternative Medicine on Trial*. London: Corgi.

Spray, E.C. 2011. "Health and medicine in the Enlightenment." In Mark Jackson (ed.) *The Oxford Handbook of the History of Medicine*, 82–93. Oxford: Oxford University Press.

Stolberg, H., Norman, G. and Trop, I. 2004. "Randomized controlled trials." *American Journal of Roentgenology*, 183.6: 1539–44.

Stoller, P. and Olkes, C. 1987. *In Sorcery's Shadow. A Memoir of Apprenticeship among the Songhay of Niger*. Chicago: University of Chicago Press.

Taussig, M. 1980. "Reification and the consciousness of the patient." *Social Sciences and Medicine*, 14B: 3–13.

Thomas, W.I. and Thomas, D.S. 1928. *The Child in America: Behavior Problems and Programs*. New York: Knopf.

Thompson, R.F. 1983. *Flash of the Spirit*. New York: Vintage Books.

Turner, V. 1995. *The Ritual Process: Structure and Anti-Structure*. New York: Aldine de Gruyter.

Voeks, R. 1997. *Sacred Leaves of Candomblé: African Magic, Medicine, and Religion in Brazil*. Austin: University of Texas Press.

Part II
Socio-medical narratives

6   Voices in medicine

Ethics, human rights and medical experimentation

Jennifer Greenwood

The crimes against humanity committed by Hitler's Nazi party have been well-documented, as have those of the Tuskegee Untreated Syphilis trials, although to a lesser extent. Even so, the question persists as to how putatively highly educated professionals can perpetrate violations of human rights: "Gas chambers built by learned engineers. Children poisoned by educated physicians. Infants killed by trained nurses" (A Head Teacher qtd in Pring 2004a, 24). This chapter analyses these well-known cases, specifically to address the potential disconnect between education and human understanding, and the impact that this disconnection has had historically by enabling unethical human scientific experimentation that is justified as medical scientific research. Unlike the other essays in this collection that address fictional representations of such scientific behaviour, such as Mary Shelley's *Frankenstein* (1818), these case studies are crucial because of the very fact that they are well known and still a part of living memory for survivors and perpetrators. The chapter does more than provide an explanatory framework for this disconnection, however; it also, importantly, provides pedagogic guidelines to ensure that education "make[s] our children more human" in the words of the Head Teacher above, by obviating, or at least mitigating, the privileging of one voice, even if that one voice is the voice of science, in medical (indeed, in all professional) education. My argument requires the creative synthesis of a range of insights from different disciplines, including history (Tuskegee, Nazi medical experimentation), philosophy (Plato, Kant) and education (Oakeshott, Pring). Ethics break down when one voice is privileged to the exclusion of others. I will argue, therefore, that all ethically acceptable discourses, including medical discourse, should represent three conceptual schemes, or "voices" and, further, that the indiscriminate privileging of one voice can result in behavioural atrocity.

The purportedly scientific studies leading to the human rights violations addressed in this chapter were the result of privileging the pursuit of scientific truth, supported by the dogged adherence to cultural stereotypes and personal mythologies, despite or, even more disturbingly, possibly because of the obvious human suffering it caused. This kind of monocentric discourse dehumanises its objects by failing to recognise and respect the rational autonomy which is the *sine qua non* of personhood or distinctly human being: "man, and in general every *rational being, exists as an end in himself*, not merely as a means for arbitrary use by this or that will" (Kant [1786] 1964, 428, emphasis added). In this context, autonomous, rational human beings recognise that others are also rational and autonomous and, as such, their autonomy should also be respected. What this implies is that personhood or personal identity is intersubjectively constructed. To treat another human being merely as a *means* – as merely an instrument for one's own purposes – is to ignore her identity as a human being. It is, in other words, to dehumanise her. This Kantian maxim attracts almost universal assent (if not observation) and has been enshrined in The Golden Rule of at least 11 major religions: "Do unto others..." (Mizzoni 2009, 49). It has also been enshrined in the Universal Declaration of Human Rights (UDHR), which states that everyone is born free and equal in dignity (Article 1), with rights to life, liberty and security (Article 3), with freedom from torture and degrading treatment (Article 5) and with rights to seek and enjoy asylum in other countries, free from persecution (Article 14). The UDHR was signed by signatory states on 10 December 1948; yet since then, by the end of 2015, 65.3 million people worldwide had been forced to leave their homes as a result of conflict, persecution, violence and human rights violations (Amnesty International 2017).

Education that makes people more human should result in a profound respect for people's human rights and their different ways of living, provided they do not impede the human rights of others. All cultures have religious beliefs, regulations governing human relationships and property, ways of recreation and so forth. What cultures have in common is more important than how they differ individually, and this is key to the humanising education I discuss below.

Dehumanisation does not have to be as obvious and extreme as that exemplified in Tuskegee and National Socialist Germany; it can be much subtler but still dangerous. The process of dehumanisation in the two studies described below was augmented by the rhetorical devices deliberately employed in the scientific discourse of the scientists involved (Solomon 2000). The Tuskegee Untreated Syphilis Study and the Nazi medical experiments demonstrate the dangers of "scientific" pursuit at any cost. Plato's typology of rhetorical styles provides a useful analytic device to explicate the dangers of monocentric discourse, which occurs when the privileging of only one voice, as in these cases, leaves such behaviour unchallenged. A liberal education (in the most general sense) is a humanising education because it promotes the knowledge and values characteristic of the rational autonomy of all distinctly human agents. In this way, it stands in opposition to the kinds of scientific experimentation that violate human rights by refusing to recognise the humanity of the objects of experimentation.

Plato famously characterised human discourses as requiring three distinct rhetorical styles ("voices") to represent them: *logos*, the analytic voice of critique, of science, philosophy and truth; *thymos*, the voice of the outraged oppressed, disempowered and marginalised; and *mythos*, the personal voice, the voice of narrative, autobiography, cultural mythology and literature. Plato's mission was to promote pure or unpolluted logos in the pursuit of truth and to discredit mythos, in particular, as leading away from truth. Plato construed logos and mythos as diametrically opposed. Thymos takes on a variety of different meanings in Plato and it is difficult to find an exact English translation (Carlson 1998, 548), but Plato presents it as a complex mix of components of the human psyche. These include indignation, courage, self-determination and survival instinct or "spirit." Importantly for this essay, Carlson notes that Hegel famously construed thymos, in his story of master and slave, as the voice that calls out for recognition, resistance and social justice. Thymos drives the slave to assert his rights as an equal, to be treated with respect and not as a second-class citizen or be reduced to an instrument of another's purposes. The critique which follows from feelings of outrage at injustice generates a new truth (logos) about a more equitable and humane world that recognises humanity in difference. Once the Tuskegee and Nazi experimentation scandals were made public, the thymic response resulted, respectively, in the establishment of Scientific Research Ethics Committees in all Western democracies and in the Helsinki Declaration of Human Rights, leading to national and international ethical advance.

The socio-political background of the studies

It is important to recognise at the outset that the sort of systematic unethical behaviour represented in the studies discussed below does not arise *de novo*; rather, general socio-political views and the particular views they engender – for example, concepts of racial difference and current concepts of science – are mutually informative. It cannot be over-emphasised that race, as a social category, has been created and creates differing kinds of medical assumptions and practices that historically have affected definitions of humanity and treatment protocols (Reverby 2000; Savitt 1982). What this in turn implies, and *pace* Plato, is that there are no unpolluted logoi. The scientific received views of the day (logoi) are inevitably influenced by the attitudes and values of working scientists and these, in turn, are influenced by the prevailing socio-political values of the cultures in which they are embedded. The two cases of human rights violation to be discussed demonstrate that the prevailing socio-political views of the early to mid twentieth century enabled medical and other health professionals to take advantage of opportunities for what we now conceive of as unethical practices. The Tuskegee studies took advantage of the availability of research subjects, and Nazi human experimentation took advantage of both the availability of research subjects and of the equipment and trained personnel to carry out Hitler's Final Solution to "the Jewish Problem."

The Tuskegee study involved the complicity of black physicians and nurses and large numbers of white physicians, some of whose predecessors, before the abolition of slavery, had bought sick slaves solely for scientific experimentation (Weld [1839] 2011, 170). In Nazi Germany, more than 38,000 physicians (over 50 per cent of their number) had enrolled in the National Socialist Party *before* Hitler came to power. It is also worth noting that the Tuskegee scandal had to await the press to make it public and arouse a public thymocentric response, while the Nazi crimes had to await the Allies for prosecution. The staggeringly small number of prosecutions was, again, due to the prevailing socio-political situation in the USA and Europe. Nonetheless, it is salutary to note that these crimes were actually *made possible* by the prevailing socio-political climate, which was conducive to them. The same is true of present-day violations of human rights and will continue to be true of them in future.

Tuskegee Untreated Syphilis Study (1932–72)

On 25 July 1972 Jean Heller broke the news of the Tuskegee experiment in *The Washington Star*, bringing to an end the longest running non-therapeutic study in medical history (Caplan 1992). The experiment was conducted under the auspices of the United States Public Health Service with the full cooperation of the Alabama State Department of Health, the Tuskegee Institute (a prestigious black health institute), the Tuskegee Medical Society and the Macon County Health Department. The study, which began in 1932, continued for 40 years, despite clearly violating the existing health policies in Alabama that all communicable diseases, including venereal diseases, be notified to the health authorities *and treated*. It involved tracking the natural disease progression of untreated syphilis in African American men in Macon County, Alabama. The sample included 399 infected subjects, all positive serologically for syphilis, and 201 uninfected controls. The study sought to follow all these subjects until they died. Their deaths were then to be followed by autopsy to investigate the results of the disease on body organs, even though scientists already knew at the time what caused syphilis, how it was transmitted, its symptoms and its progression.

It was asserted by the medical establishment in Alabama that African Americans were much more susceptible to disease, including syphilis, because of genetic weakness, poverty and risky lifestyles, and that they responded differently to syphilis infection than the white population. It was claimed by one eminent physician from Johns Hopkins University (Ernest Zimmerman) that African Americans were much more likely to suffer bone and cardio-vascular complications. Zimmerman's claims were based on clinical data only; there was no definitive evidence of such. On the contrary, one previous study, conducted in Oslo, Norway and reported in 1929 (Brandt 2000, 19) suggested that central nervous system complications were more commonly suffered in white populations. Even so, as Jones states, "[s]uch theories no doubt influenced many clinical diagnoses and [stand] as a powerful reminder of how racial attitudes could influence the medical profession's perceptions" (Jones 1981, 28).

There was no formal research protocol in Tuskegee. Procedures included regular serological and physical examinations and spinal taps. The study involved no testing of new treatments and no testing of the efficacy of existing treatments. The experiments were solely to produce data on the results of syphilis in black males. Contrary to claims in 1972, subjects were not given any information about what they were being investigated for (Edgar 2000, 491); indeed, they were told that they were being investigated and treated for "bad blood" (Reverby 2000, 1). This, it was claimed, was a term these illiterate men could understand; it covered everything from stomach pains to rheumatism. Treatment variously included some minimal and temporary treatment for syphilis, initially as part of a previous syphilis control demonstration in rural populations. The syphilis control demonstration study was first established by the Rosenwald Foundation, a philanthropic foundation established to improve the plight of desperately poor rural African Americans. It provided $50,000 in 1930 to seed-fund a syphilis control demonstration study. This demonstration study sought to investigate if syphilis could be controlled (rendered non-infectious) using intensive arsenicals and mercury together with health education. Subject compliance was low due to toxicity and social mobility. Funding was not renewed after one year, but this was due to the fiscal emergency of the Great Depression, rather than any concerns regarding human rights. It was while compiling his final report that Dr Taliaferro Clark spotted a unique opportunity:

> the thought came to me that the Alabama community offered an unparalleled opportunity to study untreated syphilis…. Macon County has the highest incidence of syphilis that the PHS has uncovered anywhere in the South … an incredibly high incidence rate … 35%.

He knew that of the 1,400 admitted to the study, only 33 had received any treatment at all (Jones 1981, 92).

Subjects were all volunteers – a problematic term for vulnerable people who were poor enough to find the participation incentives attractive. They were offered access to a physician regularly, which, for most participants, was the first time ever; they were given a hot meal on the day they attended for examination; they were prescribed pink aspirin and "blood tonic" when they complained of any malaise or symptom; they were given burial insurance, which was, again, a first for them: they were promised $50 burial stipends for their survivors, to be modestly adjusted for inflation; and they had a black nurse, first Eunice Rivers until she retired in 1970 and then Elizabeth M Kennebrew. The role of these nurses was to track subjects and facilitate relationships between the doctors and research subjects, to ensure that they attended for examination, and to oversee their welfare. Research subjects considered themselves members of a burial and social club called "Miss Rivers' Lodge" (Jones 1981, 6).

The rationale behind the withholding of treatment was that existing therapy – mercury and arsenic compounds – were toxic and painful, and of dubious efficacy. It was also assumed that black men did not take the disease seriously and that their purported susceptibility to the disease was both genetic and environmental (Brandt 2000, 16). The prevailing racially biased narratives construed them as genetically susceptible because of their weak physical constitution and exaggerated and largely uncontrollable libido (for which there was no scientific evidence), and environmentally susceptible because of their appalling living conditions in terms of nutrition and sanitation. This fails to explain, however, why penicillin was withheld from 1947 onwards when it became the treatment of choice for syphilis and was widely available. Instead, when penicillin became available free from clinics, including mobile clinics, the lists of subjects' names were sent to them with instructions *not* to treat. When news of the study broke, critics were quick to point to the racial and class implications involved. All the subjects were black and all of them extremely poor. In terms of race, physicians in the southern state were almost all white middle and upper-class men indoctrinated with the racial stereotypes of their time.

It is not known exactly how many men died, perhaps as many as 100 (Jones 1981, 2). How many of their wives and other women became infected, and how many children were born with congenital syphilis, remains unknown. The lawyer representing the subjects, Fred Gray, was black and fought the case on racial grounds; no black institution or individual was mentioned as complicit or culpable at the hearing. Gray filed for $1.8 billion (class action) but settled out of court for about $100 million (Bell 2000, 38). Survivors of the study and infected children received compensation, $37,500 and $15,000 respectively. Surviving control subjects and their heirs were also compensated, $16,000 and $5,000 respectively (Gray 2000, 487). The world had changed in the 40 years since the study began, and questions were raised regarding the separation of races effectively into human and not human. Civil Rights was a political priority, and by this point, the Nazi atrocities were well known. At the same time, interest in the protection of human subjects in medical research was burgeoning. The Tuskegee study provoked outrage in the general population and in many physicians because of its lack of ethics. Physicians involved in the study, however, were adamant that ethics had not been compromised; if there were any weaknesses at all in the study these were scientific, due to early partial treatment of some subjects.

It is disturbing, however, that 13 "progress reports," which included details of the research protocol and its devastating results, were published in prestigious medical journals during the life of the study. These reports failed to generate criticism from the medical community (Solomon 2000, 251–52), possibly because analysis of them shows four features of scientific investigation which are reflected in scientific reporting: the scientific method encourages the perception of distinctions/differences and the investigation of their significance; objectivity and detachment are systematically pursued; science construes knowledge as a primary value; and, the scientific method is consistent across subject matter areas. These features of scientific practice are supposed to minimise prejudice and bias, but they can also dehumanise subjects by distorting scientists' perceptions of salient features in the realities they seek to investigate.

Analysis of the Tuskegee reports shows that they depicted research subjects not as human beings but as "contexts," "hosts" and "syphilitics" in which the disease process was being played out, and physicians as separate, noble agents systematically observing this process in pursuit of scientific truth. It is the disease itself which ravages the "context" or "host." Also, in a scientific community that emphasises difference, the focus on a difference, such as skin colour, masks any real recognition of significant resemblances such as common humanity. The use of third-person scientific terminology serves to further depersonalise and support objectivity. "Male Negro," with its associated construals of physical weakness, sexual promiscuity and inferior intellect, depersonalises and dehumanises subjects, conspiring to obscure the moral and ethical implications of scientific practice (Solomon 2000, 261).

The Tuskegee study highlighted the need to protect society from scientific studies that ignored the rights of human subjects to respect, autonomy, informed consent and treatment. As the Editor of the *Atlanta Constitution* (1972) put it,

> Sometimes with the best of intentions, scientists and public officials and others working for the benefit of all, forget that people are people. They concentrate so totally on plans and programs, experiments and statistics – on abstractions – that people become objects, subjects on paper, figures in mathematical formulae or "impersonal subjects" in a scientific study.
>
> (Jones 1981, 14)

The editorial continued: "moral judgment should always be a part of any human endeavour," including "the dispassionate search for scientific knowledge." Following the Tuskegee outrage, scientific ethical progress emerged in the National Health Act of 1974, which required the establishment of Institutional Review Boards to oversee the conduct of all federally funded research involving human subjects (Heintzelman 2003). The Act also established The National Commission for the Protection of Human Subjects of Biomedical and Behavioral Research of the Department of Health, Education and Welfare (DHEW). This eventuated in the Belmont Report of 1978 which identified three ethical principles that all research studies are required to observe and their primary areas of application: respect for persons; beneficence; and justice. Primary areas of application are informed consent, assessment of risks and benefits, and selection of subjects.

Nazi medical experimentation

It is common knowledge that the Nazis murdered 6 million Jews during World War II (WWII). The socio-political system that preceded this slaughter and initiated it is, however, known mainly to war historians. This ignorance, too, is due to countervailing socio-political views. The same Social Darwinism that fuelled the miscegenation legislation in the USA prevailed in Germany, but the inferiors in the German case were any non-Aryans, especially Jews. The social and economic plight of the German people following WW1 was blamed mainly on the weakening of the Nordic races by interbreeding with inferior non-Nordics. Marriage and sexual relations between Aryans and non-Aryans were prohibited (1933) and laws were passed to ensure the development of racial hygiene (*Rassenhygiene*).

Crucially, medical scientists of the era were not forced to adopt these policies; rather racial hygiene was invented and operated *by* medical scientists and physicians. Racial hygiene was taken up by National Socialists as a means of biologising perceived social problems to the extent that National Socialism was considered a form of applied biology. This emphasis on biology attracted doctors who joined the National Socialist party in greater numbers than any other professional group. By 1942, over 38,000 were members – that is, over half the profession in Germany. In addition, as early as 1937, 7 per cent more doctors were members of the SS than any other group of employed males (Proctor 1992, 18). In 1929, the National Socialist Physicians League coordinated the Nazi medical policy to cleanse German medicine of "Jewish Bolshevism," the purported cultural dominance of Jews in Europe (Proctor 1992, 19). Physicians held differing views concerning answers to the Jewish problem. Some suggested deportation to Madagascar, others suggested forced sterilisation; but gassing became the method of choice as the equipment and trained personnel who could operate it became available. Racial hygiene was an umbrella term used to refer to the policies and processes of Nordic purification which protected Nordics from non-Nordic genetic pollution. Racial hygiene, therefore, was rhetorically positioned as a means to purify humanity.

Racial hygiene was enacted through the results of three policy initiatives: the Sterilisation Law (1933); the Nuremburg Law (1933); and the euthanasia operation. The Sterilisation Law forced the sterilisation of anyone with a physical or mental weakness or defect, while the Nuremburg Law required the physical examination of engaged couples (to ensure they were racially pure) and prevented Aryan-Jew intermarriage. These laws were considered public health measures and were largely initiated by physicians. The euthanasia operation began in 1939 when Hitler decreed that a "mercy death" should be given to anyone whose life was deemed not worth living, including people with incurable diseases, those with mental health problems, and children with congenital abnormalities. By 1941 over 70,000 inmates of mental institutions had been murdered. They were gassed or killed by phenol injection, administered by a physician. Medical scientists developed and tested the efficacy of different gases and oversaw the construction of gas chambers in mental hospitals. This systematised killing enabled the freeing up of beds for the war casualties and the elimination of these "useless" people (Aly 1994) who were "unnecessary eaters" (Proctor 1992, 39). By 1941 euthanasia was both banal and popular. In 1941, a psychiatric hospital in Hadamor celebrated the cremation of its 10,000th euthanasia victim. Every doctor, nurse, technician and secretary was given a bottle of beer to celebrate the occasion (Procter 1992, 25). The gas chambers used in these hospitals were dismantled and sent to Auschwitz and other concentration camps, together with the doctors, nurses and technicians who operated them, to solve the Jewish Question (as well as the Question of gypsies, criminals, homosexuals, political dissenters and some prisoners of war).

Doctors were active and enthusiastic in developing and implementing the racial hygiene policies. They selected subjects for transportation, for execution and for work duties. Their numbers swelled, their status and pay increased and, in the 1940s, 59 per cent of university presidents were doctors (Proctor 1992, 27). In addition, killing Jews freed up 60 per cent of medical practices in Berlin, providing unprecedented employment opportunities for Nordic doctors. What the Nazi political and military machines accomplished was the rendering of mass murder banal and ordinary by the medicalisation of killing. It viewed killing as a therapeutic imperative to purify the German race and produce the Master Race. As one doctor opined when questioned, he would remove a gangrenous appendix from a body if he found one and, in the same way, he removes Jews because "The Jew is a gangrenous appendix on the body of mankind" (Lifton 1986, 15). Gassing was apparently chosen by physicians as the mechanism of choice for mass murder because it separates the victim from the victimiser and thus minimises the psychological problems associated with mass shootings. Many soldiers suffered serious psychological trauma after shooting some 1.4 million Jews in Eastern Europe (Lifton 1986, 16). That some soldiers experienced serious psychological trauma after committing mass murder demonstrates that separating humans from non-humans conceptually and acting accordingly is not as clear-cut as the Nazis imagined.

The euthanasia policy and the concentration camps provided abundant subjects for human experimentation and material for necropsy. In terms of the euthanasia operation, neuropathologist Julius Hallervorden, from the Kaiser Wilhelm Institute for Brain Research, ordered hundreds of brains from euthanasia killings from a local killing hospital for his research. It was reported anecdotally that when he heard of the proposed mass killings he said to the killers "look here now, boys, if you are going to kill all those people, at least take the brains so that the material can be utilized" (Pross 1992, 36). When asked how many brains he wanted, he replied, "The more the better." It is telling that experiments in the concentration camps included studies that involved procedures that had been specifically banned, in November 1933, in experiments involving animals (Pross 1992, 45). If anything demonstrates the complete dehumanisation of Jews and other concentration camp inmates by National Socialism, this does. Certain categories of people were denied the rights afforded to non-human animals. Hypothermia, infection, sterilisation, transplant and multiple other inhumane studies were performed. It was these atrocities that the Allies concentrated on when they brought perpetrators to trial, despite the central role doctors played in the planning and execution of mass genocide. This focus was politically motivated.

Eugenic policies were popular in America and in Europe at the time, and the Allies wanted to take advantage of some of the research that had been undertaken in the camps and elsewhere in German scientific institutions. The war in the Pacific was ongoing and the Allies hoped that this research would assist in defeating the Japanese. In light of this agenda, it was considered unwise to criticise the entire German scientific community. It was also claimed that it was difficult to distinguish between war crimes, politically sanctioned killings and legitimate research (Weindling 2002, 62). Considering this, General Telford Taylor, Chief Prosecutor, cautioned that exposure of facts should be careful in order not to jeopardise the validity of clinical experiments. The dilemma was solved by the introduction of a new category of war crime, "medical war crimes," a term coined by Dr John West Robertson Thompson in November 1945. "Medical war crimes" were characterised as "crimes of a medical nature" (Weindling 2001, 42). Only 23 defendants were tried at Nuremburg by the Americans, of which 20 were physicians. Fifteen were found guilty and seven were acquitted. Seven were hanged on 2 June 1948 at Landsberg Prison in the American Sector, 12 were given life sentences, and the remainder were sentenced to between 10 and 20 years: "It can never be said that the quality of American justice was strained" (Mitscherlich and Mielke 1992, 106). The Nuremburg Code was enumerated as part of the judgement against the defendants; it contained 10 points relating to ethical research and stressed the importance of informed consent. It is embodied in most if not all subsequent ethical codes and informed the Helsinki World Medical Assembly Code of 1964 (Helsinki 1) and the subsequent revisions of 1975, 1983 and 1989 (Perley *et al.* 1992, 149).

Voices in education

The Tuskegee study and the Nazi medical experimentation illustrate the dangers of privileging one voice, the voice of science, in medical discourse. The "objective" voice of science, spoken and heard in the appropriate socio-political context of the American South and Europe respectively, enabled large-scale racially motivated atrocities. Male Negroes and Jews were construed in the prevailing culture as subhuman (host, syphilitic) or non-human (gangrene), which rendered them ideal subjects for the untempered pursuit of scientific truth. Subjects were involved in research studies that would be considered unacceptable for fully human beings. The irony of using purported non-human research subjects in studies to investigate human health problems was apparently missed or ignored, evidence of the metaphorical deafness in the mid twentieth-century scientific community to the heterogeneity of voices in society. The idea of voices, or utterance, has been used extensively by philosophers and educational researchers to speak to the capacity to recognise human agency because the capacity to speak has been positioned as the faculty that distinguishes humans from animals.

In his thought-provoking "Poetry in the Conversation of Mankind," Oakeshott (1962) takes this idea further by using conversation as a figure for human social development. Education formed through conversation between multiple voices, therefore, is central to his premise. He suggests that a number of philosophers consider human utterance as essentially involving a single mode; they distinguish different tones of utterance and a variety of expressions but hear only one authentic voice: "We are urged, for example, to regard all utterances as contributions (of different but comparable merit) to an inquiry, or a debate among inquirers, about ourselves and the world we inhabit" (Oakeshott 1962, 197). This view appears to accommodate a variety of voices but, in fact, recognises only one, namely, the voice of science. All other voices are acknowledged only insofar as they imitate this voice. Yet this univocality is not the only or the true construal of human intercourse. The appropriate construal of human intercourse is not an inquiry, but a conversation in which multiple voices feature and are acknowledged as valuable and equal.

Oakeshott's discussion of conversation is worth quoting at length:

> It is the appropriate image of human intercourse – appropriate because it recognizes the qualities, the diversities and the proper relationships of human utterances. As civilized human beings, we are the inheritors neither of an inquiry about ourselves and the world, nor of an accumulating body of information, but of a conversation, begun in the primeval forests and extended and made more articulate in the course of the centuries. It is a conversation which goes on in public and within each of ourselves. Of course, there is argument and inquiry and information, but wherever these are profitable they are to be recognized as passages in this conversation, and perhaps they are not the most captivating of the passages. It is the ability to participate in this conversation, and not the ability to reason cogently, to make discoveries about the world, or to conceive a better world, which distinguishes the civilized man [*sic*] from the barbarian ... *Education, properly speaking, is an initiation into the skill and partnership of this conversation in which we learn to recognize the voices, to distinguish the proper occasions of utterance, and in which we acquire the intellectual and moral habits appropriate to conversation.*
>
> (196, 199–200, emphasis added)

Oakeshott claims that this sort of education is a humanising education, where all the voices are recognised and respected as legitimate and equal. Richard Pring (2004a, 2004b) agrees with Oakeshott, although he is a little less abstract in his theorising. He characterises education as an essentially moral and political activity. Education is a moral activity because both its aims and the means to its pursuit are value-laden; the values it reflects are those considered worthwhile and good by those forming the curricula. It is political because it furnishes the young with the kind of knowledge and attitudes they need to make intelligent, alternative choices. Liberal education, properly conceived, frees the educated person from ignorance and barbarity. Pring sees this end as requiring a critical dialogue between students' mythocentric concepts and the logocentric concepts of their culture, involving

> making links between ... the public meanings we have inherited (and which are embodied within the subjects of physics, mathematics, history and literature) and ... the personal strivings of each and every one to make sense of their experience and to find their own identity within it.
>
> (Pring 2004b, 28)

It is, in other words, to render personally significant that which is presented in an impersonal form to all, "the inheritance of previous generations, refined by previous argument, scholarship and criticism, and to be found in textbooks and artefacts of various kinds" (28).

According to Pring, therefore, to be educated is to be in possession of those understandings, skills and attitudes whereby one can make sense of the human world: for the physical world to be understood through the sciences and mathematics; the ways in which we are embedded in a social and political world that shapes our lives and perspectives; and the moral world of ideals and responsibilities and the aesthetic world of beauty and style through which we find pleasure and delight. Pring observes, crucially, that

> entry into those different worlds is more than a making sense of that which is inherited from others. It gives access to the ideas and thus the tools through which the learner's own distinctive personal development might actively take place.
>
> (Pring 2004b, 27)

In short, teaching involves an interpersonal transaction, or critical dialogue, between the personal knowledge and understanding (mythos) of students and the impersonal world of ideas (logos) embodied in particular cultures. This requires that the concepts and conceptual frameworks of both personal knowledge and impersonal science, in the broadest sense, be continuously cross-examined.

Establishing a critical dialogue between the personal logos and mythos and the embedding cultural logos and mythos requires what I have previously characterised as single and double loop learning from feedback (Greenwood 1998). Single loop learning results from examining the results of an activity or procedure in light merely of its aims. How efficacious was my experimental surgery? Or my hypothermia experiment? How might these be performed in future where time and economy are improved? How efficient is our tracking system to prevent accidental penicillin treatment of syphilis patients? Double loop learning, however, requires that the values and motivations behind the activity or procedure be examined. Are the prevailing cultural values and stereotypes rationally defensible? Why or why not? And are they ethically defensible? Why or why not? In what respects are Male Negroes and Jews different from whites and Nordics? Are these characteristics actually relevant to ascriptions of humanity? Why or why not? Why did I subject human beings to experiments expressly prohibited on non-human animals? What criteria did I use? Are they valid? Why am I withholding treatment for syphilis when I already know almost everything about it? Is the discovery of scientific knowledge ever worth the cost of human lives? If so, on what grounds (and are these valid)?

Conclusion

This chapter has reported two familiar cases of medical atrocity, which highlight the danger of privileging one untempered voice in human discourse. In addition, they show that they were made possible by the socio-political climate at the time. As much as they may be separated out as scientific scandals, it cannot be ignored that the Tuskegee and Nazi medical experiments were enabled by the racial hygiene/eugenics policies that were already well established in Europe and North America. They also demonstrate that biomedical sciences (and, presumably the sciences more generally) are not merely passive, apolitical innocents, merely responding to external political forces; they are in the vanguard if not actually leading the initiation, administration and execution of public health service policy, some of which is deeply unethical. It was certainly the case that over 20 institutes of racial hygiene were established in universities *before* Hitler came to power.

Fortunately, both cases resulted, eventually, in ethical advance. The privileged *logos* and *mythos* of the perpetrators were eventually challenged by the *thymos* of the larger population, and remedial and preventative measures were implemented. The message to medical and other health professional educators, therefore, is clear. The *logos* and *mythos* of each individual within a culture are typically consistent with the prevailing socio-political values in which the individuals are embedded and, given this factor, double-loop reflection should be facilitated to take account of these values. Such socio-political values, together with individual logos and mythos of students, should be brought to the surface, clearly articulated, examined for adequacy, accuracy and propriety and, where necessary, elaborated, refined and revised.

Reference list

Aly, G. 1994. "Medicine against the Useless." In *Cleansing the Fatherland: Nazi Medicine and Racial Hygiene*, edited by G. Aly, P. Choust and C. Pross, 22–99. Baltimore, MD: Johns Hopkins University Press.

Amnesty International. 2017. *Understanding Human Rights: Free and Equal*. supporter@ amnesty.org.au.

Atlanta Constitution, 27 July 1972. 30A.

Bell, S.E. 2000. "Events in the Tuskegee Syphilis Study." In *Tuskegee Truths: Rethinking the Tuskegee Syphilis Study*, edited by S.M. Reverby, 34–40. Chapel Hill: University of North Carolina Press.

Brandt, A.M. 2000. "Racism and Research: The Case of the Tuskegee Syphilis Experiment." In *Tuskegee Truths: Rethinking the Tuskegee Syphilis Study*, edited by S.M. Reverby, 15–33. Chapel Hill: University of North Carolina Press. briandeer.com/mmr/ lancet-summary.htm.

Caplan, A.L. 1992. "Twenty Years after: The Legacy of the Tuskegee Syphilis Study: When Evil Intrudes." *Hastings Center Report*, 22: 29–32.

Carlson, D. 1998. "Finding a Voice and Losing Our Way?" *Educational Theory*, 48.4: 541–54.

Edgar, H. 2000. "Outside the Community." In *Tuskegee Truths: Rethinking the Tuskegee Syphilis Study*, edited by S.M. Reverby, 489–94. Chapel Hill: University of North Carolina Press.

Gray, F. 2000. "The Lawsuit." In *Tuskegee Truths: Rethinking the Tuskegee Syphilis Study*, edited by Susan M. Reverby, 473–88. Chapel Hill: University of North Carolina Press.

Greenwood, J. 1998. "The Role of Reflection in Single and Double Loop Learning." *Journal of Advanced Nursing*, 27.5: 1045–53.

Heintzelman, C.A. 2003. "The Tuskegee Syphilis Study and its Implications for the 21st Century." *The New Social Worker*, 10.4. www.socialworker.com/feature-article-article/ethics-article/TheTuskegeeSyphilisStudyanditsImplicationsfortheTwenty-FirstCentury/.

Heller, J. 1972. "Syphilis Victims in United States Went Untreated for 40 Years. Syphilis Victims Got No Therapy." Associated Press. *New York Times*, 26, 1 July.

Jones, J.H. 1981. *Bad Blood: The Tuskegee Syphilis Experiment.* London: The Free Press.

Kant, E. [1786] 1964. *Groundwork to the Metaphysics of Morals.* Trans. H.J. Paton, New York: Harper & Row.

Lifton, R.J. 1986. *The Nazi Doctors: Medical Killing and the Psychology of Genocide.* New York: Basic Books.

Mitscherlich, A. and Mielke, F. 1992. "Epilogue: Seven Were Hanged." In *The Nazi Doctors and the Nuremburg Code: Human Rights in Human Experimentation*, edited by G.J. Annas and M.A. Grodin, 105–08. Oxford: Oxford University Press.

Mizzoni, J. 2009. *Ethics: The Basics.* Chichester: Wiley-Blackwell.

Oakeshott, M. [1962] 1992. "Poetry in the Conversation of Mankind." In *Rationalism in Politics and Other Essays*, 167–97. London: Methuen.

Perley, S., Fluss, S.S., Bankowski, Z. and Simon, F. 1992. "The Nuremburg Code: An International Overview." In *The Nazi Doctors and the Nuremburg Code: Human Rights in Human Experimentation*, edited by G.J. Annas and M.A. Grodin, 149–73. Oxford: Oxford University Press.

Plato. 1974. *The Republic.* Trans. D. Lee. London: Penguin Books.

Pring, R. 2004a. "Education as Moral Practice." In *Philosophy of Education: Aims, Theory, Commonsense and Research*, edited by R. Pring, 9–25. London: Continuum.

Pring, R. 2004b. "Educating Persons." In *Philosophy of Education: Aims, Theory, Commonsense and Research*, edited by R. Pring, 27–41. London: Continuum.

Proctor, R.N. 1992. "Nazi Doctors, Racial Medicine, and Human Experimentation." In *The Nazi Doctors and the Nuremburg Code: Human Rights in Human Experimentation*, edited by G.J. Annas and M.A. Grodin, 17–31. Oxford: Oxford University Press.

Pross, C. 1992. "Nazi Doctors, German Medicine, and Historical Truth." In *The Nazi Doctors and the Nuremburg Code: Human Rights in Human Experimentation*, edited by G.J. Annas and M.A. Grodin, 32–52. Oxford: Oxford University Press.

Reverby, S.M. 2000. "Introduction. More Than a Metaphor: An Overview of the Scholarship of the Study." In *Tuskegee Truths: Rethinking the Tuskegee Syphilis Study*, edited by S.M. Reverby, 1–14. Chapel Hill: University of North Carolina Press.

Savitt, T. 1982. "The Use of Blacks for medical Experimentation and Demonstration in the Old South." *Journal of Southern History*, 48: 331–48.

Solomon, M. 2000. "The Rhetoric of Dehumanisation: An Analysis of Medical Reports of the Tuskegee Syphilis Project." In *Tuskegee Truths: Rethinking the Tuskegee Syphilis Study*, edited by S.M. Reverby, 251–65. Chapel Hill: University of North Carolina Press.

Weindling, P.J. 2001. "The Origins of Informed Consent: The International Scientific Commission on Medical War Crimes and the Nuremburg Code." *Bulletin of the History of Medicine*, 75.1: 37–71.

Weindling, P.J. 2002. "The Ethical Legacy of the Nazi Medical War Crimes: Human Experiments and International Justice." In *A Companion to Genethics*, edited by J. Burley and J. Harris, 53–69. Oxford: Blackwell.

Weld, A.D. [1839] 2011. *American Slavery as It Is: Testimony of a Thousand Witnesses.* Columbia: University of South Carolina Press.

7 The cost of efficiency in Great War nursing literature

M. Renee Benham

In British literature from the 1880s and 1890s, sympathy was considered the most desirable quality for nurses. Literature from the early twentieth century, however, claimed that nurses needed to control, mask and even forsake sympathy to be efficient professionals. Florence Nightingale had wanted efficient nurses during the Crimean War (1853–56), but the profession did not obtain this standard until decades later.[1] By this time, the nursing profession was one of many industries striving for efficiency. Jennifer Karns Alexander (2008) states there was "an efficiency craze" throughout Europe and the United States in the first few decades of the twentieth century that established efficiency as a household name and applied it to numerous non-mechanical areas, including the control of people (1–2). It is difficult to provide an exact definition of efficiency because its meaning varies depending upon context; it is both a measurement and a metaphor, a tool and an objective (Alexander 2008, 4). Efficiency was first a philosophical concept, but after the Industrial Revolution the word referred to "increasing the output of a machine or organization through the elimination of waste" (Cobley 2009, 6). During the twentieth century, however, its usage extended to numerous non-mechanical areas: "Efficiency became promiscuous, describing activities of all sorts, including marriage, fuel consumption, use of leisure time, and political and moral behavior" (Alexander 2008, 2).

Literature not only reflected this increase; according to Evelyn Cobley (2009), it "shaped the public reception of the efficiency calculus" (16). Expanding on Cobley's claim, I argue that literary portrayals of nursing from 1900–18 mirror the contradictory encouragement of, and discomfort with, the notion of efficiency in broader society. This emphasis on efficiency effectively downgraded sympathy because it hindered the effectiveness of the medical machine. *The Red Cross*, the official magazine of the British Red Cross and Voluntary Aid Detachment (VAD) organisation, reflects this increasing emphasis on efficiency in the nursing field, as does E. Charles Vivian and J.E. Hodder Williams' novel *The Way of the Red Cross* (1915) and Frank Moore's *The Romance of a Red Cross Hospital* (1915).[2] These texts praise efficiency unabashedly, even when sympathy is sacrificed. Memoir and novel authors writing after the war, however, especially after 1928, resisted the constant drive for efficiency because they felt it turned them into heartless machines. In Mary Borden's memoir *The Forbidden*

Zone (1929) and Vera Brittain's *Testament of Youth* (1933), as well as in Rad-clyffe Hall's novel *The Well of Loneliness* (1928) and *Not So Quiet* (1930) by Helen Zenna Smith, the nurses recognise that abandoning sympathy will make them more efficient, and efficiency is necessary to handle the overwhelming number of wounded men. When they lose sympathy, however, they are turned into soulless machines, and thus lose their own humanity while trying to save others.

Despite recent critical attention towards these texts, no one has compared these retrospective narratives to the pro-efficiency romances written during the war, and thus recognised that Great War fiction and memoir reflect society's increasing enthusiasm for efficiency and simultaneous devaluing of sympathy within the nursing profession. For example, historians Geoffrey Searle (1971), Martha Vicinus (1985) and Jennifer Alexander (2008) examine the increase of efficiency in early-twentieth-century society, yet do not examine how literature both shaped and helped normalise this new value system within medical care. Literary scholars Sandra Gilbert and Susan Gubar (1989) and Sharon Ouditt (1994) have analysed these classic nursing memoirs and novels, and Ouditt has noted the dehumanisation and loss of "sensitivity" in nursing care, yet links this emotional disconnection to the "motifs of literary modernism" (37–38), rather than the professionalisation of nursing or the changing public estimation of efficiency. Cobley also examines literary modernism, claiming that "modernist novels are primarily interested in dramatizing the detrimental effects of the internalization of the efficiency calculus on the consciousness of individuals and on traditional central values" (2009, 15). Much like the modernist novels that Cobley examines, the World War I nursing novels and memoirs I examine challenge the "internalization of the efficiency calculus" and its effect on nurses and on the profession. I assert that the Great War hastened the evolution of nursing into a modern profession and solidified the transition away from sympathy and towards efficiency, a shift that made nurses feel like soulless machines. In effect, valuing efficiency above all else made nurses sacrifice their own humanity to save the humanity of others. While the circumstances of war no doubt played a critical role in this progression, these memoirs reveal the cost of considering efficiency the most important objective in nursing care, both to nurses and to society.

The rise of efficiency

Fin de siècle and early-twentieth-century nursing materials frequently mentioned efficiency and debated whether efficiency or sympathy was more important in nursing care. For instance, Alice Dannatt's article "What Constitutes an Efficient Nurse?" published in *The Nursing Record* (May 1888, 87), states that nurses should strive to be "efficient" yet need "thorough-going unselfishness" to obtain it.[3] Two months later (June 1888), Miss Mollett's article "Sympathy" appeared in the same periodical and asserted that sympathy was the most important element of nursing care. Another short yet remarkable article from February

1889 uses the word "efficiency" or its cognates five times in a single paragraph describing a nursing meeting in Bristol:

> Miss Wood pointed out the change which had come over the profession of Nursing, and said many people now became Nurses who had not the training to render them *efficient* for the position.... These *inefficient* Nurses were a great danger to those they had to look after.... It was proposed in the Association that Nurses should combine for mutual improvement, and with the object of insuring professional *efficiency*. It was proposed to apply for a Royal Charter, so that Nurses who gave proof of *efficiency* might be registered, and a sort of guarantee of *efficiency* given to the world.
>
> ("The British Nurses' Association" 1889, 134; emphasis added)

Nurse training was not yet standardised; therefore, efficiency often became the distinguishing factor between qualified and unqualified nurses. The presence of these articles contemporaneously within the same nursing periodical reflects the broader discussions regarding sympathy and efficiency within the profession at the end of the nineteenth century.

This debate continued in early-twentieth-century nursing texts, which largely considered sympathy to be more important than efficiency. The manual *Home Nursing* by Margery Homersham (1900), for example, emphasises sympathy in the home nurse, stating, "A really good nurse will always regard implicit obedience to the doctor as foremost of her qualifications, but kindness and sympathy with her patient are hardly of less importance" (1).[4] This passage is consistent in all seven editions between 1888 and 1900. Similarly, a 1901 editorial in *The Nursing Record* begins with the familiar question, "What constitutes an efficient nurse?" but then relates a scenario in which the nurse was efficient but was dismissed by the patient because she was not sympathetic ("Nursing Echoes" 211). The anonymous author states, "Surely the greatest technical skill is of no avail if a nurse is fundamentally unsympathetic" (212). As the century progressed, this opinion declined.

Gradually, efficiency became more important than sympathy in nursing texts, particularly those published by the Voluntary Aid Detachment (VAD) organisation. The VAD organisation was formed in 1910 after the failures of the Boer War (1899–1902) demonstrated the urgent need for an organised system to manage volunteer nurses during war. On 16 August 1909, the War Office issued a "Scheme for the Organization of Voluntary Aid in England and Wales," which included men's and women's Voluntary Aid Detachments (Summers 1988, 247). The detachment's objective was to supplement the territorial medical service (247). VADs were organised by the Red Cross, but incorporated training and volunteers from St. John's Ambulance Association, a large and well-respected stretcher-carrier organisation (Bowser 2003). At the start of the Great War, the British government merged the St. John's Ambulance Association with the British Red Cross and added it to the War Office as the Joint Voluntary Aid Detachment. Materials published by the British Red Cross or this joint office emphasise efficiency more than sympathy in nursing care. For instance, the standard first-aid manuals by James Cantlie, a highly respected physician known for the implementation and teaching of first-aid programs (McEwan 2014, 37), state that a volunteer's primary goal is efficient service: "That this textbook may be of real help to those whose patriotic aim is to prepare themselves to render efficient help to the Red Cross in its beneficent mission to the sick and wounded, is the author's earnest desire" (Cantlie 1912, x). This manual was published when the VADs were organising for an almost unimaginable event: an invasion on British soil. As they recruited volunteers and practised mobilising auxiliary hospitals, the highest praise VAD members could receive was that they operated efficiently. Sympathy, however, was still valuable. Cantlie explains in the first chapter of his manual that "The study of First Aid ... demands intelligence, tact, observation, resourcefulness, and sympathy" (1912, 1). Though placed at the end of the list, sympathy is still mentioned, signalling its necessity, but only as an aid to fulfil the main objective of efficiency.

The Devonshire handbook for VAD workers (1910) also emphasises efficiency as the greatest objective. J.S.C. Davis explains that the third "condition of enrollment" for VADs, after having enough members and equipment, is "that the detachment will maintain its efficiency" (6). Beneath the subheading titled "Efficiency," the manual states,

> Voluntary Aid detachments can be kept in efficiency by being called out about once a month to practise their duties under their officers; but it is not intended to place any limit on the activities of detachments in rendering themselves efficient.
>
> (6)

Several paragraphs later, Davis adds, "The principal requirement in every case is efficiency, which term includes the efficiency of officers and members of the detachments" (9). The handbook mentions efficiency dozens of times, denoting its importance as the "principal requirement in every case" (9). This handbook, like Cantlie's Red Cross manual, was published when large-scale war was a remote possibility. After war began, efficiency became even more important and was the determining factor in VAD member mobilisation and advancement. When the War Department announced that they would send VAD members abroad, Headquarters advised them to become efficient immediately: "It now behooves every VAD member who desires to serve her country to make herself as efficient as possible forthwith" ("The Army Medical" 1915, 62). Once mobilised, VAD members could be awarded a "red efficiency stripe" to acknowledge excellent performance ("V.A.D.s Required" 1918, 27).

The Red Cross magazine similarly underscored efficiency, both in the praise it repeated and in its original articles. When the editors printed praise within the magazine, which they often did, invariably the compliment mentioned qualities like order and discipline rather than sympathy. For example, in an article titled "Note on the Work of the VAD Nurses in Malta" (June 1916), high-ranking

Army Medical Service Officers C.A. Ballance, Purves Stewart, Charter Symonds, A.E. Garrod and William Thorburn praise the efficiency of the VAD organisation: "They were well disciplined, alert in recognizing unfavorable symptoms, and whilst losing no time in sending for assistance, were capable themselves of rendering efficient first aid" (72). Later in the article, the doctors again state, "the great majority proved themselves highly efficient and worthy to be employed in any military hospital" (72). It is the women's efficiency (noted first) which makes them worthy of employment. Medical professionals were initially sceptical of amateur VAD nurses; thus, the doctors' praise was significant. Their comments also reveal that medical and military authorities similarly valued efficiency. Jeffrey Reznick (2004) notes that many wartime industries were interested in increasing efficiency, including factories, YMCA workers and military hospitals. When analysing YMCA canteen posters, he notes how the YMCA war posters position women as "efficient industrial workers" similar to factory munitions workers (35–36). Reznick focuses on a variety of industries during the war, and though he does include a chapter on military hospitals, he focuses on their architectural structure of efficiency rather than the individual or corporate efficiency of the nurses and doctors working there. In another example, Colonel Sir Courtland Thompson, the Chief Commissioner of the British Red Cross and Order of St. John for Malta, Egypt and the Near East Commission, praises the efficiency of VAD nurses in a dispatch, saying, "It is impossible to speak too highly of their utility, exemplary conduct and efficiency" (Thompson 1916, 104).

The Red Cross also reprinted praise from other newspapers that noted VAD efficiency. For example, they reprinted a passage from a *Morning Post* article (April 1915) declaring the care of the wounded "a splendid specimen of Red Cross efficiency" (74). A reprinted article originally from *The Times* (Saturday, 29 July 1916) agrees that "The Women's Voluntary Aid Detachments have conclusively proved their efficiency and usefulness both in the military and auxiliary hospitals" ("A Call for Women" 9). While other newspapers and magazines praised VAD nurses using sentimental language, *The Red Cross* reprints focus almost exclusively on the nurses' efficiency. This emphasis is echoed in their original articles. "The Organization of a VAD Hospital" (November 1916) advises

> A definite allocation of duties amongst the respective officers, enabling each to work in water-tight compartments, and thus to concentrate on attaining efficiency in a particular direction. Method and order are the ideals to be aimed at. *No amount of sympathy and kindness by themselves will ensure a sick man's comfort.*
>
> (143; emphasis added)

The belief that efficiency, rather than sympathy, ensures effective care is the exact opposite of the opinion printed in *The Nursing Record* 15 years previously (1901), which stated that "the greatest technical skill is of no avail if a nurse is

fundamentally unsympathetic" ("Nursing Echoes" 1901, 212). By 1916, efficiency, method and order were considered more valuable than sympathy. These
materials do not explain the cause of this transition, yet creative literature
explains some of the contributing factors.

The gradually increasing emphasis on efficiency rather than sympathy is also
evident in creative literature. Turn-of-the-century novels such as Grant Allen's
Hilda Wade (1900) and L.T. Meade's *Nurse Charlotte* (1904) advocate for sympathy in nursing, particularly to assuage the cultural concern that medical care
was becoming indifferent. As medical care professionalised throughout the
century, it became increasingly secular and impersonal.[5] For instance, patients in
hospitals were often referred to by number, rather than by name. In *Hilda Wade*,
Doctor Sebastian and Doctor Nielsen are more concerned with the advancement
of science than the patient's safety. Nurse Hilda serves as the sympathetic shield
between the cruel doctors and the patients. She insists that class and training are
not the distinguishing factors between nurses; rather, sympathy is "the really
important thing" (Allen 1900, 271). Similarly, in Meade's *Nurse Charlotte*
(1904), two Sisters at St. Christopher's hospital are "loved" or "not loved" by
the patients and staff depending upon whether they have sympathy (53–54).
Sister Winifred is a sympathetic woman who has "a gentle sort of presence. No
one ever dared to disobey her, and yet patients, probationers, and nurses all
loved her well" (Meade 1915, 53–54). Contrary to Sister Winifred, Sister Elizabeth "was not loved. She was a small, dark woman, with a vivacious face and a
quick manner. She was just as determined as Sister Winifred, but there was no
sympathy about her" (54). Though Meade values sympathy, she also recognises
the necessity of controlling sympathy both for the patient's sake and for hospital
efficiency. For example, despite being loved by the patients, the heroine Nurse
Charlotte struggles to cope with the emotionally demanding atmosphere of the
hospital. Her sorrow over a patient's death hinders her work and she is scolded
by her colleague, Nurse Jane:

> Well, I wouldn't be as soft as that if I'd given myself to be a nurse. I
> wouldn't fret when it isn't necessary. What will the other nurses say to you
> if you're not able to do your work well because one of the patients has died?
> You're not fit to be a nurse, and that's evident.

(59)

Nurse Jane believes that sympathy hinders a nurse's productivity and should
therefore be ignored. Readers in 1904 sympathised with Charlotte, but Jane's
notions gain prominence as time progresses. The sympathy that was the defining
element between good and poor nurses in literature from the 1890s is considered
a liability by 1915.

By World War I, literature reflects the increasingly common opinion that
managing cases impersonally is more valuable than sympathetic care. This shift
is evident in *The Way of the Red Cross* (1915), a collection of stories gathered
by a man as he toured the battlefield and hospitals in France and Britain. The

narrator, referred to only as "I," appreciates that nurses have learned to work without being affected by sympathy:

> There were, in those first days, nurses who fainted at the sight of blood and shuddered at the business of dressing wounds – these drawbacks were unavoidable at the outset, just as they were unavoidable in the training of nurses in large permanent hospitals. There were many who shed tears at parting with favourite patients, and regarded the work too personally, and there were some who would not make good nurses if they were kept at the business for years. But these drawbacks to the work have disappeared – the voluntary aid nurse, at the present time, is very nearly equivalent to the trained nurse. She regards a case as a case and nothing more.
>
> (Vivian and Williams 1915, 201)

This account considers nursing "personally" or with sympathy as a "drawback," and boasts that volunteer nurses have become impersonal and see patients "as a case and nothing more."

Romance in a Red Cross Hospital (1915) by Frank Moore expresses similar sentiment. This novel follows the experiences of Angela Inman, Doctor Charwood and Mrs. Thorburn as Angela sponsors and manages an auxiliary hospital in England during the war. Angela, the heroine of the story, is praised for overcoming her fear of seeing wounded men:

> But only at first did she have any sense of horror, and by the time she was able to visit her own ward she had advanced some way toward acquiring the attitude of the true nurse who is not moved by the appearance of unlimited horrors, and whose sympathy is not of a sentimental character, but most active in realization of the fact that she is doing something to lessen the suffering under her eyes.
>
> (Moore 1915, 235)

As with the previous example, the "true nurse" is the one who is "not moved" by a patient's suffering but cares for him impersonally. Moore praises Angela for reaching this point, as she is now able to face "unlimited horrors" without lowering her standard of care. Both Vivian and Moore are laymen rather than medical professionals; thus, their approval of impersonal, efficient nursing suggests a shift in popular opinion regarding nursing care. Both authors recognise that emotions make it more difficult for nurses to work effectively. To put it bluntly, weeping or vomiting upon seeing wounded men would make nurses unable to function, much less work efficiently. The new and terrifying horrors of war thus make sympathy a detriment to the "full efficiency" that is an "absolute necessity" in wartime (Vivian and Williams 1915, 84). According to Vivian and Moore, losing sympathy is necessary for productivity. Nursing memoirs, however, reveal that removing sympathy was also a coping mechanism nurses employed to deal with the psychological trauma of war.

Upon further reflection: critique on the loss of sympathy

Fictional novels and memoirs written after the war also discussed the loss of sympathy; yet, unlike literature written during the war, texts printed after 1928 questioned and critiqued the overriding emphasis on efficiency. Hattaway explains that 10 years after the war, many texts, including *Not So Quiet*, "sought to disprove the notion that adventure or romance had any place in the conflict" (Goldman, Gledhill and Hattaway 1995, 67). In addition to removing elements of romance, these novels and memoirs demonstrate how the drive towards efficiency turns nurses into machines. In Radclyffe Hall's novel *The Well of Loneliness* (1928), for example, England enrolls Stephen as an ambulance driver in France despite her homosexuality because she is "strong and efficient" and can "fill a man's place" (319). While serving, Stephen describes how the number of wounded outweigh the sympathy she might have had to offer:

> From what had once been its spacious cellar, they were hurriedly carrying up the wounded, maimed and mangled creatures who, a few hours ago, had been young and vigorous men. None too gently the stretchers were lowered to the ground beside the two waiting ambulances – none too gently because there were so many of them, and because there must come a time in all wars when custom stales even compassion.
>
> (329)

There are so many wounded men that the stretcher-carriers operate with haste rather than gentleness. Stephen attributes this change directly to the war, which undoubtedly contributed to the decrease of sympathy in nursing care. Hall's novel does not include much self-reflection about coping with the war, yet it mentions Blakeney, a driver "who had done with all feeling" (335). She is described as emotionally void until the Armistice is announced, at which time, "Blakeney, who had long ago done with emotions – quite suddenly laid her arms on the table and her head on her arms, and she wept, and she wept" (345). Blakeney's breakdown suggests that her façade of equanimity was a coping mechanism to deal with the trauma and keep working, but she was still deeply affected by her experience. Neither the characters nor the narrator comment upon Blakeney's reaction as either positive or negative, but her breakdown finishes the section, and the reader is left with tears. Blakeney's reaction suggests that there are personal consequences for abandoning sympathy, even during war.

Contrary to Hall's subtle questioning, Helen Zenna Smith's *Not So Quiet ... Stepdaughters of War* (1930) overtly criticises efficiency and the lack of sympathy during the war. *Not So Quiet* was written as a response to Erich Remarque's *All Quiet on the Western Front* (1929) and was intended to supply the "woman's war-story" (Smith 1930, 7). Though technically fictional, *Not So Quiet* is largely based upon the experiences of Winifred Constance Young, an ambulance driver in France (Smith 7). Smith's novel follows Helen Smith and a crew of ambulance drivers under the command of a Commandant they have nicknamed "Mrs. Bitch." Smith recognises efficiency as a military and nursing watchword and vilifies it throughout the novel, largely through Mrs. Bitch, who is a parody of women who seek efficiency above all else: "Commandant is dreadfully efficient. Like most dreadfully efficient women, she is universally loathed" (19). The Commandant lacks sympathy for her overworked and underfed volunteer drivers. For example, during a roll-call, the Commandant must wait until a sick girl stops coughing, "but she is merely annoyed, not concerned, at the interruption. Like all efficient machines, she has no humanity" (49). Smith aligns efficiency with the mechanical and places it in opposition to humanity. The Commandant is efficient, and since readers despise the Commandant, they also despise the efficiency for which she stands. Helen recognises that she is supposed to be impersonal so she can work effectively, yet she resists:

> I have schooled myself to stop fainting at the sight of blood. I have schooled myself not to vomit at the smell of wounds and stale blood, but view these sad bodies with professional calm I shall never be able to do.
>
> (89–90)

Even though the team members who distance themselves emotionally are better workers, readers sympathise with Helen and her desire to retain her humanity.

Despite Helen's determination to avoid "professional calm," she eventually succumbs and becomes a machine. After her friend Tosh dies in a bombing, Helen is traumatised. She leaves the service, determined never to return, but she is still unable to feel: "I do not care. I am flat. Old. I am twenty-one and as old as the hills. Emotion-dry. The war has drained me of feeling. Something has gone from me that will never return" (Smith 1930, 169). Helen's loss of emotion is not a conscious effort to increase productivity, but a result of trauma. Her equanimity, however, makes her an admirable worker when she re-enlists as a cook's assistant in the Women's Auxiliary Army Corps. Seven months into her service, she writes, "I have become accustomed to being a machine" (214). She describes the routine of her days without feeling and explains that her entire life is regulated and controlled:

> I am a slot machine that never goes out of order. Put so much rations into the slot and I will work so long, play so long, and sleep so long. The administration is perfect. Everything is regulated. Even my emotions.... I am the most equable disposition in the unit. My Administrator says so. My companions like me because I am "always the same."
>
> (214–15)

Helen is a stellar worker whom her supervisor uses as an example to others (216). Readers, however, remember when Helen was alive, and mourn her loss of humanity. At the end of the novel, Helen is one of the few people who survive an air raid, through which she remains calm. While she appears unharmed, the narrator explains, "Her soul died under a radiant silver moon in the spring of 1918 on the side of a blood-spattered trench" (239). The trauma of war turns Helen into an efficient machine but causes her to lose her soul – something irreparable and tragic.

Mary Borden's memoir *The Forbidden Zone* (1929) reveals a similar struggle and loss of soul. Mary Borden was an American heiress without nursing experience, yet she offered to fund and manage her own hospital for the French Army during the war. They could not refuse. Her short memoir is written in fragmented episodes, each one compelling and heartbreaking, with simple, lyrical prose. During one segment, Borden describes a nurse going from hut to hut on rounds as a woman who has killed her senses to survive the ordeal of war:

> She is dead already, just as I am – really dead, past resurrection. Her heart is dead. She killed it. She couldn't bear to feel it jumping in her side when Life, the sick animal, choked and rattled in her arms. Her ears are deaf; she deafened them. She could not bear to hear Life crying and mewing. She is blind so that she cannot see the torn parts of men she must handle. Blind, dead, dead – she is strong, efficient, fit to consort with gods and demons – a machine inhabited by the ghost of a woman – soulless, past redeeming, just as I am – just as I will be.
>
> (43)

Borden poignantly describes the pain that nurses feel as they witness the trauma of war – pain so intense that they intentionally "kill" their senses in order to bear it and keep working. Contrary to Moore's heroine, Angela, who remained her cheerful self after losing sympathy, Borden explains that killing the senses destroys the self. Losing sympathy makes Borden "strong, efficient" and able to handle the quantity of wounded men, but it also makes her lose her soul. By abandoning emotion, she and the other nurses become machines. While this transition is lamentable, it is also necessary to continue nursing.

Vera Brittain's *Testament of Youth* (1933), like Borden's memoir, discusses the necessity of losing sympathy, yet Brittain resists the loss even as she feels it happening. When Brittain starts working at the auxiliary hospital, she is naïve and sentimental, yet these attributes disappear as she gains experience. She recognises the change she is undergoing, yet she is not able to stop it. When she witnesses her first death, she reflects:

> Although surprised at my own equanimity, I had not yet acquired the self-protective callousness of later days.... To me it is strange that I take this death – sad as it makes me feel – so much as a matter of course when only a short time ago the idea of death made me shudder and filled me with horror.
>
> (176)

Brittain's views about life and death have already altered, and though she acknowledges that "callousness" can be "self-protective," she considers it "a great revulsion of mind" (176). Later, however, when she becomes a competent dressing assistant, she remembers with "humiliation" the time she nearly fainted at the sight of an open wound (211). She admits that even though she is getting better at dealing with the gore, she does not want to turn into the cold trained nurses she sees around her:

> Sisters, calm, balanced, efficient, moving up and down the wards, self-protected by that bright immunity from pity which the highly trained nurse seems so often to possess, filled me with a deep fear of merging my own individuality in the impersonal routine of the organisation.
>
> (211)

Though the trained nurses are more capable and efficient than she is, "There is something so starved and dry about [them] – as if they had to force all the warmth out of themselves before they could be really good nurses" (211). Brittain knows that efficiency makes nurses "self-protected" and more productive, but she considers sympathy integral to her identity and humanity, and resists losing it. Her resistance, however, is futile.

Despite Brittain's fears about becoming impersonal and "indifferent to pain," the frequency and routine of her work causes her to lose the sympathy she once felt (212). She reflects,

> No sudden gift of second sight showed me the future months in which I should not only contemplate and hold, but dress unaided and without emotion, the quivering stump of a newly amputated limb – than which a more pitiable spectacle hardly exists on this side of death.
>
> (216)

After her fiancé, Roland, is killed in battle, Brittain intentionally becomes as unemotional as the trained nurses she earlier despised: "My only hope now was to become the complete automaton, working mechanically and no longer even pretending to be animated by ideals. Thought was too dangerous.... On the whole it seemed safer to go on being a machine" (450). Like Borden, Brittain sacrifices her humanity and turns into a machine because remaining human and feeling is too painful. Brittain identifies the discrepancy between the altruistic motivations that led her to nursing, and the values of efficiency that dominate while she is nursing:

> It is always so strange that when you are working you never think of all the inspiring thoughts that made you take up the work in the first instance. Before I was in hospital at all I thought that because I suffered myself I should feel it a grand thing to relieve the sufferings of other people. But now, when I am doing something which I know relieves someone's pain, it is nothing but a matter of business.
>
> (212)

Though Brittain is speaking only to her situation, the similarities between the memoirs suggest that her experience was common. She exposes the paradox of the nursing profession: the sympathy for humanity that leads people into nursing is counter-productive to the efficiency that is demanded within the medical field. Moreover, abandoning sympathy to be efficient turns nurses into machines, and sacrifices their own humanity in order to preserve others.

Conclusion

Though nursing periodicals and literature suggest that sympathy was already losing importance in the early twentieth century, the Great War hastened its exodus and may have permanently displaced sympathetic nursing in lieu of efficiency. Moore's *Romance of a Red Cross Hospital* (1915) and Vivian and Williams' *The Way of the Red Cross* (1915) agree that sympathy hinders efficiency, and thus hinders one of the primary goals of medical care. Texts written during the war praise the efficiency and the emotional hardness of nurses, but novels and memoirs published after 1928 such as Smith's *Not So Quiet* (1930), Borden's *Forbidden Zone* (1929) and Brittain's *Testament of Youth* (1933) lament the loss of emotion necessitated by the war, and the consequential loss of humanity as the women evolved into machines. I am not suggesting that the medical profession was without sympathy during the war. Indeed, Christine Hallett's book *Containing Trauma* (2009) investigated nurses' personal diaries and letters and claims that their compassion was present but intentionally masked to create safe spaces for the men to heal (16–17). Rather, I claim that Smith's (1930), Borden's (1929) and Brittain's (1933) memoirs reveal that when efficiency becomes the primary goal in medical care, sympathy is often lost, and thus removes the very element the profession is trying to maintain: humanity.

The medical profession undoubtedly became more advanced and efficient during the war, but these texts suggest that it also lost something. Despite Smith's, Borden's and Brittain's warnings, the industrialised world progressed into the twentieth century with an even greater desire for efficiency and machines. Alexander states, "Efficiency has indeed become a central value in the world's advanced industrial culture, an apparently self-evident value associated with individual discipline, superior management, and increased profits" (2008, 1). Industrialised cultures today continue to strive for cost-efficient governments, energy-efficient systems, and fuel-efficient vehicles. Yet Alexander (2008) and Cobley (2009) also reveal the dangers of this drive for efficiency. While efficiency can be celebrated as a tool of conservation and growth, it can also be "a powerful tool of repression" (Alexander 167). Alexander suggests that at its root, efficiency is about control: "its aim was to regulate behavior, natural, human, or machine" (163). For example, historic eugenics movements were motivated by the desire to increase national efficiency.[6] Large-scale factory farming is more efficient, but it has significant environmental and ethical consequences. Factory-style hospitals in high-demand areas try to treat as many people as possible, but it feels like an "assembly line" (Luo 2015, 1059). As the medical profession transitions further away from small, independent practices and towards large corporations who are influenced by large, bureaucratic health insurance companies, there are many consequences for the drive towards greater efficiency. The medical profession is keenly aware of these costs. As even a minimal perusal of medical journals can attest, there are extensive discussions about increasing cost-efficiency without losing quality of care. Eva Luo's article, for example, "Increasing Cost Efficiency in Health Care without Sacrificing the Human Touch" (2015), argues that medical industries need to balance "high-volume" with "high-touch" approaches to achieve healthier lifestyles that will, in the end, reduce costs. Fredrik Svenaeus (2015) similarly contends that though sympathy has been argued to reduce efficiency and increase "compassion fatigue" and burnout, both sympathy and empathy play a vital role in good health care and should be encouraged. As the medical profession continues to evolve, these Great War memoirs remind us that abandoning sympathy to obtain efficiency turns us into machines and sacrifices the very humanity we are trying to save.

Notes

1 Nightingale states in *Subsidiary Notes* that "Women only of the character, efficiency and responsibility of head nurses in other hospitals should be admitted into military ones" (qtd. in McDonald 2011, 22). Carol Helmstadter (2003) explains that efficient nurses did not become a reality until the 1890s.
2 The British Red Cross VAD magazine, *The Red Cross*, began in January of 1914 and continued throughout the war to chronicle local and national events and disseminate policy information.
3 *The Nursing Record* was a weekly periodical published by and for trained nurses that ran from 1888 to 1956.
4 Margery Homersham was a member of the Royal British Nurses' Association, an Associate of the Royal Sanitary Institute, and a Lecturer for the Ladies' Sanitary Association and National Health Society.
5 This concern is present in many literary texts, particularly H.G. Wells' *The Island of Doctor Moreau* (1896). For more information on the development of the medical profession, see *The Western Medical Tradition: 1800–2000* by Bynum *et al.*
6 Rachel Weiss's *Race, Hygiene, and National Efficiency* (1987) is one of many texts to examine the connections between eugenics and national efficiency.

Reference list

"A Call for Women." 1916. *The Times*, 29 July, 9. *The Times Digital Archive 1785–1985*, Gale Cengage Learning. Accessed 15 August 2016.

Alexander, Jennifer Karns. 2008. *The Mantra of Efficiency: From Waterwheel to Social Control*. Baltimore, MD: Johns Hopkins University Press.

Allen, Grant. 1900. *Hilda Wade, a Woman with Tenacity of Purpose*. London: Grant Richards.

Ballance, C.A., Purves Stewart, Charter Symonds, A.E. Garrod and William Thorburn. 1916. "Note on the Work of the V.A.D. Nurses in Malta." *The Red Cross*, June, 72. P.P.2706.kf, British Library.

"Boer War." 2017. *World History: The Modern Era*. ABC-CLIO. Accessed 1 February 2017. worldhistory2.abc-clio.com.

Borden, Mary. 2008. *The Forbidden Zone*. Edited by Hazel Hutchinson. London: Hesperus Press.

Bowser, Thekla. 2003. *The Story of British V.A.D. Work in the Great War*. London: Imperial War Museum. Catalog Number 03/954, Shelf Mark 38(41).23 [Voluntary Aid Detachments]/3. Imperial War Museum, London.

Brittain, Vera. 1978. *Testament of Youth*. Preface by Rt. Hon. Shirley Williams. New York: Penguin Books.

Bynum, W.F., Anne Hardy, Stephen Jacyna, Christopher Lawrence and E.M. Tansey. 2006. *The Western Medical Tradition 1800–2000*. Cambridge: Cambridge University Press.

Cantlie, James. 1912. *British Red Cross Society First-Aid Manual No. 1*. London: Cassel. W.P.1831/1 General Reference Collection, British Library.

Cobley, Evelyn. 2009. *Modernism and the Culture of Efficiency: Ideology and Fiction*. Toronto: University of Toronto Press.

Dannatt, Alice. 1888. "What Constitutes an Efficient Nurse." *The Nursing Record* 1, no. 8 (24 May): 87–90. *Royal College of Nursing*. Accessed 15 August 2016. www2.rcn.org. uk/development/library_and_heritage_services/library_collections/rcn_archive/historical_nursing_journals.

Davis, J.S.C. 1910. "Devonshire Voluntary Aid Organization: A Handbook for Workers." British Red Cross Society, Devonshire Branch, M.A. Rudd & Son. 07306.g.38.(1.), General Reference Collection, British Library.

Gilbert, Sandra M. and Susan Gubar. 1989. *No Man's Land: The Place of the Woman Writer in the Twentieth Century*. Vol. 2. Sexchanges. New Haven, CT: Yale University Press.

Goldman, Dorothy, Jane Gledhill and Judith Hattaway. 1995. *Women Writers and the Great War*. New York: Twayne.

Hall, Radclyffe. 1928. *The Well of Loneliness*. Commentary by Havelock Ellis. Paris: The Pegasus Press.

Hallett, Christine E. 2009. *Containing Trauma: Nursing Work in the First World War*. Manchester: Manchester University Press.

Helmstadter, Carol. 2003. "Building a New Nursing Service: Respectability and Efficiency in Victorian England." *Albion* 35, no. 4 (Winter): 617.

Homersham, Margery. [1888]. *Home Nursing*. London: National Health Society. Box B000001032940, 15192 f.5, Radcliffe Science Library. Oxford University.

Homersham, Margery. [1891]. *Home Nursing*. Second Edition. London: Allman & Son. MIC.A.7793.(5.), General Reference Collection, British Library.

Homersham, Margery. [1897]. *Home Nursing*. Sixth Edition. London: Allman & Son. Box B000001032940, 15192 f.14 (1), Radcliffe Science Library, Oxford University.

Homersham, Margery. [1900]. *Home Nursing*. London: Allman & Son. D-07686.f.2, General Reference Collection, British Library.

Luo, Eva. 2015. "Increasing Cost Efficiency in Health Care without Sacrificing the Human Touch." *AMA Journal of Ethics* 17, no. 11 (November 2015): 1059–63.

McDonald, Lynn. 2011. *Florence Nightingale on Wars and the War Office*. Volume 15 of the series *Collected Works of Florence Nightingale*. Ontario: Wilfrid Laurier UP.

McEwan, Yvonne. 2014. *In the Company of Nurses*. Edinburgh: Edinburgh University Press.

Meade, L.T. 1915. *Nurse Charlotte*. London: John Long. Kroch Library Rare & Manuscripts, Cornell University.

Mollett, Miss. 1888. "Sympathy." *The Nursing Record* 1, no. 16 (19 July): 192–93. *Royal College of Nursing*. Accessed 15 August 2016. www2.rcn.org.uk/development/library_and_heritage_services/library_collections/rcn_archive/historical_nursing_journals.

Moore, Frank Frankfort. 1915. *The Romance of a Red Cross Hospital*. London: Hutchinson. *HathiTrust*, n.d. Accessed 30 June 2016. https://hdl.handle.net/2027/nyp. 33433 112049949.

"*Morning Post* reprint." 1915. *The Red Cross*, April, 74. P.P.2706.kf, General Reference Collection, British Library.

"*Morning Post* reprint." 1915. *The Red Cross*, May, 99. P.P.2706.kf, General Reference Collection, British Library.

Nightingale, Florence. 1858. *Subsidiary Notes as to the Introduction of Female Nursing into Military Hospitals in Peace and War*. London: Harrison.

"Nursing Echoes." 1901. *The Nursing Record*, 26, no. 676 (16 March): 211–12. *Royal College of Nursing*. Accessed 15 August 2016. www2.rcn.org.uk/development/library_and_heritage_services/library_collections/rcn_archive/historical_nursing_journals.

Ouditt, Sharon. 1994. *Fighting Forces, Writing Women: Identity and Ideology in the First World War*. London: Routledge.

Reznick, Jeffrey S. 2004. *Healing the Nation: Soldiers and the Culture of Caregiving in Britain during the Great War*. Manchester: Manchester University Press.

Searle, Geoffrey Russell. 1971. *The Quest for National Efficiency: A Study in British Politics and Political Thought, 1899–1914*. Berkeley: University of California Press.

Smith, Helen Zenna. [1930] 1988. *Not So Quiet ... Stepdaughters of War*. Introduction by Barbara Hardy. London: Virago Press.

Summers, Anne. 1988. *Angels and Citizens: British Women as Military Nurses 1854–1914*. London: Routledge & Kegan Paul.

Svenaeus, Fredrik. 2015. "The Relationship between Empathy and Sympathy in Good Health Care." *Medical Health Care and Philosophy* 18 (2015): 267–77. Accessed 11 September 2016.

"The Army Medical Service and V.A.D. Members." 1915. *The Red Cross*, March, 62. RCB/6/7/3, British Red Cross Archives, London.

"The British Nurses' Association – Bristol." 1889. *The Nursing Record* 2, no. 48 (28 February): 134. *Royal College of Nursing*. Accessed 15 August 2016. www2.rcn.org.uk/development/library_and_heritage_services/library_collections/rcn_archive/historical_nursing_journals.

"The Organization of a V.A.D. Hospital." 1916. *The Red Cross*, November: 143–44. P.P.2706.kf, General Reference Collection, British Library.

"The War to End All Wars (Overview)." 2017. *World History: The Modern Era*, ABC-CLIO. Accessed 1 February 2017. worldhistory2.abc-clio.com/Topics/Display/118627 4?cid=41&sid=1186274.

Thompson, Sir Courtland. 1916. "Dispatch." *The Red Cross*, October, 104. P.P.2706.kf, General Reference Collection, British Library.

"V.A.D.s Required." 1918. *The British Journal of Nursing* (12 January): 27. *Royal College of Nursing*. Accessed 15 August 2016. www2.rcn.org.uk/development/library_and_heritage_services/library_collections/rcn_archive/historical_nursing_journals.

Vicinus, Martha. 1985. *Independent Women 1850–1920: Work and Community for Single Women*. Chicago: University of Chicago Press.

Vivian, E. Charles and J.E. Hodder Williams. 1915. *The Way of the Red Cross*. London: Hodder and Stoughton.

Weiss, Rachel. 1987. *Race, Hygiene and National Efficiency: The Eugenics of Wilhelm Schallmayer*. Berkeley: University of California Press.

Wells, H.G. 1934. "The Island of Dr. Moreau." *Seven Science Fiction Novels of H.G. Wells*, 79–182. New York: Dover Publications, Inc.

8 Negotiating wonders

Medical-triggered redefinitions of humanity in popular fiction

Anna Gasperini

On 16 November 2016, the online edition of the *Independent* (UK) featured an article titled: "DNA-editing breakthrough could fix 'broken genes' in the brain, delay ageing and cure incurable diseases" (Johnston 2016, n.p.). The article explained that the study, which was hailed as a "'holy grail' of genetics," consisted in the successful manipulation of adult DNA cells, which could, with this new technique, be "modif[ied] at will" (Johnston 2016, n.p.). While some of the views expressed in the article suggested the scientific community was cautious about the actual extent of immediate results, the article itself emphasised forcefully one of the new technique's potential outcomes: the extension of human life. One of the scientists interviewed remarked that "improvements in this type of technology … seem inevitable these days" (Johnston 2016, n.p.). The author of the article apparently harboured great faith in this inevitability, and emphatically underlined its potential contribution to the human being's fight against ageing and, ultimately, death. Suspending for a moment any moral and scientific judgement of such endeavour, I want to focus on the perceived "inevitability" of the result in the article. As decay, physical and mental, is one of the traits that defines the human being, it follows that the very concept of "human" is currently undergoing a powerful redefinition.

If we look at history, such momentous changes in the fabric of human experience have always being characterised by a certain tension between the world of science and medicine on the one side, and the general public on the other, two spheres that tend to be perceived and to perceive themselves as distinct, if at times juxtaposed. In this chapter, I will position popular fiction as the unlikely arena for confrontation between the layperson and the medical world. Its episodic, dramatic narratives translate the unintelligible medical language, analyse the mysterious figure of the scientist, and conflate the general public's interest for, and simultaneous fear of, medicine. By focusing on the resonances between nineteenth-century and contemporary fictional representations of scientists attempting to improve humanity, I will address two fundamental questions: how does popular fiction represent the tension of the human-inhuman nature of the medical scientist and their experiments; and how does the survival or discontinuation of particular narrative elements tell us about the way the wider public perceives the medical scientist set on improving human/ity? To answer these questions, I compare the rewriting of the supreme narrative of science and monstrosity, Mary Shelley's *Frankenstein* (1818), in the Victorian popular fiction series *Varney the Vampyre, or: the Feast of Blood* (1845–47) (henceforth *Varney*) and the neo-Victorian horror TV series *Penny Dreadful* (2014–16). While in general a progressive humanisation of both the scientist and the experiment emerges, in these narratives the medical man carries full responsibility for the humanity or inhumanity of its creation. This depends on whether he is willing to perceive it, and himself, as capable of fear, love, and anger. Humanity, in brief, is the direct result of the scientist's acknowledgement, or lack thereof, of feelings in the creature and himself.

Leslie Henderson (2007) explores the capability of popular fiction to embed important medical issues in its narratives for its audience. Her *Social Issues in Television Fiction* focuses on the genre of the soap opera, analysing how news stories and themes were tackled in soap operas' "'safe' viewing space," suggesting that its "unresolved narrative structure" allowed it to propose to its audience "more challenging and critical themes" (Henderson 2007, 6–7). Starting from the idea that "the function of television fiction in contemporary culture" is "culturally charged" (7), Henderson argues in favour of a connection of the two traditionally separated "'public knowledge' project" and "'popular culture' project" areas of media studies, of a merging of news and media with popular television (8). The analysis here developed makes the "cultural charge" of popular fiction its premise and compares how its past and present forms incorporate critical issues related to developments in medical science in their narratives, examining how the representation of the scientist relates to the general public's degree of proximity to the medical world. The layperson's ignorance of the technical aspects of medicine makes the doctor appear inhuman, a detached being bent upon toying with humanity, life and mortality; through fictional elaboration, he becomes knowable, because he becomes human.

Since the nineteenth century, science has been progressing at an unprecedented pace, life expectancy has risen, fatal diseases have been successfully treated, and yet, the relationship between the medical world and the general public remains characterised by a lack of trust. The extraordinary medical developments of the nineteenth century were accompanied by a shift in the power relationship between patients and doctors, who underwent a loss of humanity in one another's eyes. In *The Birth of the Clinic* (1963), Foucault notes the "suzerainty of the gaze" that came to characterise nineteenth-century medicine (2003, 2), the "silent and gestureless [*sic*]" gaze that made the doctor a figure that observed and scrutinised the human form (131), while simultaneously excluding the rest of society. To prevent any impairment of their clinical gaze, surgeons strived to detach themselves from their patients, thus dehumanising them; in turn, patients perceived this detachment as lack of humanity – therefore dehumanising the medical man. The ascent of medicine as a discipline, with subsequent closure of its ranks and specialisation of its language, enveloped the medical world in a shroud of foreignness that widened the chasm between doctors and laypeople. Their language was unintelligible. Their practice included such unsavoury aspects as dissection and vivisection, while surgery was considered akin to butchery for a substantial part of the nineteenth century. However, traces of the troubled relationship of the surgeon and the human body have resurfaced leading into the twenty-first century, particularly when medical science intervenes in areas strictly related to the concepts of human life and death (Mulkay 1996, 1).

Inhuman medicine and dehumanised patients: history and fiction

Since the early nineteenth century, popular fiction has engaged with the dehumanised and dehumanising aspects of medicine. While traditionally sensation fiction, which developed during the second half of the nineteenth century with Wilkie Collins as its foremost figure, is the most renowned for discussing issues of medicine and morality, I contend that this practice began at least 20 years before Collins, specifically with the rise of that allegedly unsavoury chapter in the history of Victorian fiction: the penny bloods. An earlier form of the infamous penny dreadfuls, the bloods were cheap serialised fiction for the working class that developed between the 1830s and the 1860s, and were sold at the diminutive price of 1 penny per issue. Characterised by gory plots and sensational woodcut illustrations, they were not bound to the moral and aesthetic restraints that characterised genres that were more socially acceptable; therefore, they could tackle medicine's disquieting traits, including the unsettling change in the patient-doctor relationship examined by Foucault, which drastically impacted the readership of the penny bloods from the onset. Shortly after the passing of the 1832 Anatomy Act, which destined the bodies of the poorest among the poor, those unable to pay for their own funeral, to become dissection material to train medical students in human anatomy, representations of dehumanised patients and "inhuman" medical men started appearing in the emerging genre of the penny bloods. In the 1840s, in one of the most sensational episodes of the enormously successful serial *Varney*, a medical student bribes London's common hangman to obtain the body of a hanged felon for his galvanism experiment. In the 2010s, when developments in medicine are once more redefining the idea of diseased body and are focusing on prolonging human life, popular fiction is again showing a marked interest in medical men experimenting with dead bodies, one of the latest examples being *Penny Dreadful. Varney* and *Penny Dreadful* share several traits, among which the rewriting of two iconic figures of anxiety about experimental medicine: Dr Victor Frankenstein and his Creature.

In Shelley's novel *Frankenstein – or, The Modern Prometheus* (1818) a surgeon attempts to create the "perfect" body, unleashing a monster on humanity. *Varney* and *Penny Dreadful* rewrite the Frankenstein figure, interlacing the concept of "medically improving humanity" with anxiety about the potential "inhumanity" of both the product and the medical scientist: one can be simultaneously superior being *and* monster, the other portentous healer *and* madman. Such persistence in rewriting the Frankenstein figure over two centuries suggests that popular fiction continues to rewrite and readapt tropes stemming from the nineteenth-century patient-doctor divide to confront momentous readjustments in the fabric of the human experience.

My choice of *Varney* among the hulking corpus of penny-blood fiction is based on its long-lasting fame and success. Penned, most likely, by the prolific and elusive James Malcolm Rymer,[1] this series was issued weekly over two years, and was later reprinted in volume form. Within the world of cheap serialised fiction, where selling figures were paramount and unsuccessful series were unceremoniously ended, such features attest to *Varney*'s success among its intended readership and beyond: the 2008 Zittaw Press reprint of Rymer's mammoth series, edited by Curtis Herr, made it to non-academic bookshops' shelves, thanks to the recent vampire literature revival. Even more recently, *Varney* surfaced again in *Penny Dreadful*. The series, directed by John Logan, consciously adapts and revivifies the penny blood/dreadful genre, from the gory, swashbuckling and graphic plot to the cliff-hangers that characterise episode and season endings. Featuring vampires, werewolves, demonic possession and witchcraft, the series includes characters from gothic literature that made it to the general canon, such as Dracula, but it also recurrently refers to penny dreadful literature, especially to *Varney*. This connection makes these two popular narratives particularly well-suited for a comparison of their two Frankenstein figures, *Varney*'s Dr Chillingworth and *Penny Dreadful*'s Victor Frankenstein.

Michael Mulkay analyses the use of the Frankenstein figure in public and political debate on embryo research in the UK in the 1990s, suggesting that laypeople resort to "narrative structure[s] that [are] already available" to fill in the gaps in their knowledge of a subject, particularly a disturbing one (Mulkay 1996, 158). He contends that "when the practical consequences of some widely discussed scientific innovation are as yet unclear," the "mad scientist" narrative will resurface in public debate to support anti-scientific arguments (159). This chapter intervenes in this argument by observing how the mad scientist narrative itself works and develops. I would also venture that the Frankenstein narrative is used not merely as a "homil[y] on the evil of science," as argued by Christopher Toumey in his scathing critique of the genre (Toumey 1992, 411), but as a tool to bring the figure of the scientist and its experiments closer to the layperson for examination. When the layperson can explore the figure of the medical scientist against the background of the extremely human experience of failure – failure to achieve his grand goal, failure to control his own creation – the tension between the concepts of humanity and inhumanity applied to medical-scientific developments can ease, and subsequently be faced by the general public. Lacking the knowledge to understand the technical aspects of medicine, laypeople (re)create a narrative that allows them to perceive the alien figure of the medical scientist as human.

Dr Victor Frankenstein, the fictional character that came to be identified with distrust in medical experimentation, was himself the product of a moment of change in medical science: in the story, the young doctor assembles his Creature using parts of fresh bodies stolen from cemeteries, a meaningful detail for audiences at the time. In the early nineteenth century, the number of medical students had been steadily increasing since the Company of Surgeons had become independent from that of Barbers in 1745 (Hurren 2012). According to a 1742 Act of Parliament, teachers and pupils were allowed to perfect their surgical skills and knowledge of human anatomy on the bodies of hanged murderers (Richardson 1987). The number of bodies obtained through this channel, though, was insufficient, which led to the practice of stealing fresh bodies from graves and the rise of the professional bodysnatcher, or resurrection man. Despised by the wider community and barely tolerated by the medical fraternity, bodysnatchers had as their prime target the bodies of the poor, which rested in fragile coffins laid in shallower graves than those of wealthier people. For the poor, then, the dread of death included also the dread of dissection, which represented the impossibility of resurrecting in body and soul on Doomsday. The medical fraternity's disregard for this dread implied that, both in life and in death, the pauper was somewhat less human than other members of society.

Political action sanctioned the condition of the pauper before medicine as a "lesser human" early in the century: in the 1820s, the Benthamites, a progressive political group led by the philosopher Jeremy Bentham, backed the medical fraternity in Parliament, suggesting solving the problem of shortage of bodies by making the pauper who died in workhouses and hospitals a legal supply of teaching material for anatomists. The debate unfolded for about a decade, until on two separate occasions the remunerative anatomy sale business led to serial killings. Burke and Hare, two Irishmen who posed as resurrectionists but were in fact serial murderers, killed between 14 and 16 people in Edinburgh between 1828 and 1829 to sell them to Dr Robert Knox; in 1831, occasional resurrectionists Bishop and Williams were tried in London for the murder of three victims (the ascertained ones). Three of the murderers were sentenced to death by hanging and dissection.[2] The Burkers cases (from Burke's name, as he allegedly invented the practice of killing to sell the body to an anatomist) were exploited by the Benthamites in Parliament, particularly the London case: in 1832, the Anatomy Act was voted in.

Dehumanisation also characterised anatomy training proper, and worked in both directions, affecting both the corpse and the living medical student. To overcome any religious or superstitious fear of the dead while performing dissections, medical students learned to detach themselves from their feelings, beginning with disconnecting from the body on the dissection slab: what they were cutting was not a person, but a "subject," a status that deprived the dead of humanity in the eyes of the surgeon-in-training (Rosner 2010, 155). Pranks and jokes on (and sometimes using parts of) their subjects were also part of the process of becoming a skilful surgeon (Rosner 2010; Wise 2004). This detachment, however, particularly when it manifested itself with disrespect for the dead, exacerbated the general public's relationship with the medical fraternity. The working class's subjected position in this relationship constituted a particularly delicate point: the poor were dependent on charity treatment, which meant that their bodies functioned as training material for students, even in death, due to bodysnatching. Richardson notes that when the pauper sought "hospital treatment at all [it was] a measure of the desperation generated by serious illness or injury. To many, to enter the hospital was synonymous with death" (1987, 44). She connects this to the fact that "much of the therapeutics, as well as the surgery, practised upon the poor was known to be experimental" (44), and she uses the example of the pauper Stephen Pollard, who died of a simple lithotomy operation performed by a sadly incompetent surgeon, who, upon extracting Pollard's stone, was more interested in showing it to the students, rather than taking care of the patient. The paupers' anxiety about the impact of medicine on their bodies extended to death: Hurren illustrates the pauper's practice of "chalking" the dead relative's name on the coffin lid to make sure it was really interred (2012, 10). She also cites cases of corpses being detained by the family, notwithstanding the discomfort and health hazard, either to gain some time to collect the money for a proper funeral, or out of sheer despair arising from the awareness of being unable to afford one. Thus, the idea that patients undergoing charitable treatment might actually be subjected to "experimentation and prurient interest" on the part of medical students became a serious public concern (Hurren 2012, 83), and anatomy training contributed to this impression. After all, William Hunter himself, one of the most influential figures of British medical history, stated that the discipline's purpose was that of "familiariz[ing] the heart to a kind of necessary inhumanity" (Hunter 1784, 67).

Arrogance and madness: Varney's unsupervised scientist

Frankenstein pre-dates the Anatomy Act by fourteen years, yet the young doctor's obsession with revivifying dead matter and bodysnatching practices reflects the concern that was taking shape in the mind of the early nineteenth-century British public about the medical fraternity. If they thought nothing of hacking a corpse into pieces, if they really did perceive themselves above the moral code of the rest of the community, as their relationship with bodysnatchers and, in some cases, with burkers suggested, what would happen if they decided to undertake unsupervised experiments? *Frankenstein* enacts on the page the worst-case scenario – that is, a medical student who undertakes the taboo endeavour, the reversion of death. Traditionally, hubris is a core theme in readings of *Frankenstein*: the subtitle of the novel itself, "the Modern Prometheus," suggests as much. Victor would be god, create a new species of fair, invincible humans and be regarded as their father; as soon as his Creature comes alive, though, he flies before its horrific features. His flight makes abandonment and rejection the Creature's very first experience, catalysing the dramatic development of the novel. The Creature is indeed hideous, his nature as revivified corpse apparent; yet, it is obvious that initially he has the potential to be either good or bad. His first actions tend to goodness, but repeated rejection and the absence of the creator that should have taken care of him finally turn him vengeful. He manages to track Frankenstein, demands from him a female companion, and threatens to destroy him if he will refuse. Terrified at the thought that the two creatures might procreate, starting a new species that would ultimately overcome humanity, Frankenstein destroys the female. The Creature then kills Frankenstein's bride, and the two begin a chase that will end with Frankenstein's death.

Chris Baldick (1987) notes how nineteenth-century popular culture quickly "assimilated and accepted" the Frankenstein story "as the contemporary form of the Faust myth," simultaneously "experimenting" with it, reworking and readapting its plot for a variety of contexts (142). It is therefore unsurprising to find a version of the Frankenstein figure in a penny blood such as *Varney*. *Varney* is a perfect representative of its genre: its plot is a stream of highly sensational events that, gory chapter after gory chapter, relate the adventures of the vampire baronet. In two years of publication, the readers see Varney resurrecting repeatedly; the most sensational instance, though, is when he is galvanised back to life by the Frankenstein-like Dr Chillingworth.

Although the peak of medical men's appearance in literature would come a bit further into the century (Sparks 2009), doctors were becoming fashionable characters in narrative, and Chillingworth is an early example of this phenomenon. *Varney* opens with the story of the Bannerworths, a formerly rich family of good breeding and kind disposition; the fair Flora Bannerworth is viciously attacked by the vampire in the very first instalment, and it is later discovered that Sir Francis Varney, the vampire, who has recently moved to the neighbourhood posing as a human being, plans to drive the family out of their mansion to search for the late Marmaduke Bannerworth's treasure. Marmaduke, Flora's father, had been Varney's accomplice in his days as a highwayman, but had escaped with their loot, leaving Varney to be tried and hanged. Coincidentally, this happened when Dr Chillingworth, then a mature medical student, was learning his trade in London.

The doctor, now a countryside practitioner, is compelled to reveal his ties with Varney to the Bannerworths, who are both family friends and patients to him. The doctor explains that, as a student, "there was nothing connected with [his studies] which [he] did not try to accomplish" (*Varney* 1: 327), and his greatest ambition was to bring a dead person back to life through galvanism. Of course, he mentions the issue of scarcity of dissection material, explaining that "all sorts of schemes had to be put into requisition to accomplish so desirable and, indeed, absolutely necessary a purpose," meaning dissection (327–28). In his case, this meant bribing London's common hangman to obtain the body of a hanged felon to use for his experiment, with the assurance that the hangman will "let him down gently, so that he shall die of suffocation, instead of having his neck put out of joint," which would prevent the success of the experiment (328). In the footnotes to this chapter in the Zittaw edition, Herr notes that this additional cruelty casts doubts on the doctor's professional integrity (310) – a medical man is supposed to relieve people from suffering, rather than inflicting further pain on them – and soon the narrative questions the doctor's mental balance as well. He describes his mental state as "inflamed" and "mania[cal]" (328) at the thought of his experiment. And yet, when the hangman asks him whether he has thought about what to do with the dead man, once he has come alive, Chillingworth simply replies: "Not I" (330). His only thought, he states, was "the success or the non-success, in a physiological point of view, of [his] plan for restoring the dead to life" (330). The hangman's attempt to reframe the corpse as human, as some*one* in need of Chillingworth's care, is resisted by the doctor. His answer is the supreme expression of clinical detachment, it denies both the subject's and the surgeon's humanity, aligning Chillingworth with the general public's perception of the effects of clinical detachment on medical students, and therefore medical practitioners.

The figure of the medical scientist in *Varney*, though certainly not as magisterially penned as in Shelley's novel, includes all the key elements of the Frankenstein figure: professional and personal arrogance, borderline pathological single-mindedness, and the perception of the dead body as an object of experimentation. While Shelley's Victor Frankenstein intended to be a guide for his new Creature and be regarded as its Creator, Chillingworth only seeks professional recognition. The new, or renewed, life that will result from his experiments is irrelevant. This shift in the representation of the scientist's work from ill-guided good intent to unfeeling professional arrogance bespeaks three decades of debate around the controversial ethics of anatomy studies, marked by the passing of the Anatomy Act. *Varney*, as literature for the pauper, responded to what was perceived as gross disregard for the pauper's feelings with an appropriately unfeeling – inhuman – fictional doctor.

To Chillingworth's already rather unkind portrait, *Varney* adds a morbid detail, hinting that the former medical student might have entertained necrophilic thoughts about the corpse, as Chillingworth compares his impatience in waiting for the "dead body" to that of a lover waiting "for the arrival of the chosen object of his heart" (*Varney* 1: 329). As soon as the hangman arrives, he runs down the stairs "to meet what ninety-nine men out of a hundred would have gone some distance to avoid the sight of, namely, a corpse livid and fresh from the gallows" (330). The narrative endeavours to single out the doctor's behaviour as peculiarly inhuman, highlighting his departure from the human instinct to recoil from death and decay. The tension between the doctor's lack of feelings about the living man, made explicit by his reply, "Not I," and his attraction for the dead body, the object of experimentation, sets him apart as an alien being. His attitude announces the consequences of his experiment: whatever feelings he might have entertained for the corpse, and however strong his obsession for his experiment, the moment in which Varney comes back to life with a scream Chillingworth follows the pattern traced by Shelley's Frankenstein: he runs away from the man he has just revivified, abandoning him.

It is unclear if Varney's vampiric nature influenced Chillingworth's experiment, or if he would have been revivified anyway, eventually; still, it is obvious that the galvanic experiment resuscitates him. Unlike Shelley's Creature, Varney is (re)born in a state of vengefulness: the first words he shouts in Chillingworth's terrified face are "Death, death, where is the treasure?" (330) Chillingworth, true to his word, does not feel the least commitment to the resuscitated man, not even when he appears to be dangerous. By openly declining any responsibility towards the being that his experiment brought into the world, he unleashes a vengeful fiend on his friends and patients, and on himself. Chillingworth's arrogance and levity bespeak the anxiety of the mid-to-lower social strata about a selfish medicine concentrated solely on the experiment, uninterested in the actual human they are trying to cure, or to improve. This detachment is perceived as unnatural, and therefore its results must be likewise unnatural. Merging and sensationalising in Chillingworth the traits that problematised the image of the medical man in the eyes of the general public – detachment and contact with dead bodies – *Varney* enacted for its readers the terror evoked by the idea of a scientist free from any moral restraint or supervision from the authorities.

Coping with trauma: *Penny Dreadful*'s Frankenstein

Penny Dreadful's twenty-first-century rewriting of Victor Frankenstein necessarily differs from that of the nineteenth-century *Varney*. The doctor is still a brilliant mind, ahead of his times. He shows remarkable clinical detachment and, like Chillingworth, he performs galvanic experiments on corpses. However, he represents a departure from the traditional Frankenstein figure, as his dominant trait is not hubris, but fragility, which entails an audience inclined to think that such extreme experiments must be rooted in something deeper than a mere wish for glory.

While perceiving himself above common people, the young doctor shows signs of social awkwardness and, although professional arrogance is still a prominent trait of his character, the story justifies his attempts to restore the dead to life, not with mere thirst for knowledge and professional ambition, but with trauma. Flashbacks show Victor as a pensive, sensitive child strongly attached to a mother who dies of tuberculosis very early in his life, an event that the narrative connects with Victor's obsession for revivifying the dead. Like Shelley's Frankenstein and Chillingworth before him, he builds a creature whose traumatic and terrible birth is a grotesque reflection of an actual birth: in episode 3, Caliban[3] (a name that the creature receives later in the story) describes his as "a difficult birth" (00:07:50). Covered in blood, completely bald, screaming wordlessly, he is "born in sheer, terrified agony" (00:07:52–00:07:55). According to tradition, Caliban's birth horrifies the young scientist, who flies, triggering Caliban's feelings of abandonment and revenge. He is not, however, the only result of Frankenstein's endeavours.

While *Varney*, closer to Shelley's work in this respect, suggests that the vampire's rebirth gives Chillingworth a shake sufficient to cure him from his obsession for revivifying the dead, *Penny Dreadful*'s Frankenstein engages in a series of trials and errors. Caliban's birth, though horrible, seems to prompt Victor to improve his technique, and indeed his following experiments are far more successful. The appearance of increasingly rewarding multiple attempts in the traditional Frankenstein narrative denotes a cultural change in the perception of the failed attempt: having such a strong motive as trauma, as opposed to the professional arrogance of his Victorian antecedents, allows twenty-first-century

Frankenstein to overcome the experience of failure and build upon it. When his secret laboratory first appears, the audience immediately recognises the experiment: a corpse criss-crossed with stitches, an operating table and electrical paraphernalia. Yet, when the Creature comes alive, his aspect is not too terrifying: the stitches can be easily concealed under clothes that Frankenstein promptly provides, and his true nature only shows in the eyes, which are a startling tone of yellow, a reminder of Shelley's Creature's yellow eyes. He is quite docile, he chooses for himself the name Proteus, and the doctor appears to be very caring. The explanation for this departure from the typical Frankenstein's plot is offered when Caliban sensationally steps onto the scene, destroying Proteus: the audience has witnessed not the first, but the second experiment, the fruit of an improved technique. Following the original *Frankenstein* plot, Caliban demands a bride from Frankenstein. The result of this third experiment, Lily, is virtually perfect: the stitches are even less showing than Proteus's, and her bright yellow eyes are the only uncanny detail in an otherwise perfectly lifelike Creature. In yet another departure from the original story, the female creature lives. Soon enough, however, *Penny Dreadful*'s Frankenstein, like *Varney*'s Chillingworth, develops feelings for the object of his experiments, the revivified corpse Lily. His attachment to the un-dead female Creature again appears to be connected to his child trauma: to separate Lily from her previous identity as the prostitute Brona, he dyes her red hair blonde, like his mother's. In the end, though, Lily refuses to be a bride, either to Caliban or to Frankenstein. It is then that Frankenstein attempts to destroy her, only to discover that he has indeed created the perfect Creature, as Lily cannot be killed with common weapons, and she spitefully rejects him both as creator and as man. It is in this moment that the roles of the characters with respect to in/humanity emerge vividly: Lily, the supposedly improved human, displays non-human features. Conversely, Frankenstein, the supposedly detached scientist, is unable to resist, or properly express, his feelings of love, longing and rejection, and appears at his most human when confronted with the inhumanity of his own Creature.

By looking at how *Varney* and *Penny Dreadful* rewrite the Frankenstein figure, it emerges that both attempt to bring the figure of the doctor closer to their audience, though in different ways. In *Varney*, the secretive, aloof Victorian scientist, revered for his knowledge and dreaded for his godless practices, is brought down to the level of common human beings through that intrinsically human experience that is failure. Failure characterises the original scientist of Shelley's novel, and the fact that a popular fiction narrative continued this trait in its rewriting of the classic story suggests that it would be meaningful for its audience. Besides the sensational component in the image of the mad scientist, which suited the penny blood genre, I would venture that to *Varney*'s working-class readership, whose position in the health care system was that of charity-dependent patients and therefore study material, the figure of Dr Chillingworth represented a double catharsis. On the one hand, he performed the much-feared unsupervised experiments with the amoral attitude that was perceived to be a direct consequence of the training in clinical detachment medical students received. On the other hand, one wrong experiment is sufficient to awaken his dormant moral scruples and make him refrain from carrying on his plans any further. He is reformed and becomes aware of his own madness. Chillingworth describes his former self as a madman, implying that he acknowledges that his ideas were wrong. The "mad scientist" Chillingworth was certainly, to an extent, in Mulkay's words, part of an "anti-science fiction" story that the British public was adopting to cope with the "yet unclear" "practical consequences" (Mulkay 1996, 159) of the Anatomy Act. However, I would argue that the narrative makes a point of showing Chillingworth-before versus Chillingworth-after the experiment, and the second one is characterised by failure and shame for his past actions, two experiences with which the readership of *Varney* could identify. Chillingworth, therefore, was not simply a manifestation of the tension between medical science and the general public: he allowed the readers to face anxieties about a distant and disquieting medical community, while simultaneously reassuringly suggesting that scientists, like all humans, are affected by experiences such as failure and shame.

   Penny Dreadful takes a more sympathetic approach towards the humanisation of the mad scientist: instead of being a vague, general "madness" stemming from professional arrogance and amoral practices, the twenty-first-century Frankenstein is characterised by an identifiable psychological issue rooted in childhood trauma. While his behaviour towards both Caliban and Lily is not beyond reproach, by linking his obsession for revivifying the dead to trauma, the cold and proud Frankenstein becomes a human being with whom the audience can sympathise and whose motives they can understand. I would suggest that *Penny Dreadful*'s Frankenstein, in a way, embodies an attempt to understand the desire of our own age for defeating death: the scientist is not engaged in a war against death as a philosophical concept, but rather in the process of defeating a personal experience of disease and mortality, of improving what he perceives to be the malfunctioning of a mechanical process. While *Varney* openly criticised the attitude of the men of science in approaching death and the dead body – especially the "unclaimed" body, where "unclaimed" was the condition that made a body fit for the dissection slab – *Penny Dreadful* is more lenient towards the scientist while simultaneously questioning his scientific endeavours. *Penny Dreadful*'s Frankenstein's experiments are all successful, and yet, they present fatal drawbacks: none of his Creatures can lead a normal life and the two who survive are extremely dangerous. Perhaps, being allowed to continue his experiments, Frankenstein would finally achieve his goal, but the series seems to question whether the collateral damage would be worth the achievement.

Facing man-made inhumanity: the Creatures

The Creatures themselves in these texts embody the contradictory nature of science in the anxious gaze of the layperson: planned to be wonders, the proof that man can defeat death, they turn out to be monsters. The main component of their monstrosity is their failing to meet the scientist's expectations in some respect. Shelley's Frankenstein clearly states that in his intention the Creature should have been beautiful (39); yet, when it comes to life Frankenstein flies before its repulsive aspect and, though the Creature shows no sign of being a threat, its ugliness causes constant rejection along the narrative. Therefore, the Creature grows bitter and finally vengeful. The Creatures in *Varney* and *Penny Dreadful* share some features with Shelley's Creature: they are all superhumanly strong, and almost all of them are characterised by malevolence and anger, either intrinsic, as in Varney's case, or developed, like Caliban and Lily. This distinctive trait can be directly linked to the attitude of the scientist-creator, who either abandons the Creature or attempts to subject it, threatening its individuality. The only incognitant is Proteus: in his brief second life, he appears to be meek and driven by gentle impulses. His contact with Frankenstein is so short and the doctor's behaviour so caring, that malevolence never emerges. However, we do not know what he might have become, had he lived; Caliban is certain that the world would have changed Proteus, as he tells a horrified Frankenstein: "Aborting your child before it could know pain? It is a mercy!" (00:11:59–00:12:03). This remark implies that there is no place for meekness among manmade Creatures: be they physically repulsive or not, they are subjected to either rejection or enslavement, and only a truly hardened Creature could survive. Lily confirms this trend: while she initially appears to be docile and hapless, she later reveals herself to be a cold murderer.

Unlike Shelley's Creature, both the vampire and *Penny Dreadful*'s Creatures are endowed with some form of charm: Varney can "fascinat[e] when he lik[es]" (*Varney* 2: 792); Lily is beautiful; Proteus is full of childlike gentleness; even Caliban, the one that is physically most like Shelley's Creature, has an endearing love for poetry, so much in fact that he chooses the name of the poet John Clare as his alias. Charm both humanises and underlines the inhuman traits of the revivified corpses, highlighting the tension between their wish to be human, and their inability or unwillingness to accept the moral code of the human community in which they act. Actually, the driving force of the revivified bodies from both the Victorian and Neo-Victorian popular narrative is revenge. Varney wants revenge from the family of the man who betrayed him and left him for dead, his coming back for the treasure being a literal representation of the vengeful dead come back to claim a stolen property. Caliban wants revenge for the suffering and loneliness he experienced and that he blames on his "Creator," as he makes a point to call Victor, and Lily wants revenge over men, who exploited her as Brona and would exploit her again in her new life.

Anger, monstrosity, and humanity are tightly interconnected in Varney, Caliban and Lily. Before Varney awakens, crying in rage for his treasure, the hangman asks, "Doctor, have you duly considered what you mean to do with this fellow, in case you should be successful in restoring him to life," and when Chillingworth replies in the negative, he observes: "you can do as you like; but I consider that it is really worth thinking of" (*Varney* 1: 330). The implicit statement is that, while the doctor answers to no one and can do "as he likes," he is not considering that a successful experiment would make him responsible for a living human. While the hangman highlights the humanity of the resurrected body, Chillingworth reacts with in-human coolness: he is only interested in the "success or the non-success" of his experiment (330). This contrast between Varney's humanity and Chillingworth's inhumanity can be better understood within the context of the original penny blood: *Varney's* readership would have readily identified with the unclaimed felon subjected to medical experiments. I would venture that the vampire's subsequent resurrection in a state of rage, therefore, would have functioned partly as a sensational element, but also partly as a just punishment befalling the arrogant scientist: his refusal to consider Varney's humanity is rewarded with the awakening, not of a human, but of a vengeful monster.

Caliban and Lily, given their genre, are far more complex characters than the Victorian vampire baronet, yet the same connection exists between their anger and vengefulness, and their human traits. While he is murderous, the audience can sympathise with Caliban's profound loneliness and need to belong somewhere and to someone. As for Lily, it is unclear if she is simply duplicitous, or if her gradual recollection of her previous life triggers in her cruelty and serial killing; still, the link between men's tendency to use her body as an object to bed and/or wed, and her spite for mankind is very clear. The negation of her right to be her own woman, her own person, is at the basis of her homicidal rage, a very human response that the audience can understand, if not condone. Although not as outspoken as Chillingworth, *Penny Dreadful's* Frankenstein also fails to understand his Creature's humanity. Like his eponym from Shelley's novel, he cannot overcome the horror that Caliban's birth inspires in him, and he leaves him to die. While he certainly makes progress in this point with his following experiments, he does so only to a point: he ultimately fails to see Lily as an individual, as she is first the means to get rid of Caliban and then a potential partner. Thus, the Creatures that should attest for the supremacy of science fail to do so because their humanity, their individuality, is denied by their very same aspiring Creators.

By comparing the two popular narratives examined, it emerges that the rewriting of the Frankenstein trope taps into a very specific anxiety: what if the scientist's attempt at improving humanity are fundamentally devoid of humanity? As samples of horror fiction, both rewritings here examined envisage the worst-case scenario: the scientist is basically irresponsible, his attempt to improve human beings is basically inhuman, and disaster is the outcome. However, it is possible to notice a development of the concept of humanity related to the experiment in the two narratives: written in a context in which improvements of the human body were still at a very experimental stage, the Victorian series conveys the concept of humanity and lack thereof through the corpse. The medical practices, and later the laws that impacted on the bodies of the (destitute) patient, dehumanised the individual both in life and in death, and were perceived as inhuman. Consequently, to be under observation is the medical scientist's attitude towards the corpse, his in/ability to see it as more than experiment material. The contemporary series, instead, envisages an experimental medicine that could succeed repeatedly in its goals. With the advancements in gene manipulation, embryo research and creation of artificial living tissues, the ethical problem raised by the Frankenstein figure includes the possibility that the work of the medical scientist could produce multiple living creatures, characterised by different degrees of success respect to the experiment's goals, and that the scientist himself will need to learn to interact with the result of his experiments.

We could therefore conclude that, as Henderson suggests in relation to soap operas, the Frankenstein trope is used by both series to bring to the audience's attention a sensitive social topic, the ethical debate around the human body in science. The way each series performs this operation reflects the state of medical development and the circulation of knowledge around medical experimentation of the respective historical moment, as well as the degree and complexity of the moral component attached to medical experimentation by the intended public. The Victorian narrative addressed an audience that occupied a position of subjection with respect to medicine, and therefore represents the medical man's attempt at improving humanity as fundamentally wrong, both in its premises and in its results. The contemporary narrative instead, being intended for an audience of mixed cultural levels but with a generally higher degree of instruction and not systematically subjected to medical study, goes beyond the clear-cut condemnation of the experiment, exploring the reasons behind it and its impact on the Creatures.

It is also possible to observe a development in the figure of the medical scientist. *Varney*'s representation confirms Foucault's analysis of the patient-doctor relationship as increasingly distant in the nineteenth century, presenting a medical man whose disconnection from the dread of the dead affected his compassion and kindness, and whose obsession with the "physiology" (330) of the human body makes his experiments unethical. A blind pursuer of professional recognition, the early Victorian medical scientist is portrayed as unable to see beyond the length of his dissection scalpel. *Penny Dreadful*, on the other hand, presents Frankenstein's experiments as rooted in the supremely human experiences of bereavement and anxiety about incurable disease. Showing the human side of the medical scientist, the narrative tries to operate an inversion of the Foucauldian dehumanisation process: the "suzerainty" of the gaze that Foucault identified as a specific attribute of the Victorian clinician (2003, 2) is appropriated by the spectator, who observes, "silent and gestureless" (131), an emotionally distraught medical scientist. While most of the contemporary audience probably lacks specific medical knowledge, which in Foucault was the barrier between Victorian doctors and the general public, they might be able to reconnect to the universal experience of death and disease. The "mad scientist" narrative, therefore, does indeed fill the gaps in the audience's knowledge of medical experimentation, as Mulkay suggests, but in this case tries to do so by suggesting that any attempt at improving humanity arises from the painful human experience of disease and death. Frankenstein's methods and actions are still under scrutiny, but his trauma makes him more human. This detail suggests a shift in the representation of the medical man in the popular mind: if the general public can now empathise with this figure, to recognise itself in him, to an extent, then we are accepting that, underneath his detachment, the medical scientist is still human, and that he might produce monsters as well as wonders.

Notes

1 In the world of cheap serialised popular fiction, works were published anonymously and authors were easily replaced if unavailable. Consequently, making any conclusive statement regarding authorship is extremely difficult, and *Varney* itself had been for a long time attributed to Thomas Peckett Prest, one of the most famous penny-blood writers. Recent stylistic studies, however, most notably Helen R. Smith's study *New Lights on Sweeney Todd* (2002), have produced convincing data to argue that J.M. Rymer, and not Prest, is the author of *Varney*.
2 Hare turned King's evidence against Burke to escape death.
3 The obvious Shakespearian reference in Caliban's name ties him to his namesake in *The Tempest*, reverberating not only with the monstrous physicality associated with the name, but also with the wish for vengeance and resentment towards a father figure. This connection also impacts Frankenstein's character: as the magician Prospero fails to be a father to the monstrous Caliban, whom he adopted with a view of ruling upon him, so does Frankenstein fail in his purpose of becoming a Creator. He cannot see any humanity in the deformed Caliban and, like Prospero, all he can achieve is a resentful rejected son.

Reference list

Baldick, Chris. 1987. *In Frankenstein's Shadow – Myth Monstrosity, and Nineteenth-Century Writing*. Oxford: Clarendon Press.
Foucault, Michel. [1963] 2003. *The Birth of the Clinic*. London: Routledge.
Henderson, Leslie. 2007. *Social Issues in Television Fiction*. Edinburgh: Edinburgh University Press.
Hunter, William. 1784. *Two Introductory Lessons Delivered by Dr. William Hunter to His Last Course of Anatomical Lectures, at His Theatre in Windmill Street*. London: J. Johnson.
Hurren, Elizabeth T. 2012. *Dying for Victorian Medicine – English Anatomy and Its Trade in the Dead Poor, C. 1834–1929*. London: Palgrave Macmillan.
Johnston, Ian. 2016. "DNA-Editing Breakthrough Could Fix 'Broken Genes' in the Brain, Delay Ageing and Cure Incurable Diseases." *Independent – UK*. N.p., 14 June 2017. www.independent.co.uk/news/science/gene-editing-breakthrough-fix-broken-genes-delay-ageing-cure-incurable-diseases-a7421596.html.
Logan, John. 2015. *Penny Dreadful*. DVD. Showtime.
Mulkay, Michael. 1996. "Frankenstein and the Debate over Embryo Research." *Science, Technology, & Human Values* 21.2: 157–76.
Richardson, Ruth. 1987. *Death, Dissection and the Destitute*. Chicago and London: University of Chicago Press.
Rosner, Lisa. 2010. *The Anatomy Murders*. Philadelphia: University of Pennsylvania Press.
Rymer, James Malcolm. [1845–47] 2008. *Varney the Vampyre; or: The Feast of Blood*. Ed. Curtis Herr. Crestline, CA: Zittaw Press.

Rymer, James Malcolm and Thomas Peckett Prest. [1845–47] 1973. *Varney the Vampyre or The Feast of Blood*. Ed. E.F. Bleiler. New York: Dover.

Shelley, Mary. [1818] 2008. *Frankenstein*. Ed. Marilyn Butler. Oxford: Oxford University Press.

Smith, Helen R. 2002. *New Light on Sweeney Todd, Thomas Peckett Prest, James Malcolm Rymer and Elizabeth Caroline Grey*. London: Jarndyce.

Sparks, Tabitha. 2009. *The Doctor in the Victorian Novel*. Farnham: Ashgate.

Toumey, Christopher P. 1992. "The Moral Character of Mad Scientists: A Cultural Critique of Science." *Science, Technology, & Human Values* 17.4: 411–37.

Wise, Sarah. 2004. *The Italian Boy – Murder and Grave-Robbing in 1830s London*. Pimlico 20. London: Jonathan Cape.

9 The human ideal and the real

Artistic vision and anatomical sight

Corinna Wagner

Early in his tenure as Oxford's first Slade Professor of Fine Art, John Ruskin gave a series of 10 lectures "On the Relation of Natural Science to Art," which were subsequently published in 1872 as *The Eagle's Nest*. Although he described art and science as "parallel studies," these lectures reveal a growing disillusionment with the relationship between disciplines and, as is well known, express a strong antipathy towards evolutionary theory, scientific materialism, and, in particular, anatomy (Ruskin 1872, 101). In the eighth of his lectures, on "The Relation of Art to the Sciences of Organic Form," Ruskin made no bones about his position: anatomy had, much to society's "degradation and misfortune, usurped the place, and taken the name, at once of art and of natural history" – and it is worth noting that by "natural history" Ruskin meant the meticulous but sensitive and at times Romantic study of living things and their environments that characterises his early science writing (Ruskin 1872, 156).[1]

I am concerned here with three points that Ruskin makes consistently in his lectures, about the fraught relationship between art and anatomy.[2] First, Ruskin asserts that artistic vision, the source of the social and cultural power of art, is very different from the type of vision associated with anatomy and the life sciences it gave rise to; second, he argues that the study of anatomy had degraded or weakened the artist's vision; and, third, he claims that as a result of this loss of vision, a troubling uniformity had crept into visual representations of human and animal bodies.

Since at least the Renaissance, anatomy was celebrated as the science that would unveil Nature: it would reveal the previously unseen details of the internal body and make visible the fine discriminations between living things. However, it seemed to Ruskin and other nineteenth-century observers that anatomy was having exactly the opposite effect: it had led to the *obscuring* of categorical differences in science and in art. Anatomy was the foundation of comparative anthropological and evolutionary theories that conflated differences between horse and ape, African and European, human and animal. As we will see, Ruskin argued that anatomy, and the theories it gave rise to, had effectively stripped the cultural skin from living things, atomised them, mixed them indiscriminately, and conflated their genealogies. Along with critics and connoisseurs, even some anatomists complained that the eye of the anatomy-trained artist had become *less* rather than more attuned to the finer points of physical, behavioural, and moral differences between races and species. Like Ruskin, many of them argued that such visual indiscriminateness both reflected and promoted degraded ideas about what it meant to be human.

Indiscriminate representations

There is a particularly provoking passage in Ruskin's lecture on "The Relation to Art of the Sciences of Organic Form." In it, he takes aim at illustrations in natural history books, and in particular at a set of images in the first pages of Étienne Geoffroy Saint-Hilaire and Frédéric Cuvier's multi-volume 1824 *Histoire Naturelle des Manmiferes*:

> You will find the law hold universally that apes, pigs, rats, weasels, foxes and the like, – but especially apes, – are drawn admirably; but not a stag, not a lamb, not a horse, not a lion; the nobler the creature, the more stupidly it is always drawn, not from feebleness of art power, but a far deadlier fault than that – a total want of sympathy with the noble qualities of any creature, and a loathsome delight in their disgusting qualities. And this law is so thoroughly carried out that the great French historian of the mammalia, St. Hilaire, chooses, as his single example of the highest of the race, the most nearly bestial type he can find, human, in the world. Let no girl ever look at the book, nor any youth who is willing to take my word; let those who doubt me, look at the example he has given of womankind.
>
> (Ruskin 1872, 156–57)

For Ruskin, one law links two otherwise separate criticisms, about the muddled representations of animals and about the bestial portrayal of "womankind" (by which he means the images below, in Figures 9.1 and 9.2, of Sarah Baartman, the Khoisan woman brought from South Africa to Europe and exhibited as "the Hottentot Venus" in the early 1800s).

The "law" that universally guides modern artists and natural scientists like Geoffroy is anatomical knowledge. Anatomy links these instances of genealogical intermingling, or the confusion of species and races. Importantly, the passage above comes immediately after a section in which Ruskin criticises anatomical training for artists. A number of things could be said about Ruskin's derogatory statements about Baartman: the tradition of drawing links between African and animal bodies, of objectifying and exhibiting "exceptional" bodies, of prejudicial scientific theories of race, of the racial biases of Western aesthetics. But my focus here is on the anatomical context to his comments – a context that makes sense, for instance, of why he characterises the ape, the species closest to the human, as ignoble, for it was through dissection that Darwin and earlier comparative anatomists had identified skeletal similarities and likenesses between the muscles and organs of various species.

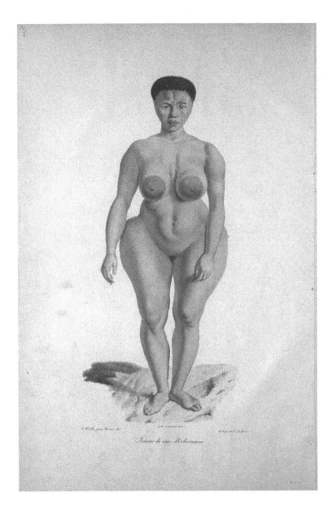

Figure 9.1 Léon de Wailly, "Frontal view," "Femme de race Boschismanne," *Histoire de naturelle mammifieres*, 1824.

As Jonathan Smith observes, Darwinism "enfolded" a taxonomy of separate species "into an evolutionary genealogy," which encompassed wider cultural categories, including aesthetics (Smith 2006, 27). Indeed, Smith's use of the word "enfolding" captures precisely what was at stake for Ruskin: the indiscriminate mixing of categories and the problem of proximity – between species, races, anatomies, morals and values – in the visual arts as much as in anatomy-based sciences. Among others, Jonathan Smith and Rachel Teukolsky have detailed how Darwin's supporters and the popularisers of his theories threatened not only religious and moral structures and "the very basis of Ruskin's aesthetics" (Smith 2006, 27). Even further, evolutionary theories and a sub-field best described as "the sociobiology of aesthetics" – headed by popular writer

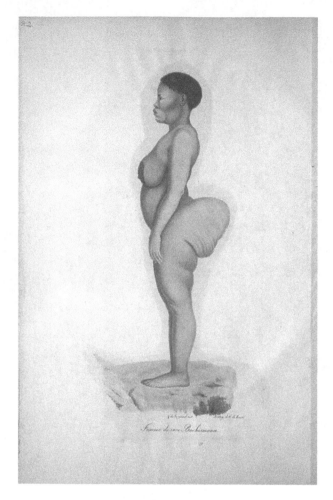

Figure 9.2 Léon de Wailly, "Side view," "Femme de race Boschismanne," *Histoire de naturelle mammifieres*, 1824.

Grant Allen, who applied Darwin's theories to the realm of taste and art production – threatened foundational ideas about what it meant to be human. In Ruskin's view, such applications had, as Teukolsky describes it, "potentially frightening and inhuman connotations" (Teukolsky 2009, 163). Among the frightening connotations that are expressed in the long passage above, it seems to me, is a belief that a loss of specificity or distinctiveness between living things devalued the human and led to moral breakdown.

Ruskin's identification of, and contempt for the wider cultural effects of anatomical knowledge also explains why, looking back from the 1870s to the natural history of the 1820s, he only targets Geoffroy for including the Baartman images in the *Histoire de naturelle mammifieres* (1824). No mention is made of

Geoffroy's co-author Frédéric Cuvier, which is surprising as it was his older and more famous brother Georges Cuvier who had not only dissected Baartman's body and classified her race as nearest the apes, but had also solely authored the chapter in the *Histoire* that included the Baartman images. Ruskin likely singled out Geoffroy because of his theory, anticipating Darwin, of a "unity of plan" that posited anatomical similarities between living things. In the famous 1830 scientific debates, Geoffroy opposed the more politically, religiously and scientifically conservative Georges Cuvier's firmly functionalist view of life, which emphasised the distinctiveness of each animal's anatomy. Following instead the transcendentalist approach of German comparative anatomists who identified structural similarities between different parts of the *same* animal, Geoffroy went a step further by identifying structural similarities between *different* animals. So, for example, the leg bones – femur, tibia, tarsals – of lizards and men may have adapted to different environmental stimuli, but they were essentially homologous in form (Appel, 1987; Desmond, 1989).

These structural resemblances indicate descent from a common evolutionary ancestor, suggesting what Adrian Desmond describes as "a serial stacking of organisms, all reducible to a common composition" (Desmond 1989, 59). This reduction or conflation of species – and the anxieties it inspired – are illustrated plainly by J.J. Grandville's 1842 caricature of an ape-like Geoffroy, which bears more than passing resemblance to later lampoons of Darwin (Figures 9.3 and 9.4). As these popular images illustrate, Geoffroyans, Lamarckians, and Darwinists may have produced a wide array of work, but their evolutionist models inspired very similar anxieties. There was opposition to their image of an autonomous, determining nature, to which humanity and its values were subordinate.

Realism and the abstract ideal

Art historian Charles Cramer observes that the Cuvier-Geoffroy debate "exactly parallels" key artistic struggles that went on within and outside the Royal Academy for some decades (Cramer 2006, 111). Cuvier's emphasis on ordered, distinctive taxonomies in the animal kingdom translated into an artistic emphasis on particularisation and verisimilitude. With his distaste for brush techniques that obscured the differences between species, or which made it impossible to tell if an animal in the foreground was "a pony or a pig," Ruskin was allied with Cuvier (Ruskin [1843] 1903, 3:35). In the century before this, the classical idealism of the Royal Academy's first president, Sir Joshua Reynolds (from 1768–92) was aligned with Geoffroy's transcendentalist unity of plan. I want to be cautious about oversimplifying what were often overlapping and/or changeable positions (Ruskin was notoriously inconsistent and Reynolds could be contradictory).[3] Moreover, there are many points of agreement between the two men; for instance, like Reynolds, Ruskin advocated art that encouraged viewers to aim for ideals, though not via the classical universalised forms of Reynolds' grand style. With these caveats in mind, Cramer's alignments helpfully draw

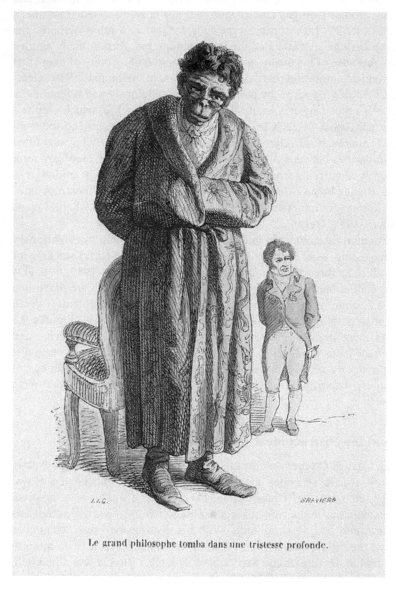

Le grand philosophe tomba dans une tristesse profonde.

Figure 9.3 P.J. Hetzel, *Scenes de la vie privee et publique des animaux vignettes par Grandville*, 1842.

attention to the tugs-of-war between generalisation and specificity, idealism and realism, and abstraction and naturalism in the arts as well as sciences.

In the late eighteenth century, these contests over style of representation and ways of viewing the world were entangled with deliberations about the role of anatomy in art education and practice. As might be imagined, proponents of

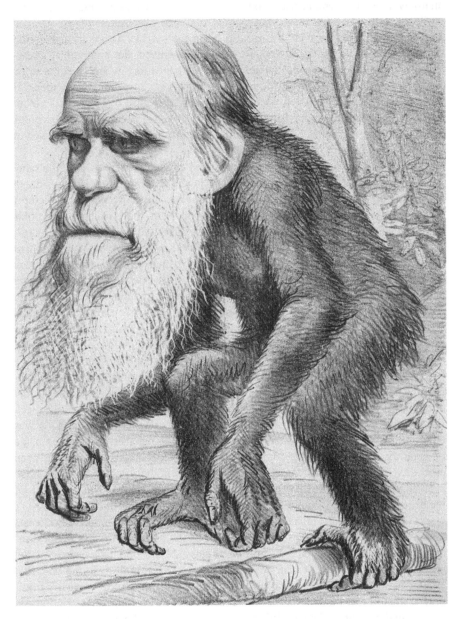

Figure 9.4 "A Venerable Orang-outang": A Contribution to Unnatural History, *The Hornet*, 22 March 1871.

anatomy tended to emphasise – but not always – specificity and naturalism, while opponents tended to be theorists of classical abstraction who portrayed idealised notions of the body beautiful in their own work. Although invested in the classical model of abstraction, Reynolds recognised that anatomical knowledge could address "a principle defect" in art education: when students drew from life models, they drew "according to their vague and uncertain ideas of beauty" so that they depicted "what they think the figure ought to be," rather than what they actually *saw* (Reynolds [1769] 1891, 61). Accordingly, Reynolds oversaw the appointment of the anatomist William Hunter as first Professor of Anatomy at the Royal Academy (from 1769–83).

Martin Kemp traces how, although Reynolds and Hunter were part of "the same basic enterprise" at the Royal Academy, the incompatibility of their views about imitation and representation of the body is obvious in their competing lectures (Kemp 1992, 77). Even before his first Discourse at the Academy, Reynolds lamented that "there is one maxim universally admitted and continually inculcated": to *"Imitate Nature"* (Reynolds [1769] 1891, 112). The problem was that "every one takes it in the most obvious sense" so that objects and figures were painted to "seem real" (112). This "mechanical" art was devoid of "understanding and imagination"; if artists did not interpret the rule of imitation to go beyond straight naturalism, art could not be "liberal" nor could it "claim kindred with poetry" (112–13). In his fifth Discourse, Reynolds clarified this maxim further, as he expatiated on the challenges of executing the human figure in the grand manner style. *"The art of seeing nature"* might be "the great object," but it should be represented "in the abstract"; moreover, human figures should embody "the character of its species" rather than the idiosyncrasies and flesh-and-blood realities of the body (93). What Reynolds means by "character" here might not be what we expect, for anything coarse, deformed, idiosyncratic or even ordinary about the body was out, while solely idealised abstract qualities were in. Character is "an assemblage of contrary qualities" of "the highest form of perfection," which was not even embodied "in the Hercules, nor in the Gladiator, nor in the Apollo," but only in the near-impossible sculpture that "partakes equally of the activity of the Gladiator, of the delicacy of the Apollo, and of the muscular strength of the Hercules" (89).

As these comments indicate, Reynolds is a theorist of abstraction, who insists that art should turn nature into an object of beauty, and a theorist of generalisation, who holds that human and animal figures should be characteristic of the species. He is not, however, an advocate of anatomical realism in the way that Hunter was. Reynolds' aesthetic principles are part, though, of an earlier tradition of anatomical illustration that melded the classical idiom and period styles with a medical idiom. This tradition can be traced from the 1543 publication of Andreas Vesalius's *De humani corporis fabrica* forwards, but Bernhard Siegfried Albinus' magisterial 1747 *Tabulae sceleti et musculorum corporis humani* is a particularly good example of the melding of aesthetic and medical priorities. Drawing from several bodies to make one composite image, Albinus and artist Jan Wandelaar emulated the ancients who had sculpted one perfect limb from the study of a number of admirable examples (Figure 9.5). As Albinus indicates

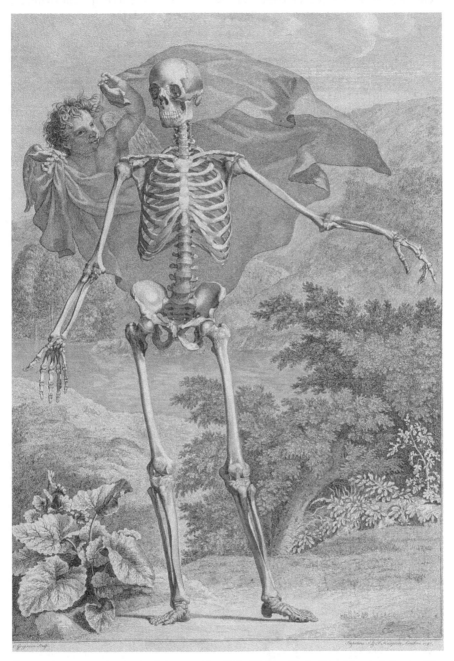

Figure 9.5 Engraving by C. Grignion after B.S. Albinus, A skeleton, front view, standing with lift arm extended, in a pastoral setting, 1747. Credit: Wellcome Images.

in his text, he did not see a conflict between the visual idiom of ancient sculpture and an anatomical science that emphasised literalness and transparency.

William Hunter's graphic style, which signals something of a watershed in the history of anatomical illustration, was distinctly at odds with the methods and styles of Albinus and with the grand manner style of Reynolds. It was true that as early as 1685, the anatomist Govard Bidloo illustrated his belief that "perfect" illustrations of human anatomies were "without ornamental or misleading representations" and were "naer het leven," portrayals "after life" (in Knoeff 2007, 123). But the strikingly uncompromisingly realistic images of Hunter's famous 1774 atlas of the *Anatomy of the Human Gravid Uterus* leave behind all of the classical or Renaissance artistic idiom that even Bidloo included. Hunter depicted the human figure "exactly as it was seen" rather than "under such circumstances as were not actually seen, but conceived in the imagination" (Hunter 1794, Preface). Composite representations of the body may have "elegance and harmony" but the image that is taken directly from the single, dissected body "carries the mark of truth," rendering the image "as infallible as the object itself" (Hunter 1794, Preface). This principle of anatomical illustration also informed Hunter's Academy lectures for artists: on the question of "how far the artist should copy Nature herself precisely; or how far this work should be the copy rather of what his own poetick or creative mind makes out in imitation of nature," it was realism that ultimately won. Reynolds had equated the artist who portrayed "the minute discriminations which distinguish one object of the same species from another" with the lowly "collector of shells" (or, one surmises, the anatomist), but for Hunter, those minute discriminations were endlessly fascinating and beautiful (Reynolds [1769] 1891, 93).

Historians often point to Jan van Rymsdyk's engravings for Hunter's *Anatomy of the Human Gravid Uterus* as manifestations of the Enlightenment commitment to truth to nature.[4] Aris Sarafianos categorises them as "hypernaturalism," while Martin Kemp places them in the "flesh and blood school" that heralded a new "'proto-photographic' method" in anatomical imaging (Kemp 2010, 202; Sarafianos 2009, 5). In spite of the emphasis on realism, another of Hunter's famous Royal Academy productions might seem to belong more to the classically informed Albinus school. The écorché, sculpted by Agostino Carlini and nicknamed Smugglerius, is copied from the famous Roman sculpture, the *Dying Gaul* or *Dying Gladiator* (Figure 9.6). Yet this is not a composite but was cast from the dissected body of an executed criminal (thus the nickname), selected by Hunter for his well-developed musculature. Moreover, while the classical idiom is apparent here, it is a form that shows off all the minute particulars of the body beneath the skin on display, without drapery or abstraction. The perfection comes from precision, exactitude and truthfulness, not from an ideal.

The problem of uniformity

At the turn of the nineteenth century, something was profoundly wrong with art. The physician, philosopher and sometime art critic Thomas Cogan observed that

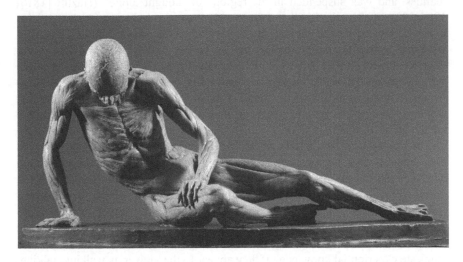

Figure 9.6 Smugglerius, cast by William Pink from original cast of 1776 supervised by
Agostino Carlini RA, Smugglerius, *c*.1834.

Source: photographer Paul Highnam. © Royal Academy of Arts, London.

lovers of art had noticed that a kind of uniformity had taken over painting
(Cogan 1794). It seemed to those who attended the Academy shows that modern
artists were merely imitating established models; they produced "very few
works" that were "exempt from gross imperfections" in "the delineation of
different animals" and in representations of the human (Cogan 1794, v). How
then should artists represent the complex taxonomy of the living world? What
about the types of individuals excised from Reynolds' art: the anomalous, the
deformed, the unusual, or the banal?

The generation that came after Reynolds expressed a dissatisfaction with a
uniformity often seen as an inevitable byproduct of generalisation and idealisa-
tion. William Hazlitt took issue with Reynold's argument, made early in his
career, that the artist must remove "what is particular and uncommon" from representations of the human figure and his instruction that the human subject in art
should rise "above all singular forms, local customs, particularities, and details
of every kind" (Reynolds [1770] 1891, 85). In his 1814–15 essays on Reynold's
Discourses, Hazlitt discerned these principles in paintings of people that were
"all equally young, blooming, smiling, elegant, and insipid;" their bodies and
faces "confound[ing] all difference of sex or passion" (Hazlitt [1815] 1904, 225).
Just as all colours were reduced to a muddy leaden shade, so all bodies were
composites that exhibited "an absolute negation of all expression, character, and
discrimination of form and colour" (225).

Hazlitt's dissatisfaction with a lack of realistic detail in portrayals of the
human figure is an expression of a wider movement against the Reynoldian
view of art as "the superstructure" that "towered by degrees above the world of

realities, and was suspended in the regions of thought alone" (Hazlitt [1816] 1904, 332). For Hazlitt, it was not the world of realities *or* beauty. As he explains in his 1816 essay on the subject, the Elgin marbles demonstrated these qualities were compatible: the marbles were colossal, monumentally romantic figures, but their forms were taken from nature. The Greeks had so expertly sculpted the veins, wrinkles, muscles, finger joints and nails, that even a modern anatomist would be impressed (329). The grandeur of the Elgin marbles exists in the fact that they "find no place in the theory of *ideal* art," which abstracts or generalises human features (329).

The charge of a lack of discrimination goes beyond dissatisfaction with the grand manner style of representing the human body; it is also a dissatisfaction with the current role of art in society. Art should aim to communicate what it means to be human, or as Hazlitt puts it, the "essences" of human experience – and by "essences" he means thoughts or emotions that might be general to humankind, but are distilled through the prism of individual bodies and characters (Hazlitt [1816] 1904, 340). Figures in paintings and sculpture can only communicate experiential knowledge if they appear to the viewer as walking, talking, eating, fighting, embracing and breathing individuals. This was only possible if the painter translated "the internal machinery" of the human body into "a flexible machinery" that breathed with motion and emotion (342). This is how art arouses sympathy (in the widest sense of that word, as common feeling). Good art inspires the viewer to wrestle with those experiences that make us distinctly human, such as the destructive power of jealousy, the fearful anguish of disease, the torture of hunger and the desperation of poverty. And art – at least art for the new century – simply could not do so without referring to the realities of living in a body. The "insipid mediocrity" of generalised representations of a human form that did not naturally exist were not enough (341). Whether or not the Elgin marbles have natural human "proportions" was debated – the anatomist and artist Sir Charles Bell, for example, argued that classical artists had *avoided* what was human in their sculptures precisely because they were interested in embodying the universal, the ideal, and the divine (Bell [1806] 1865, 30). Yet there was agreement on the point that representing human experience; indeed, *humanness* required a knowledge of not just the external form of the body, but also its interior.

Reynolds' style of excising all that was idiosyncratic or distorted from depictions of the human became increasingly out of step with wider cultural changes. In the life sciences, anatomy had branched into pathology and anthropological biology, and these developments invariably inflected aesthetics. A diverse group of Romantic poets (Blake, for instance), gothic writers (such as Mary Shelley), and Victorian novelists of realism and sensation fiction (including Dickens, Zola, Wilkie Collins, George Eliot and George Gissing) were interested in precisely what Reynolds urged art students to exclude: individual character, local customs, particularities, details and "deformities." Similarly, nineteenth-century realist painters were more interested in capturing physical idiosyncrasies, the particularities of human expression, and the ways in which the body testified to the realities of everyday life.

As idealism and generalisation became increasingly at odds with new ways of representing what it meant to be human in a modernising world, the proto-photographic presentation of the human body both challenged and promised to revive art. Hunter's scrupulous, systematic attention to anatomical detail in all its fleshy reality could be translated from the realm of science into something distinctly modern in painting and sculpture. The idea was, as Cogan put it, that learning "the *minutiae* of anatomical knowledge" – rather than simply obtaining a sense of the general forms of the body – would lead to greater "elegance, character, expression, and precision" in the delineation of human and animal figures (Cogan 1794, vii). Cogan made these remarks by way of introduction to his translation of the Dutch comparative anatomist and artist Petrus Camper's lectures on *The Connexion between the Science of Anatomy and the Arts of Drawing, Painting, Statuary* (1794). Cogan advocated Camper's argument that artists must penetrate more deeply into the branches of osteology and neurology. The knowledge of the cranial bones would allow artists to paint signs of age, to portray individual characteristics, to more convincingly represent the emotions, *and* to more accurately delineate species and national character (or race).

Black in colour only: delineating human difference

For those who rejected uniformity and called for finer delineation of physical and cultural difference in the representation of human bodies, the issue of race presented a number of challenges. Artists and anatomists had noticed that in the history of art, black subjects had darker-skinned versions of European bodies and faces. Camper recalls how, as an art student, he had been instructed to copy a Van Tempel painting. He noticed that, as in many other pictures, the African figure was black only in colour, while his "features were European" (Camper 1794, 2). This was the case in portrayals of the Eastern Magi in nativity pictures, including those by Peter Paul Rubens, such as the one below (Figure 9.7). On this issue (if not others), Charles Bell was in agreement; as he put it, "sculptors and painters have been too commonly content to characterize an inhabitant of the East by a tuft of hair on his crown; or an African by a swarthy face" (Bell [1806] 1865, 66).

European artists had difficulty because they were steeped in grand manner portraiture and they looked through the lens of Western aesthetics. Moreover, they could not distinguish between "accidental" (or cultural) differences and the "national" (or anatomical) indicators of race (Camper 1794, 14, 95). The solution to the lack of verisimilitude lay in anatomy, and especially osteology. Knowledge of the facial and cranial bones – "the truest basis" of the portrait – would prevent the artist from incorrectly blending the features of different races (96). Toward that end, Camper measured his own collection of skulls, including those of "apes, orangs, Negroes, the skull of a Hottentot, Madagascar, Celebese, Chinese, Monguller, Calmuck (Kalmyk), and diverse Europeans" with the hope that "differences might become more obvious" (50). From these activities,

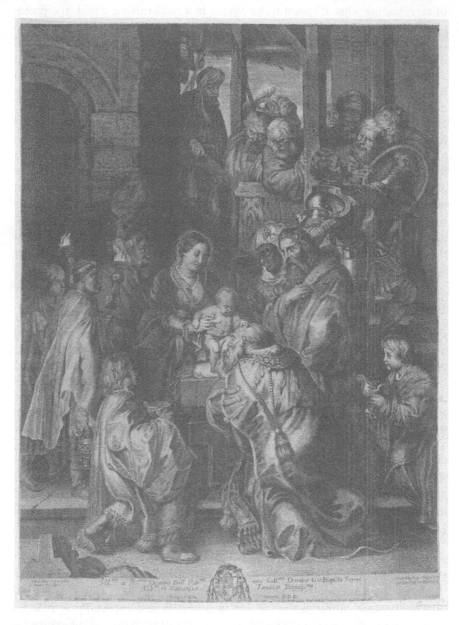

Figure 9.7 Engraving by Nicolaes Lauwers, after Peter Paul Rubens, *c*.mid-1700s,
Adoration of the Magi.

Source: © The MET, The Elisha Whittelsey Collection, The Elisha Whittelsey Fund, 1951.

Camper formulated his well-known facial angle theory: the faces of classical Greek sculptures he measured at a 100-degree angle, while Roman sculptures were about 95; by comparison, the real-life European averaged at 80, the Kalmyk and Angolan at 70, the Orangutan at 58, and the tailed monkey at 42 (see Figures 9.8a and 9.8b).

We mostly know of Camper today because his facial angle theory was used to support scientific racism (by Georges Cuvier, for example), yet he had a pre-dominantly aesthetic rather than anthropological purpose. Camper's aim could be summarised as an investigation of the physiological basis of the aesthetic ideal. His aim was to understand how the Greeks had adapted nature to create an ideal, to determine if there was an inborn or universal definition of beauty, to explore differences in national tastes, and more to the point here, to establish an empirical foundation for classical idealism. Wessel Krul rather handily labels Camper's twofold artistic mode as "stylised realism or naturalising classicism" (Krul 2015, 239). In this respect, there are points of comparison between his project and Albinus' and to a lesser extent, Reynolds'.

However, while Camper aimed to understand difference in national taste and ideals of beauty, as well as anatomical difference based on race, his dissections had the effect of effacing diversity. Critic Paul Youngquist is right to describe Camper's "aesthetics of intelligibility" as a theory that subordinated "singularity to general, geometrical rule" (Youngquist 2003, 68). As Youngquist explains, the process of collecting, dissecting and categorising skulls "for the purposes of accurate measurement" is in fact an act of "defacement" (68). While Camper

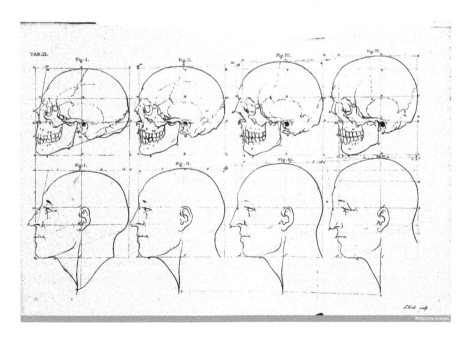

Figure 9.8a Petrus Camper, *Facial Angle*, 1792. Credit: Wellcome Images.

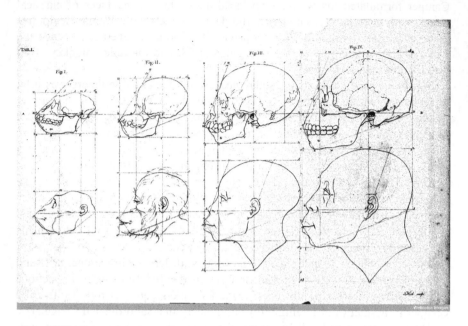

Figure 9.8b Petrus Camper, *Facial Angle*, 1792. Credit: Wellcome Images.

insisted his approach would make sense of what he described as the "amazing variety" of races and species, he subsumed them into homogeneous categories – even though his arguments about race were often creditable and even forward looking. This is particularly the case in his arguments for a shared racial genealogy that linked all of humanity. In "On the Origin and Color of Blacks" (1764), Camper describes how his autopsies revealed uniformity beneath the skin: the blood of a black Angolese boy proved to be "very much like ours and his brains as white, if not whiter;" another set of dissections, in which he compared a Moor's skin with that of an Italian, disproved superstitious theories about biological markers of racial difference, such as that soot or mercury and sulphur in the blood produced black skin. Anatomy revealed that humans were descended from a common stock and only altered by environment. "We are," Camper states simply, "white Moors" (Camper [1764] 1997, 6, 9). "Craniofacial morphology" – difference in form – was only apparent on the body's surface; beneath the skin there was evidence of "uniformity" (3). That word "uniformity" indicates an unanticipated effect of this anatomical investigation: Camper's otherwise commendably monogenist view of race has the effect of assimilating uniqueness to uniformity, difference to similitude. In this case, dissection reveals biological uniformity, rather than the finer gradations of difference.

Ruskin and anatomy, that "ghastly toil of bone-delineation"

These doubts about the cultural and scientific effects of anatomical study fuelled a growing opposition to the role of anatomy in art. As early as 1809, the Irish portrait painter and academician Martin Archer Shee described how "Anatomy extends her aid to Art," but had gone too far, so that although once the arts and sciences had been "allies," they were now "enemies" (45). Artists were "so occupied ... in taking the machine to pieces, and examining its minuter parts," Shee wrote, that they could not represent the whole. The human was stripped, fragmented, and denuded of its humanity – a point made consistently in the mid-century by the anatomist and art critic Robert Knox. In his *Manual of Artistic Anatomy* (1852) he targeted members of "the Anatomical school of art," which included Sir Joshua Reynolds (for his advocacy of Hunter), Sir Charles Bell (for insisting on the anatomical foundations for representing expression), Benjamin West (whose human figures had "a charnel-house look") and Benjamin Haydon (an admirer of Albinus). After several decades of anatomical training at the Royal Academy and in private lecture rooms, where they had access to living models, atlases, écorchés, skeletons, specimens and cadavers, artists now viewed the human being *as* a body. When they look at "the living," Knox wrote, they only "see the dead, that is, the interior" (Knox 1852, 9). That there should be something of a parting of the ways between art and anatomy could not be expressed more clearly than in Knox's statement that "the exterior belongs to art, the interior to science and to philosophy" (77).

Ruskin draws comparable conclusions 20 years later, although he admits in the "Preface" to the Oxford lectures that his unequivocal statement "the study of anatomy is destructive to art" must "appear most startling" to his readers (Ruskin 1872, vii).[5] Casting his eye over several centuries of art history, he identifies artists who were "polluted and paralyzed by the study of anatomy"; they were, he wrote, so consumed with "the ghastly toil of bone-delineation" that their artworks resembled "surgical diagram[s]" (viii). Although he had previously admired the portraits of the fifteenth-century Italian painter Andrea Mantegna, Ruskin now judged the insidious influence of anatomy in Mantegna's portraits. Even the painter's best works were "entirely revolting to all women and children" (just as he judged the images of Sarah Baartman to be) (viii).[6] Ruskin had also once praised Albrecht Dürer's decisive drawing style, but with few exceptions (one being the draped female figure of Dürer's *Melancolia I*, reproduced here as Figure 9.9), there was as little beauty in the hideously skeletal bodies of the Nuremberg-er's engravings as the Italian's paintings (see Figures 9.10 and 9.11).

Contrary to earlier expectations, the study of anatomy had, in Ruskin's words, "produced the most singularly mischievous effect on the faculty of delineation with respect to different races of animals" (Ruskin 1872, 156). Not only would "anatomy ... not help us draw the true appearances of things," but in spite of its methods of dissection and empirical observation, it will also "not add to our intelligent conception of their nature" (156). More than offending women, the infiltration of anatomy had caused real damage to aesthetics and to morality, and

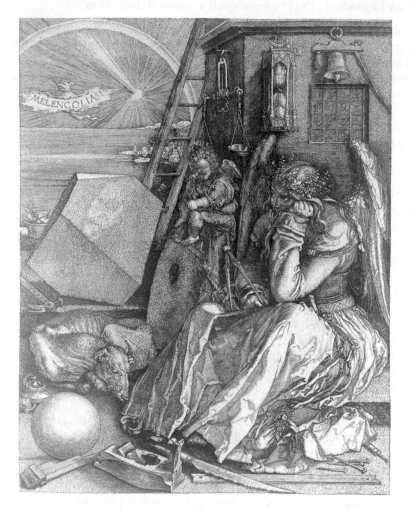

Figure 9.9 After Albrecht Dürer, *Melancolia I*, 1514. Credit: Wellcome Images.

it had led medicine and science into avenues that had devalued human life, so that men and women were reduced to apes or even pigs and rats. Along the way, too, anatomy had jeopardised the artist's greatest skill – the ability to *see* and to understand the nature of things.

Anatomical vision vs artistic vision

Different ways of seeing are profoundly at stake in Ruskin's project. As Dinah Birch points out, he consistently made the point that the main role of the artist "was not to analyse, nor to theorise, not to argue, persuade, fantasise, decorate or even instruct, but simply to see, and to communicate what has been seen" (Birch

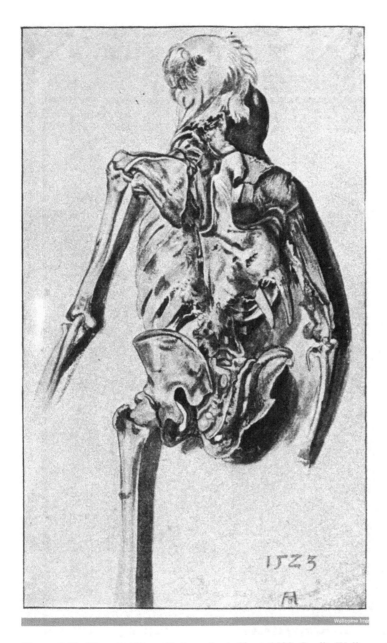

Figure 9.10 Albrecht Dürer, *Skeleton Study Sheet*, 1523. Credit: Wellcome Images.

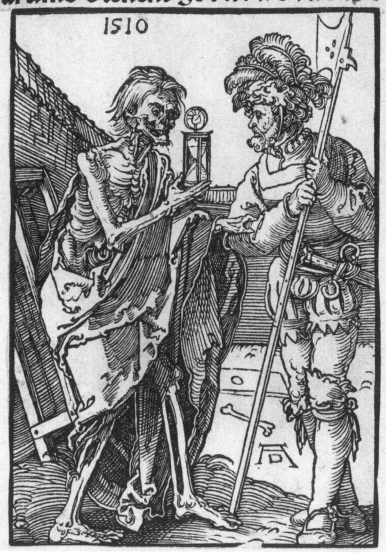

Figure 9.11 Albrecht Dürer, *Death and the Landsknecht*, 1510; The Metropolitan Museum of Art, New York.

2000, 135). But what was to be done to recover that artist's sight in the age of anatomy, scientific materialism and evolution? In *The Elements of Drawing* (1857), Ruskin offers something of a solution: "the innocence of the eye" must be restored; the world must be studied with "a childish perception" or viewed "as a blind man would see ... if suddenly gifted with sight" (Ruskin [1857] 1904, 27). With this newly innocent and spiritually revitalised sight, artists could represent the human figure in ways as arrestingly as the Greeks had. Like their classical predecessors, bodies in modern paintings could embody virtue, suffering, moral strength and creative possibility. Artists who could re-learn to *see* properly, deeply, could also learn to create artworks that *spoke* to their viewers.

Was it desirable or even possible that artists could any longer look with innocent eyes at the human body? For, by Ruskin's time, the internal body had been explored, mapped and for several centuries, represented two-dimensionally in atlases and treatises, and three-dimensionally in wax, wood, plaster and terracotta. Inevitably, this medical mapping had shaped artistic aims, styles and techniques. There were those, like the evolutionist Grant Allen, who accused Ruskin of espousing vague and nostalgically religious, unscientific aesthetic theories.

But Ruskin's solution takes this into account, for his writing on this topic is neither blindly nostalgic nor naïve; he did not shrink from modernity or deny the importance of scientific discovery. Ruskin's views are informed by Enlightenment science and, as Rachel Teukolsky points out, he also adapted something of the "experimental method" of early Victorian comparative anatomists, which "located truth in the empiricist proof of the eye" (Teukolsky 2009, 36). Ruskin may have adapted some of the careful investigative methods of medics and scientists, but there is a key difference between that way of looking and the artistic version. As Teukolsky explains, Ruskin's "mode of nonintrusive scientific looking presumed that an object could be perfectly, visibly legible" and thus "discerned by the eye without penetration to interiors or causes" (36). Ruskin advocates an artistic vision that is empirical but which refuses to dissect, to disassemble, or to copy mechanically.

These lines of influence are clearly discernible, it seems to me, in Ruskin's appropriation of the term "anatomy" in *Modern Painters*. With curious, receptive, exploratory eyes, artists should investigate, he argues, the anatomy of architecture, the anatomy of clouds and trees, "the sea's anatomy," "hill anatomy," or more to the point here, "the animal anatomy." Crucially, though, artists gain intimate knowledge about human bodies – of the "distinct and fixed" laws of "the animal frame" – without dissection and "without knowledge of the interior mechanism" (Ruskin [1843] 1903, 3:425). These fixed laws are the fine gradations of physical and moral difference, and differences of character between species and races, which fit together in a "highly fragmented taxonomy" (Cramer 2006, 111). So Ruskin redefines "anatomy" to refer to the precise and minute study of the external forms of objects and bodies, with close attention to how the interior structures affect that form.

Ruskin unequivocally insisted upon authenticity of form, or to use a phrase he consistently used, "a truth of species." Artists should, and in fact, had a duty to represent the formal distinctiveness of subjects and objects. Trees should appear *as* trees, with all the details of their leaves, rather than as a spot of green paint. Bodies and faces should be more than a smear of pink or red paint. Bodies and faces must pulse with physicality and movement; they should communicate character and emotion; they should be differentiated and speak to occasion. But a truth of species did not translate into transparently naturalistic images, as Ruskin's impassioned arguments for the greatness of Turner's sublimely impressionistic Romantic vision of nature indicates. In fact, the basis of Ruskin's advocacy of Turner was his meticulous study of the subject and his ability to translate this precision into colour and movement. The greatness of Turner, or of any artist, could not come from anatomical dissection. Anatomy was the science of disassembly and fragmentation, and the logic of its primary method, dissection, was mechanistic. As a result, artistic representations were likewise fragmentary, imitative, and mechanistic, and the anatomically accurate body parts did not communicate a sense of wholeness, or the *idea* behind the artwork. A great artist was not a "neat imitator of the texture of a skin" but instead combined specificity of form with higher ideas and deeper meanings, which could only come from seeing the world with artistic, rather than with anatomical vision (Ruskin [1843] 1903, 3:89).

Already in *Modern Painters I*, in a section on "Vital Beauty," Ruskin had expatiated on how the two types of vision manifested themselves in visual representation. "We are impressed, uplifted, enlightened by the sight of a graceful or powerful animal in movement," he writes,

> but if we were to see the inner mechanisms involved in that same movement – the jerking ligaments of an ostrich's joint or the up-and-down movement of the "peg" of the shark's dissected dorsal fin – we would *only* be impressed by that mechanism.
>
> (Ruskin [1843] 1903, 3:155)

"When we dissect the animal frame, or *conceive it as dissected*," we cease to experience "the pleasure of the animal" and instead only think of "the neatness of mechanical contrivance" 3:155). This is the "moment we reduce enjoyment to ingenuity," Ruskin continues, and it is also the "instant all sense of beauty ceases" (3:155). When we see the joints and ligaments everything becomes just that: a uniform, indiscriminate collection of physical fragments that are devoid of aesthetic and moral meaning. Differences of essential character between species are obscured. Dissection strips the cultural skin – the form, the colour, the expression, the character, and all value and beauty – from the body. And it is impossible that this interior view of animal bodies (or similar views of the interior of human bodies) can rouse us to higher contemplation about what it means to be ostrich or shark (or human, for that matter).

In the past, artists and anatomists had often shared aims, methods and representational styles, but by the mid-nineteenth century, they had diverged over these very things. A crucial issue for Ruskin was that "modern science" had "entirely cease[d] to understand the difference between eyes and microscopes" (Ruskin [1883] 1903, 3:158). Ruskin urges, and also speaks for, critical changes underway in artistic production and taste in the last half of the nineteenth century. There had been a growing sense that artists had to take off the anatomical lenses that they had adopted, and had to view the world through alert, curious, searching, knowledgeable, but also innocently "artless" eyes. Only then could they participate in that grandest of enterprises: identifying and communicating what was worthiest about being human. As we have seen, some saw this as an enterprise in which anatomy had failed to take part. Anatomy had revealed the body's internal structures and functions, but it had obscured rather than clarified what it was that separated humans from animals. Anatomy had failed, too, to expose all the finer differences between species and races; instead, it had given rise to a genealogical enfolding of species and races in science and art.

This realisation – or perception – gave impetus to a split between art and anatomy. Art branched off from the scientific enterprise of making nature and its laws transparent, and left the realist enterprise to medical illustrators and anthropological photographers. Photography promised to provide an objective inventory of human variety and access to authentic identities, but fine art offered something best encapsulated by Ruskin's deification of Turner's sublime impressionistic art. Turner's eye captures the finer discriminations of things, yet his art offers something much more than the daguerreotype or photograph's indexical record. While there is a truth to nature in his paintings, they fuse naturalism with emotion and idea; Ruskin's famous elegy to Turner's *Slave Ship* captures the unique ability of art to communicate truths about being human in ways that immediately resonate for the viewer. This painting is based on "truth" and is technically perfect – the colour, the tone, the composition on the canvas, the accuracy of drawing – but that accuracy is combined with a "fearless" spirit; truthfulness is blended with "daring conception" (Ruskin [1883] 1903, 3: 572). This is modern art that aims for the human "ideal in the highest sense of the word" (3: 572). Importantly, as Turner's sketchbook studies of Dürer's human figures reveal, the anatomical view of the human informs but also is transformed into a modern, impressionistic vision of the human body in the modern world.

Notes

1 Ruskin had three articles published in *Loudon's Magazine of Natural History* in 1834.
2 It is unusual to use the word "consistent" with reference to the notoriously changeable Ruskin, and critics acknowledge that, as Jonathan Smith puts it, "characterizing Ruskin's aesthetics is a complicated matter," as "he variously reaffirmed, modified, repudiated, and contradicted his earlier positions" (2006, 24). Rachel Teukolsky reminds us that over the course of 40 years, Ruskin "adopted a bewildering array of positions on art and aesthetics" (Teukolsky 2009/2013, 27).
3 See note 1 regarding Ruskin's changeability; likewise, as Günther Leypoldt points out, "most commentators on Sir Joshua Reynolds's critical writings have grappled with the argumentative inconsistency of his *Discourses on Art*" (Leypoldt 1999, 330).
4 See, for example, Kemp, 2010, 192–208; Daston and Galison. 2007; C. Wagner, 2017.

5 In *The Stones of Venice*, Ruskin called anatomy "a true science" and in *Modern Paint-ers III* (1856), he criticised Wordsworth for failing to understand "that to dissect a flower may sometimes be as proper as to dream over it" (Ruskin [1856] 1904, 359).
6 Ruskin had once described one of Mantegna's portraits as "a perfect type of the schools of delineation in Italy" in *Works*, xxi, 24; qtd. in *Correspondence*, f. 1, 198, "Letter to Charles Eliot Norton, 8 July 1870," 198.

Reference list

Appel, Toby A. 1987. *The Cuvier-Geoffroy Debate: French Biology in the Decades before Darwin*. Oxford: Oxford University Press.
Bell, Sir Charles. 1865. *The Anatomy and Philosophy of Expression as Connected with the Fine Arts*, 5th edn. London: Bohn.
Birch, Diana. 2000. "'That Ghastly Work': Ruskin, Animals and Anatomy." *Worldviews: Global Religions, Culture, and Ecology*, 4.2: 131–45.
Camper, Petrus. 1794. *The Works on the Connexion between the Science of Anatomy and the Arts of Drawing, Painting, Statuary*. Trans. T. Cogan. London: C. Dilly.
Cramer, Charles. 2006. *Abstraction and the Classical Ideal, 1760–1920*. Newark: University of Delaware Press.
Cogan, Thomas. 1794. "Letter 18." *The Rhine, of a Journey from Utrech to Francfort; Chiefly by the Borders of the Rhine, and the Passage Down the River, from Mentz to Bonn* (2 vols), vol. 1, 184–97. London: J. Johnson.
Daston, Lorraine, and Peter Galison. 2007. *Objectivity*. New York: Zone Books.
Desmond, Adrian. 1989. *The Politics of Evolution Morphology, Medicine, and Reform in Radical London*. Chicago: University of Chicago Press.
Hazlitt, William. 1903. *The Collected Works of William Hazlitt*, vol. 9, edited by A.R. Waller and Arnold Glover. London: J.M. Dent.
Hazlitt, William. 1904. *The Collected Works of William Hazlitt*, vol. 11, edited by A.R. Waller and Arnold Glover. London: J.M. Dent.
Hunter, William. 1794. *An Anatomical Description of the Human Gravid Uterus, and its Contents*. London: J. Johnson and G. Nicol.
Kemp, Martin. 1992. "True to their Natures: Sir Joshua Reynolds and Dr. William Hunter at the Royal Academy of Arts." *Notes and Records of the Royal Society of London*, 46: 77–88.
Kemp, Martin. 2010. "Style and Non-Style in Anatomical Illustration: From Renaissance Humanism to Henry Gray." *Journal of Anatomy*, 216: 192–208.
Knoeff, Rina. 2007. "Comparison of Mennonite and Calvinist Motives in the Anatomical Atlases of Bidloo and Albinus." In *Medicine and Religion in Enlightenment Europe*, edited by Ole Peter Grell and Andrew Cunninghamm, 121–43. Farnham: Ashgate.
Knox, Robert. 1852. *Great Artists and Great Anatomists: A Biographical and Philosophical Study*. London: Van Voorst.
Knox, Robert. 1852. *A Manual of Artistic Anatomy, for the Use of Sculptors, Painters and Amateurs*. London: Renshaw.
Krul, Wessel. 2015. "A Slight Correction: Petrus Camper on the Visual Arts." In *Petrus Camper in Context*, edited by Klaas van Berkel and Bart Ramakers, 215–42. Verloren: Hilversum.
Leypoldt, Günther. 1999. "A Neoclassical Dilemma in Sir Joshua Reynolds's Reflections on Art." *British Journal of Aesthetics*, 39.4: 330–49.

Meijer, Miriam Claude and Petrus Camper. 1997. "Petrus Camper on the Origin and Color of Blacks." *History of Anthropology Newsletter*, 24: 2. http://repository.upenn. edu/han/vol. 24/iss2/3.

Reynolds, Sir Joshua. 1797. *The Works of Sir Joshua Reynolds*, vol. 1, edited by Edmond Malone, 2 vols. London: T. Cadell, Jr. & W. Davies.

Reynolds, Sir Joshua. 1891. *Sir Joshua Reynolds' Discourses*, edited by Edward Gilpin Johnson. Chicago: A.C. McClung.

Ruskin, John. 1880. *The Eagle's Nest. Ten Lectures on the Relation of Natural Science to Art, Given before the University of Oxford in Lent Term*. Orpington, Kent: G. Allen.

Ruskin, John. 1903. "Modern Painters I." *Works of John Ruskin*, vol. 3, edited by E.T. Cook and Alexander Wedderburn. London: G. Allen.

Ruskin, John. 1903. "Modern Painters II." *Works of John Ruskin*, vol. 4, edited by E.T. Cook and Alexander Wedderburn. London: G. Allen.

Ruskin, John. 1904. "Modern Painters III." *Works of John Ruskin*, vol. 5, edited by E.T. Cook and Alexander Wedderburn. London: G. Allen.

Ruskin, John. 1905. "Relation of Art to Religion," *Lectures on Art* [1870]. *Works of John Ruskin*, vol. 20, edited by E.T. Cook and Alexander Wedderburn. London: G. Allen.

Sarafianos, Aris. 2009. "The Politics of 'Prodigious Excitement': Art, Anatomy, and Physiology for the Age of Opposition," *Center and Clark Newsletter*, 50.

Shee, Martin Archer. 1809. *Elements of Art*. London: Miller.

Smith, Jonathan. 2006. *Charles Darwin and Victorian Visual Culture*. Cambridge: Cambridge University Press.

Smith, Lindsay. 1995. *Victorian Photography, Painting and Poetry: The Enigma of Visibility in Ruskin, Morris and the Pre-Raphaelites*. Cambridge: Cambridge University Press.

Teukolsky, Rachel. 2009. *The Literate Eye: Victorian Art Writing and Modernist Aesthetics*. Oxford: Oxford University Press.

Wagner, Corinna. 2017. "Replicating Venus: Art, Anatomy, Wax Models, and Automata," *19: Interdisciplinary Studies in the Long Nineteenth Century*, 24. doi: http://doi. org/10.16995/ntn.783.

Youngquist, Paul. 2003. *Monstrosities: Bodies and British Romanticism*. Minneapolis: University of Minnesota Press.

10 Medical imaging and the intrusive gaze

Catherine Jenkins

While useful in medical diagnostics, and "informative and even reassuring" to patients, images that intrude into an individual's interior space can also be troubling (Blaxter 2009, 776). Flat images are used to educate medical students to work with living, breathing, bleeding patients – subjects who may or may not be as cooperative, compliant, or anatomically average as their virtual counterparts. The distance created is not only psychological but spatial. Furthermore, the use of diagnostic images is now so common that patients themselves rarely consider the implications of their medical images being mapped onto flattened cadaveric information. This chapter examines the impact of medical imaging on patients in a diagnostic era that often privileges disembodied data over the patient voice and, arguably, by extension, the patient's humanity.

Visual representations of the human body began with artistic renderings, but with the advent of medical imaging in 1895, human images took on new and different meanings. Since anatomist Andreas Vesalius (1514–1564), accurate renderings have created permanent records, allowing the medical gaze into once-hidden human interiors, and providing images that still haunt living medicalised bodies. Wilhelm Röntgen's (1845–1923) application of X-rays to the human body entrenched an intrusive medical gaze into the living patient. Although early X-rays were perceived as an unsettling photographic novelty, they were rapidly facilitated in medical contexts. Since the 1970s, medical imaging technologies, including ultrasound, computed tomography (CT), and magnetic resonance imaging (MRI), have become the diagnostic norm in Western medical practice. The rapidity of this shift, which renders the human body a flattened data set, outstrips the consideration of the implications of applying such technologies to living patients. Advanced medical imaging technologies reinforce a reductionist biomedical model, over the holistic patient- or person-centred model that acknowledges the patient's experience of illness and their human subjectivity. This chapter explores the human and psychological impact on patients confronted by high-tech images of their bodily interiors, and how the objective medical image may be rectified with the subjective physical body.

Foucault and the "clinical gaze"

Much medical humanities research relies on concepts elaborated by Michel Foucault (1973), specifically the "medical gaze" or the "clinical gaze," which includes all physician-gathered sensory data: the "sight/touch/hearing trinity" (1973, 9; 103; 202). The clinical gaze includes not only observation, but also palpation, percussion and auscultation. In its most reductive form, the clinical gaze causes patients to feel objectified: "in relation to that which he is suffering from, the patient is only an external fact; the medical reading must take him into account only to place him in parentheses" (Foucault 1973, 7). Foucault, however, also allowed for a more complex understanding, stating that the gaze "establishes the individual in his irreducible quality" (1973, xv). In other words, the clinical gaze can simultaneously objectify and create the patient; for Foucault, object and subject are not mutually exclusive, and can occupy the same spatial and temporal moment: "The *object* of discourse may equally well be a *subject*, without the figures of objectivity being in any way altered" (1973, xv).

To perceive symptoms, the physician must observe the patient through a medical gaze. Foucault suggests that the patient's ailment "became an object of investigation, a thing invested with language, a known reality: it became, in short, an object" (2006, 443). It is not the patient, but the disease or disorder that is the object of the medical gaze; the patient loses their humanity and becomes merely the vessel containing the object of enquiry. The individual patient, as Foucault writes in *The Birth of the Clinic* (1973), must be subtracted from this engagement (15). But, as he notes, this objectifying subtraction of the individual implemented by the medical gaze, "could only be accomplished with the complicity of the patients themselves" (Foucault 1973, 77). Although patients are complicit in their objectification, living patients also want to be seen, heard and respected as subjects: to have their human agency recognised. The key for physicians is to avoid an objectifying, reductive medical gaze, and allow the subjective patient to co-create the diagnosis, a conception that resembles the therapeutic alliance formed in an ideal patient-centred approach. Unfortunately, patients often encounter physicians' biomedical bias, shifting power towards the physician.

Additionally, different types of medical gazes establish different patients, diagnoses, treatments and outcomes. The patient established in humoural medicine differs from the patient established in contemporary Western medicine, just as the patient established in acupuncture differs from that established in chiropractic, and so forth. Each medical gaze establishes its own patient by virtue of observing specific norms associated with that particular practice, training and experience. Each practice constructs its patients in unique ways, offering a medical perspective with a unique truth, and a specific lens through which to gaze; in this way, each constructs a different patient body – and each has its own limitations and blind spots – and these limitations have very real implications for the human agency of the patient within the medical context. Medical imaging is simply another form of this flawed and fragmented medical gaze.

Röntgen and the intrusive medical gaze

In 1895, physicist Wilhelm Röntgen discovered a use for X-rays, or Röntgen rays, a form of electromagnetic radiation, while experimenting with a Crookes vacuum tube. The first X-ray image was that of Anna Röntgen's hand, complete with her wedding ring (Cartwright 1995, 111). She reportedly exclaimed, "I have seen my death!" alluding to the uncanny sense many non-clinicians felt at the advent of X-rays (Kevles 1997, 38). X-rays were adopted for medical imaging within weeks of Röntgen's publication, and several journal articles appeared in early 1896. At the end of World War I (1918), X-ray machines were considered specialised equipment in some hospitals and medical offices; by World War II (1939–1945), their use had been accepted as standard practice in hospitals, as well as medical and recruiting offices.

Beyond pure curiosity, the public was quick to see potential medical and legal uses for X-rays. X-rays were taken of broken bones, recently set bones, and post-surgical patients, and to discover the skeletal structure underlying malformations. In this sense, they could contribute to the ordering of human society. They were first used as evidence in court in 1896, in Canada, the US, and UK. Yet while X-rays could seemingly prove malpractice, they were also subject to interpretation, and sometimes misrepresentation, in court. In 1897, surgeon Harvey R. Reed suggested there was a "halo of uncertainty" in X-ray images; foreign bodies, such as bullets, might escape imaging, and yet be locatable surgically. Images might be misinterpreted due to shadows, magnification, or distortion. Kevles notes that "Early X-rays had … been confusing, even to doctors who were supposed to be familiar with anatomy" (1997, 229). Yet physicians, notably surgeons, became so concerned about the possibility of malpractice suits, that they began taking pre- and post-surgical X-rays as proof that they had performed the necessary operation, even when such images were not medically necessary (Reiser 1978, 66–67).

While physicians did not suggest that X-rays should replace established hands-on examination techniques, or that X-rays should reduce physician contact with patients, the new imaging technology did have these objectifying, distancing effects. As with other medical technologies, X-rays removed vital information from the patient so it could be examined and discussed objectively by a group of physicians in consultation. During the first half of the twentieth century, the routine use of medical X-rays increased, with the unfortunate side effect that patients might receive 5 to 10 times more X-rays than were diagnostically necessary. Between 1920 and 1950, the number of X-rays taken in the UK doubled every five years; from 1938 to 1958, there was a six-fold increase in the number of X-rays taken in American hospitals. A 1971 study indicated that for every 16 X-rays taken, only one fracture was diagnosed, and that about one-third of X-rays were unnecessary. X-rays, and other routine testing, revealed little useful information, duplicated existing information from patient records, and placed patients in potential harm from excessive radiation exposure (Reiser 1978).

Advanced medical imaging and the human body as data

In the late 1950s and early 1960s, computed tomography, also known as CAT or CT, scanners combined X-rays to render three-dimensional images. Due to the algorithmic complexity of mapping a three-dimensional image from a dense interior, it was impossible to build a successful CT prototype until advanced computer technology was available. While physicians and radiologists had become comfortable reading flat X-rays, CT images were considerably more complicated, requiring more advanced interpretive skills. Since 1993, the use of CT scans has more than tripled. This is potentially problematic because CT scanners multiply the number of X-rays taken, thus subjecting patients to many times the amount of radiation of regular X-rays. A study published by Baumann *et al.* (2011), suggests that undergoing two or three CT examinations in a lifetime is roughly equivalent to the radiation exposure experienced by a Hiroshima survivor, yet few patients are aware of this risk. The study also found that nearly 75 per cent of patients underestimated CT radiation levels, and only 3 per cent of patients agreed with the statement that CT exposure over life could increase cancer risk. This lack of patient knowledge was particularly unsettling when further investigation indicated that over 80 per cent of the study's patients had previously received CT scans. Another study showed that although the number of emergency and hospital admissions remained stable, CT use rose from 6 per cent to 15 per cent between 1998 and 2007 in American hospitals (Korley *et al.* 2010, 1465). A 2007 American study suggested that 1.5 per cent to 2 per cent of cancers are likely caused by radiation overexposure from CT scans (Brenner and Hall 2007). Still another study extrapolated that, based on current levels of CT use, 1 per cent to 3 per cent of future cancers, or 29,000 cases in the US, will be caused by CT radiation exposure in 2007 (Berrington de González *et al.* 2009). Such studies indicate the increased risk of future health problems due to CT scan overexposure, and the ongoing lack of patient understanding of this risk that is indicative of the breakdown of communication within the patient-physician relationship. Importantly, there seems to be a correlation between the increased digitalisation of patient images – the conversion of human patients into data – and the breakdown of this relationship. Reiser notes, for instance, a tendency for physicians to "cut short their customary diagnostic examination when using it [CT]" (1978, 161). Thus increased dependence on advanced technology is related to decreased communication with patients; yet patients collude with physicians to create this potentially dangerous situation. As Baumann concludes, "patients' confidence levels in their medical evaluation increased with increasing use of technology, with the inclusion of CT yielding the highest degree of patient confidence in a medical evaluation" (2011, 7). Increasingly, patients trust technologically supported diagnostics more than they do the training and experience of their physicians.

While computer assistance improved imaging, not all medical imaging developed during the twentieth century required radiation; sound and electromagnetic imaging technologies were also invented. Ultrasound, the use of high-frequency sound waves for detecting mass, was used to capture diagnostic images by the 1940s, and by the 1960s it was generally accepted and commercialised.[1] Magnetic resonance imaging (MRI) uses magnetic fields to alter the alignment of the body's atoms, rendering three-dimensional images of the soft tissues, largely excluding the bones. Although the physics necessary for MRIs was conceived in the 1920s, the machines were not in common medical use until the late 1970s. As with other advanced scanners that digitally reconstruct the body's interior, MRIs required advanced computer algorithms to function. Physicians, spoiled by the advanced imaging capabilities of CT scanners, found MRI images lacked clarity (Kevles 1998).

Patients' uncritical trust of technology, alongside physicians' dependence on imperfect visualisation tools, illustrates the problem of mapping the human figure onto a flat plane, whether the image is two- or three-dimensional. Within this context, ideas of abnormality must be questioned. According to a 2011 report in the *New York Times*, MRIs are often overused, with negligible clinical effect. Most MRIs will indicate some abnormality, but most abnormalities are of no clinical consequence. A study by Dr. DiGiovanni at Brown University concluded that 90 per cent of MRIs are unnecessary and that 50 per cent of MRI interpretations are either incorrect or inconsequential. He also observed that "Patients often feel like they are getting better care if people are ordering fancy tests, and there are some patients who come in demanding an M.R.I." (Kolata 2011, np). It is often the patient who drives the demand for more, and often unnecessary, imaging. Images that reveal even benign abnormalities tend to increase patient anxiety, and may lead to demands for unnecessary interventions, with the potential to create new problems. Increasingly since the 1970s, imaging has become foundational for Western medical diagnostics. More complex technologies require more training for both technicians and radiologists. As a spokesperson for the Radiological Society of North America stated in 1985, "the difference between using MRI and conventional X-ray techniques, including computed tomography CT scans, is like the vast difference between operating a 747 jet and an automobile" (cited in Kevles 1998, 222–23). While medical imaging holds clear patient benefits, mediation by advanced technologies also troubles the patient-practitioner relationship, as well as posing very real physical threats to the body.

Objective medical images and subjective patient bodies

With the aim of improving patient outcomes, imaging technologies enable physicians to diagnose health problems efficiently, helping to guide treatment and surgical procedures. As Kevles notes, however, "While there is general agreement that imaging accelerates early detection, there is a good deal of disagreement over whether early detection makes any difference in terms of deaths from disease" (1998, 258). Despite this tension, both patients and physicians engage with medical imaging fairly uncritically. Sociologist Mildred Blaxter suggests, "A picture provided by a machine carries with it a sense of objectivity and authority" (2009, 772). Yet to accept medical imaging uncritically is to disregard the patient's experience as an object of medical imaging, the subjective element introduced by the physician's interpretation of images, as well as the necessary communication between patients and physicians regarding medical images. In *The Transparent Body* (2005), José van Dijck comments that "the myth of total transparency generally rests on two underlying assumptions: the idea that seeing is curing and the idea that peering into the body is an innocent activity, which has no consequences" (6–7). Van Dijck articulates the distancing between the patient and physician that is mediated by an image that is not objective or "innocent," but ironically active in creating a myth of healing through observation: that "seeing is curing." The popular notion is that more finely tuned technological instruments lead to deeper and more accurate information; from a patient perspective, better technology suggests more insightful diagnosis, which translates into faster treatment, higher rates of cure, and almost guaranteed survival. This unrealistic expectation creates unreasonable pressure on physicians and can lead to disappointment when the physician is unable to deliver.

Imaging advances increase the quantity of objective information available to doctors, further reducing their reliance on patient narratives. Medical technologies encourage doctors to isolate affected areas of the body for examination, rather than considering the patient holistically. This fragmentation tends to draw the patient's focus away from signals from the rest of their body, and may cause them to disregard the psycho-emotional impact of trauma. Increasing reliance on technologies leads doctors to believe that medical instruments are more reliable diagnostic tools than subjective information gathered from patients. As a result, doctors may be less confident in their own clinical judgement; during the twentieth century, many became managers and interpreters of information between patients and specialists or technicians. Reiser comments that "the patient was less a person and more an object of study, and the doctor more a biologist than a physician" (1978, 166). Once X-ray technology and biochemical tests permeated practice, the patient exam and earlier technologies like the stethoscope were viewed by many physicians as irrelevant, imprecise and time-consuming.

However, increasing reliance on diagnostic medical technologies actually increased the number of medical errors, causing patients harm or even death. A seven-year study at the Veterans Administration Hospital in Washington, in which 1,106 deceased patients were autopsied, found that 6 per cent had been misdiagnosed, and that the rate of misdiagnosis increased from 1.5 per cent in 1947 to 9 per cent by 1953 (Gruver and Freis 1957). The primary cause of misdiagnosis, affecting 45 per cent of these cases, was the lack of a patient history (for reasons including patient inebriation, confusion, weakness, shock, coma, or aphasia). In other cases, the imaging results were normal, diverting the physician from a planned course of action by incorrectly ruling out a suspected cause. Although subsequent examination found no error either technically or interpretively, the X-rays simply failed to reveal necessary information for the correct diagnosis. The study's authors, Robert Gruver and Edward Freis, suggest that medical technologies create a "false sense of security engendered by misleading negative laboratory reports, particularly x-ray films which did not disclose the lesion" (1957, 118).

While there is no doubt that advances in medical technologies have extended many lives, they also raise an inconvenient problem: interpretation. Technologically derived evidence is perceived by both patients and most doctors as objective data, and therefore accurate and correct. All data must, however, be interpreted, and this interpretative step is subjective. As medical anthropologists Margaret Lock and Vihn-Kim Nguyen observe, "it is commonly assumed in the medical sciences that the human body is readily standardizable by means of systematic assessments" (2010, 20). This sort of standardisation, or normalisation, might be referred to in Foucauldian terms as a disciplining of patient bodies. Raw objective data requires a human interpreter, someone to decide whether a health problem exists, and if so, how it should be treated. The imperfections of the technology itself aside, interpretation of data destabilises the notion that technologically derived data is purely objective, and inserts a human actor who may make errors. The accuracy of technologically supported medical diagnostics was further destabilised by several studies undertaken from the 1950s to the 2000s providing evidence of observer error, subjective misinterpretation, mechanical error, lack of lab training or regulation, incompetence, or poor inter-professional communication.

The explosion of available medical technologies in recent decades is a double-edged sword for patients and physicians, offering previously unavailable solutions, but also new problems. Nursing instructor Pascal Lehoux admits that "technology is dehumanizing," not because it is technology, but because of the ways it can be used (2006, xvi). Technologies require and allow medical personnel to distance themselves from ailing strangers. In a contemporary hospital setting, where staff are overburdened and efficiency demanded, monitors support the simultaneous observation of several patients from a central console. There is, however, a risk that patients can become nothing more than objective data on a screen. Rozzano Locsin suggests, "Technique marginalizes the incorporation of subjective and non-technical phenomenon (e.g., human experience) by either negating its importance or framing it within rational and organized order" (2005, 29). Medical technologies tend to create vast quantities of "bodiless information," flattened datasets of minutiae that are only tangentially attached to the living patient's body through barcodes (Hayles 1999, 22).

Interpreting the visual has been, and continues to be, problematic for the medical understanding of images. While issues are sometimes attributed to radiologists being overworked, or their age leading to diminished visual acuity, Doug Cochrane, Chair of the B.C. Patient Safety and Quality Council comments that "The technology in some ways has outstripped our ability to learn on the job" (CBC 2012). The importance of the accurate interpretation of medical imaging becomes paramount when it is a primary diagnostic tool; these are, after all, what Catherine Waldby calls "operative images," images upon which decisions are made that "materially order the living body," transforming human bodies and human lives (2000, 109).

Concerns regarding accurate X-ray interpretation began as early as the 1920s. An accidental finding in Carl Birkelo's 1947 tuberculosis study was significant in the critical analysis of X-ray interpretation. To the researchers' surprise, when five specialists reviewed 1,256 X-rays, their interpretations did not always agree; colleagues' assessments differed in about one-third of cases, and even a second viewing by the same specialist produced different findings in about one-fifth of cases (Birkelo *et al.* 1947). Birkelo concluded their study with the recommendation that "all survey films be read independently by at least two interpreters," a recommendation that has been echoed many times, but is still not practiced in all jurisdictions due to cost and the availability of radiologists (1947, 365). This lack of a second interpretation has potentially serious patient consequences when a finding is grossly misinterpreted or missed. Elizabeth Krupinski's survey article of chest, bone and mammographic radiological studies indicates that on average, there is a false positive rate of 2 per cent to 15 per cent, and a false negative rate of 20 per cent to 30 per cent. Accounting for the false positives, Krupinski notes that overlying anatomical structures can be misconstrued; false negatives are more difficult to comprehend. While an area may seem abnormal, a radiologist may not perceive it as problematic, so it remains unreported (Krupinski 2000).

Clearly human subjectivity enters into the accuracy of imaging data interpretation. While a radiologist's decision to mark something as suspicious is in part a matter of training and experience, van Dijck (2005) and physician James Potchen (2006) agree that interpretation is also affected by the radiologist's personality; some individuals are more inclined towards risk, while others are more cautious. Kevles (1998) suggests that computer-aided radiography (CAD), available since 1992, was designed to reduce the subjective interpretive component; however, Krupinski (2000) suggests that while CAD may help draw a radiologist's attention to neglected areas of an image, some lesions require humans for detection. The dual effect of CAD has been to make radiologists sometimes lazy in their own judgements, as well as causing a tendency to over-diagnose (Nodine in Kevles 1998). While over-diagnosing may be preferable to under-diagnosing, it contributes to unnecessary patient stress and cost.

In addition to studies of interpretive error, some researchers have explored the results of omitting or adding elements to images to determine professional perception. In a 2006 American study, radiologists were asked to separate 60 chest X-rays into two piles: normal and abnormal. Unbeknownst to the participants, some films were duplicated; surprisingly, 5 per cent to 30 per cent of the time, radiologists placed one image in the normal pile and its twin image in the abnormal pile. Also included in the set was one X-ray in which the left clavicle was obviously missing; 58 per cent to 60 per cent of the radiologists classified the X-ray as normal (Potchen 2006). Even professionals trained to critically view such images often miss or dismiss the unexpected. The results of inattentional blindness are unclear for patients, but they must be considered.

More complex digital imaging types also introduce the additional interpretive problem of artefacts – unintentional imaging effects created by the technology itself. MRI artefacts may appear as black or white spots, duplicated or blurred images, or wavy lines. Luc Pauwels (2005) notes that medical imaging creates pictures of things we cannot perceive through direct observation; we rely on and trust the technology to take accurate pictures. The only ways to verify that the images are a correct translation of the body's interior are to repeat the imaging session or to open the patient surgically, both of which add not only stress to the illness experience, but also, potentially, physical trauma to the body. Trust and authority for accurate observation are transfered to the machine. An artefact, digital noise, something the machine accidentally produces, might be misinterpreted by a radiologist as an object of medical concern, yet even so, the digital reproduction is trusted as an objective representation. Even slight patient movement during an imaging session can produce artefacts. "Cross-talk," interference caused by tomographic slices that are too close together, appears as white dots on the image and can be interpreted as either an artefact or pathology. In all cases, the impact on the patient depends on the radiologist's interpretation of the digital error. The simultaneous trust of machines and the blindness to flaws in interpretation call into question the implications that such imaging has for the representation of the patient's condition.

Setting aside such technical aberrations, medical sociologist Kelly Joyce further examines the impact of MRIs on notions of authoritative knowledge and the physician construction of patients. Through an ethnographic analysis of imaging sites and interviews with physicians and technicians, Joyce discovers that the professionals producing and interpreting images "equate the image with the physicial body ... and authoritative knowledge" (2005, 437). In this conflation, the body and its image become interchangeable, with the image being perceived as a superior and neutral agent for expert knowledge production. A similar notion is reflected in genomics researcher Maud Radstake's (2007) work in real-time imaging, suggesting that images are more tangible and malleable to doctors than are patients' fleshy bodies. The diagnosis becomes an exchange between the physician and the image, in which the physical patient, and their psycho-emotional needs, may be disregarded. As with X-rays, MRI interpretation can be problematic; bodies are constructed as well or ill based on the interpretations of radiologists, who are usually working in isolation from patients. One of the radiologists interviewed by Prasad stated: "MRI images can give a perfect positive test but a perfect negative test is not possible," so clearly interpretation is paramount in deciding whether images indicate health problems (2005, 300).

Drawing on biotechnology theorist Donna Haraway, Prasad dubs the technological shift in the medical gaze as "cyborg visuality," in which "images have become bits of data in cyberspace that can be, and are, manipulated by human beings" (2005, 292; 310). Prasad observes that MRIs, and by extension other imaging technologies that construct images via computer algorithms, do not actually involve seeing, but rather a conversion of mathematical sequences into "spatial maps of internal parts of the body" allowing "an almost unlimited extension of the medical gaze" (309). "Cyborg visuality" seems similar to what Radstake calls "*black-boxing*," referring to the unseen computer magic that renders images from complex mathematical data measured from the patient's body (2007, 27). Waldby suggests that scanning imaging technologies that use tomography have a tendency for "calibrating living bodies according to the capacities of computer-generated space, and facilitating their surgical or orthopaedic reworking ... through a linkage with data homologs" (2000, 45). Reference to such homologs, the accepted anatomical norms of the human body, creates what Prasad dubs the radiologist's "bifocal vision" (2005, 301); the radiologist has one eye on images of the patient's body, and the other on normalising anatomical references.

Also alluding to Haraway, Waldby notes that the use of technology to reconfigure the subject body effectively blurs the historic line between human and machine, recasting the human body as purely informational. The transformation of the subject into mathematical computer data requires the body's systematic fragmentation and dismemberment, working on the assumption that the whole is, like a machine, merely the sum of its component parts (Waldby 2000). From a similar perspective, visual culture scholar Lisa Cartwright suggests that contemporary medical imaging renders notions of bodily interior and exterior obsolete, and subsumes the body into "part of a living system that incorporates the technologies of its representation" (1995, xiv). This kind of assertion is what leads sociologist Simon Williams to suggest that growing biotechnological control leads to a "moral, spiritual and existential crisis" of the corporeal body (1997, 1047). Because our bodies are increasingly plastic, can be rationalised and reconfigured almost at will, and are perceived as being at constant risk, the notion of the physical body becomes "ever more elusive and problematic" and strains to find meaning (1047). The blurring of lines between the human body and the technologically reproduced medical image supports Haraway's notion of the cyborg.

Published narratives of the imaging experience show how difficult it is to verbalise the effect of imaging on patients. Scholars experienced with using words in complex circumstances struggle with the language to effectively communicate such experiences. A review of the limited literature regarding patient imaging experiences reveals the ways in which researchers have struggled for expression. The images themselves are alluded to as mirrors (Radstake 2007, 116; Wall 2009, 139); evocative of a sense of ownership and bodily responsibility (Blaxter 2009, 771); something that "provokes simultaneously a curious sense of detachment from my own anatomy and a feeling of inhabiting, or being inhabited by, the image" (Wall 2009, 142); and reflecting the complex notion of "distributed embodiment" in which "bodies are multiplied to *include* images," simultaneously both here and there (Radstake 2007, 129; 134). Images create a strained mediation in our day-to-day entwined subject-object sense of embodiment. Medical illustrator Shelly Wall suggests that "self-objectification" through the imaging experience leads to feelings of vulnerability and violation, and that

Graphic representations of the body seem to both construct and trouble a person's sense of embodiment. They provide cognitive information that, like ill-fitting clothing, sits uncomfortably with how a person inhabits her body and alters how she moves and feels in it.

(2009, 139–40)

The othering effect of the image outside our lived-in bodies creates a unique self-consciousness.

While still-imaging types are discussed above, real-time imaging, such as ultrasound, endoscopy, fluoroscopy and angiography, raise unique problems. In *Vision of Illness* (2007), Radstake examines the experience of real-time imaging, specifically considering the impact of imaging sessions on notions of patient embodiment. While acknowledging that "medical images show everything but one's own body," at least as we usually view it, and that imaging "alienates patients from their bodies," Radstake complicates the idea of a subject-object dichotomy in the patient's experience of real-time imaging (6). While agreeing that imaging is a form of mediation, she also suggests that during real-time imaging, patients relate to their bodies both subjectively and objectively, that during such imaging sessions "bodies cannot self-evidently be distinguished from their images" (7; 6). Similar to Joyce's previously discussed finding that physicians conflate the patient body with MRI images, Radstake suggests that in real-time imaging, patients conflate their own bodies with the images. She argues that though image creation might objectify the patient, during real-time imaging, patients are simultaneously aware of their subjectivity because of communication with the physician or technician, their visual perception of the images, their embodied haptic awareness of the process, their cooperation and agency as a participant in the imaging process, and sometimes even an emotional attachment to the images. The moment of separation between subject and object body comes after the real-time imaging session, when still images from the session and the written report become fragmented data documents no longer attached to the individual patient's body, but interrogated in comparison with the norms of anatomically healthy bodies.

With the first anatomical atlas, the three-dimensional subject body became flattened, rationalised into two dimensions. Cartwright (1995) suggests that this corporeal flattening was symptomatic of a broader cultural distaste for humanity's messiness, and a desire to move towards a clearer, more rational human being. While advanced imaging technologies, such as CT, attempt to revive the body's third dimension, they still "read the body's interior as digitised information configured on a computer screen" (Waldby 2000, 5). Although the body has been technologically reinflated, imaging still tends to create a sense of

medical objectification ... which on the one hand augments and shores the status of the human, protecting subjects from the encroachments of diseased embodiment, and on the other generates its knowledges and procedures by treating the human as experimental object and passive biomass.

(Waldby 2007, 7)

X-rays, ultrasounds, CT scans, and MRIs construct images of the body's interior and in so doing, they flatten, isolate and objectify some part of the patient's anatomy. The individual human patient is unrecognisable and effectively abandoned in these images. Each imaging type offers an "objective truth," yet may not reveal the same truth as an alternative imaging type; for example, an MRI may detect different information from an X-ray, and therefore may not construct the same patient or disease state. It is not that some imaging technologies are false, but rather that technology has limitations, images are always subject to interpretation, and the subjective slippage between professionals within the field of image interpretation is surprisingly broad.

While interpretive error signals a serious problem in our trust of imaging technologies, another, more subtle problem exists: the notion that imaging is a benign activity. While it might be less obviously invasive than picking up a scalpel, it is still invasive. There is a felt intrusion on and in one's person; an intimate violation that has implications for the patient's selfhood. The gaze penetrates with the aim of gathering information to choose whether to intervene more obviously; the meaning of this gaze is that it has the potential to change the structure of the body into which it penetrates. Advanced imaging types, such as CT, PET, and MRI are more obviously intrusive; CTs may require the injection of a contrast medium, PETs require the injection of a radioactive tracer, and MRIs actively affect the body's atoms.

Drawing on Foucault, Prasad suggests that by attempting precise answers, the medical community seeks "to discipline the images and through that the human body" (2005, 301). "Disciplined" or "domesticated" images are, for Prasad, those presented and labelled in various types of anatomical atlases, as well as those presented in medical reports after they have been measured against these norms for signs of pathology. Bodies that deviate too much from these norms are considered pathological; the medical professional's role is to discipline such bodies through intervention so that they more closely meet standardised notions of human norms. To be tamed, to be rendered into a clear, coherent and unambiguous report, images must be interpreted, organised and labelled. As Potchen asserts, "The purpose of any diagnostic procedure is to diminish clinical uncertainty" (2014, 424). Prasad acknowledges that this is, however, an ideal; human bodies vary greatly according to genetics, gender, geography, demographics and age. Especially with older patients, imaging is likely to reveal numerous anomalies, and while these may deviate from the medical conception of the "normal" body, it does not necessarily mean that they are abnormal for a specific body, or that they impede function. Nevertheless, building on the existing Foucauldian notion of the medical gaze, even images that are digital reconstructions of data, rather than empirically or mechanically collected, retain and extend the power of the medical gaze.

Conclusion

The rapid growth of imaging technologies since the 1970s has led to their entrenchment in the modern hospital as a sophisticated addendum to a reductive medical gaze. Blaxter, Joyce, Waldby, Williams, and patient narrative scholar Arthur Frank all contend that because the image seems to trump everything else in contemporary medical discourse, the medical gaze has slipped into Jean Baudrillard's third order of simulacra, the hyperreal, in which the simulation is substituted for the real. Frank states that in this inverted world, "the image on the screen becomes the 'true' patient, of which the bedridden body is an imperfect replicant, less worthy of attention" (1992, 83). Unlike X-rays, which use photographic technology, more advanced digital imaging technologies render an image of which there is no "original copy," only algorithmic simulations with a variety of possible interpretations (Prasad 2005, 304). If patients no longer trust their own subjective reality, they may become even more reliant on doctors' interpretations of images to determine how they feel.

A 2013 TV Ontario panel titled "More or Less Medicine" on current affairs programme *The Agenda* explored the changing complexion of healthcare. During the panel, Dr. Doug Weir of the Ontario Medical Association asserted that a serious issue with instrumental medicine is that it can create "false reassurance … that if it's all clear, that somehow you're in good health," when this may not be the case, and may not reflect the patient's experience. For example, in adrenal fatigue, tests may indicate normal adrenal function, while the patient experiences unexplained feelings of general unwellness. If the individual patient's norm has dropped, they will notice the change, long before testing shows them outside the normal range. On the same panel, Dr. Danielle Martin, a family practitioner and Vice President of Medical Affairs and Health System Solutions at Toronto's Women's College Hospital, suggested, "perhaps we need to spend a little bit less time on the technology aspect of things and a little bit more time looking at the whole human being sitting in front of us." Technologies have enticed doctors away from listening, a foundational skill for good patient care.

The technological extension that imaging affords the Foucauldian medical gaze is, however, complex, both objectifying and constructing patients. Doctors sometimes seem unaware that a mediating biotechnological gaze can cause patients to feel objectified, to struggle to assert their subjectivity. More, better and faster imaging technologies may not lead to improved healthcare or professional relationships, and such technologies clearly problematise an already complicated site of communication between patients and physicians. Researchers agree that increased or better technologies are not the solution for the challenges of patient-practitioner relationships (Blaxter 2009; Prasad 2005). Patient-centred communication offers a way to bridge the gap between patient and practitioner, especially when such mediating technologies are used. The current direction of diagnostic medicine seems to indicate that in the not-too-distant future, physicians may more closely resemble computer technicians than healthcare practitioners, and the patient voice may be even further stifled. Rather than working to accommodate technological advances, perhaps physicians should refocus on building meaningful therapeutic relationships with their patients through improved communication.

Note

1 For a critical examination of General Electric's Vscan™, a hand-held ultrasound device, see Catherine Jenkins's "The Message in Medical Imaging Media: An Analysis of GE Healthcare's Vscan™" in *Finding McLuhan: The Man/The Mind/The Message* (Regina: University of Regina Press, 2015).

Reference list

Baumann, Brigitte, Esther H. Chen, Angela M. Mills, Lindsey Glaspey, Nicole M. Thompson, Molly K. Jones, and Michael C. Farner. July 2011. "Patient Perceptions of Computed Tomographic Imaging and Their Understanding of Radiation Risk and Exposure." *Annals of Emergency Medicine*, 58.1: 1–7.

Berrington de González, Amy, Mahadevappa Mahesh, Kwang-Pyo Kim, Mythreyi Bhargavan, Rebecca Lewis, Fred Mettler, and Charles Land. 14–28 December 2009. "Projected Cancer Risk from Computed Tomographic Scans Performed in the United States in 2007." *Archives of Internal Medicine*, 169.22: 2071–77.

Birkelo, Carl, W. Edward Chamberlain, Paul S. Phelps, Percy E. Schools, David Zacks, and Jacob Yerushalmy. 8 February 1947. "Tuberculosis Case Finding: A Comparison of the Effectiveness of Various Roentgenographic and Photofluorographic Methods." *Journal of the American Medical Association*, 133.6: 359–66.

Blaxter, Mildred. 2009. "The Case of the Vanishing Patient? Image and Experience." *Sociology of Health and Illness*, 31.5: 762–78.

Brenner, David J. and Eric J. Hall. 29 November 2007. "Computed Tomography – An Increasing Source of Radiation Exposure." *The New England Journal of Medicine*, 357.22: 2277–84.

Cartwright, Lisa. 1995. *Screening the Body: Tracing Medicine's Visual Culture*. Minneapolis: University of Minnesota Press.

Canadian Broadcasting Corporation (CBC) News. 12 April 2012. "Medical Scan Mistakes: What's Behind the Problems?" Accessed 12 April 2012. www.cbc.ca/news/canada/story/2012/04/10/canada-medical-scans-problems-review.html?cmp=rss.

Dam, H.J.W. April 1896. "The New Marvel in Photography." *McClure's Magazine*, 6.5: 403–15.

Foucault, Michel. 2006. *History of Madness*. Translated by Jonathan Murphy and Jean Khalfa. London and New York: Routledge.

Foucault, Michel. 1980. *The History of Sexuality: Volume I: An Introduction*. Translated by Robert Hurley. New York: Random House.

Foucault, Michel. 1973. *Birth of the Clinic: An Archaeology of Medical Perception*. Translated by A.M. Sheridan. London: Routledge.

Frank, Arthur. 1992. "Twin Nightmares of the Medical Simulacrum: Jean Baudrillard and David Cronenberg." *Jean Baudrillard: The Disappearance of Art and Politics*. Edited by William Stearns and William Chaloupka, 82–97. New York: St. Martin's Press.

Gladwell, Malcolm. 13 December 2004. "Annals of Technology: The Picture Problem: Mammography, Air Power, and the Limits of Looking." *The New Yorker*. Accessed 16 April 2010. www.gladwell.com/pdf/picture.pdf.

Gruver, Robert H. and Edward D. Freis. July 1957. "A Study of Diagnostic Errors." *Annals of Internal Medicine*, 47.1: 108–20.

Hayles, Katherine N. 1999. *How We Became Posthuman: Virtual Bodies in Cybernetics, Literature, and Informatics*. Chicago: University of Chicago Press.

Joyce, Kelly. June 2005. "Appealing Images: Magnetic Resonance Imaging and the Production of Authoritative Knowledge." *Social Studies of Science*, 35.3: 437–62.

Kolata, Gina. 29 October 2011. "Sports Medicine Said to Overuse a Popular Scan." *New York Times*. Accessed 29 October 2011. www.nytimes.com/2011/10/29/health/mris-often-overused-often-mislead-doctors-warn.html?pagewanted=1&_r=1&partner=rss&emc=rss&src=ig.

Kevles, Bettyann Holtzmann. 1997. *Naked to the Bone: Medical Imaging in the Twentieth Century*. New Brunswick, NJ: Rutgers University Press.

Korley, Frederick Kofi, Julius Cuong Pham, and Thomas Dean Kirsch. 6 October 2010. "Use of Advanced Radiology during Visits to US Emergency Departments for Injury-related Conditions, 1998–2007." *Journal of the American Medical Association*, 304.13: 1465–71.

Krupinski, Elizabeth A. 12 June 2000. "The Importance of Perception Research in Medical Imaging." *Radiation Medicine*, 18.6: 329–34.

Lehoux, Pascale. 2006. *The Problem of Health Technology: Policy Implications for Modern Health Care Systems*. New York: Routledge.

Lock, Margaret and Vihn-Kim Nguyyen. 2010. "Biomedical Technologies in Practice." *An Anthology of Biomedicine*, 17–31. Malden and Oxford: John Wiley & Sons.

Locsin, Rozzano C. 2005. *Technological Competency as Caring in Nursing: A Model for Practice*. Indianapolis, IN: Sigma Theta Tau International.

More or Less Medicine. 5 February 2013. *The Agenda with Steve Paikin*. TVOntario. TVO, Toronto. Television. Accessed 6 February 2013. http://ww3.tvo.org/video/187922/more-or-less-medicine.

New York Times. 29 May 1898. "Her Latest Photograph." Accessed 11 September 2013. http://query.nytimes.com/mem/archive-free/pdf?res=F10D14FD3A5D11738DDDA00A94DD405B8885F0D3.

Pauwels, Luc. September 2008. "An Integrated Model for Conceptualising Visual Competence in Scientific Research and Communication." *Visual Studies*, 23.2: 147–61.

Potchen, E. James. 2006. "Measuring Observer Performance in Chest Radiology: Some Experiences." *Journal of the American College of Radiology*, 3: 423–32.

Prasad, Amit. Spring 2005. "Making Images/Making Bodies: Visibilizing and Disciplining through Magnetic Resonance Imaging (MRI)." *Science, Technology, and Human Values*, 30.2: 291–316.

Radstake, Maud. 2007. *Visions of Illness: An Endography of Real-time Medical Imaging*. Delft: Eburon.

Reiser, Stanley Joel. 1978. *Medicine and the Reign of Technology*. Cambridge and New York: Cambridge University Press.

van Dijck, José. 2005. *The Transparent Body: A Cultural Analysis of Medical Imaging*. Seattle: University of Washington Press.

Waldby, Catherine. 2000. *The Visible Human Project: Informatic Bodies and Posthuman Medicine*. New York: Routledge.

Wall, Shelley. 2009. "The View from Inside: Gendered Embodiment and the Medical Representation of Sex." *Critical Interventions in the Ethics of Healthcare: Challenging the Principles of Autonomy in Bioethics*. Edited by Stuart J. Murray and Dave Holmes, 133–46. Farnham: Ashgate.

Williams, Simon J. October 1997. "Modern Medicine and the 'Uncertain Body': From Corporeality to Hyperreality?" *Social Science and Medicine*, 45.7: 1041–49.

Part III

Limits of medical intervention

11 The fairytale narratives of plastic surgery makeover TV shows in South Korea

Surgical metamorphosis, the "surgical gaze," and the permeability of medical knowledge

Carmen Voinea

"A miracle! A life-changing experience for women who are suffering because of their physical appearance. We aim to change lives and open doors of opportunities for women who are robbed of their confidence due to their physical appearance" (Korean Plastic Surgery Experience 2014). With these lines the audience is introduced to the universe of the reality makeover television show *Let Me In*.[1] It is a universe that promises from the very beginning a story of magical transformation and creates a world in which real people (mostly women) are relieved of their suffering and offered new opportunities in life through surgical metamorphosis. From the onset, the medium of the makeover show offers no possible outcome other than a happy ending.

Following Walter R. Fisher's proposal to re-conceptualise humankind as *homo narrans*, where "all forms of human communication need to be seen fundamentally as stories" (Fisher 1987, xi), this chapter explores the universe of medically enhanced makeover reality TV shows through narrative analysis. In this globalised, standardised and, at times, restrictive medium, medicine, with its authority and powers of bodily enhancement, meets one of the most intrinsic human needs: that of transformation, of personal and social fulfillment. At the same time, considering the innate need of humans to assign meaning to events and organise them in a coherent personal narrative, I will show how, through the surgical metamorphosis that happens onscreen, the participants of these makeover shows tell their stories of hope for a better life with narratives of overcoming their social background, of familial ties, and of beauty and femininity. Fairytale tropes are embedded in the narrative arc of the shows and in the contestants' stories. At first the participants may be seen as passive subjects of the TV producers and of the medical authority; they are put in the hands of the surgeons who create beauty and consequently prepare the patients for a successful life. These medical agents do more than just modify bodies; they teach the participants and the audience to use the medical jargon, and to see as surgeons. In this highly visual medium, the surgical or the "medical gaze" becomes dominant. However, through the inherent human need for meaning, medical knowledge becomes permeable to structures of common knowledge at a linguistic, visual and narrative level. Participants therefore restore some of their agency and actively transform expert knowledge, embedding it with their subjectivities through stories of personal suffering and transformation.

Through a narrative inquiry into the universe of the Korean makeover TV show *Let Me In*, I will highlight the underlying theme in the medium's strict structure: the surgical metamorphosis of the participants, which is causally linked to a story of transformation, of personal and social success. As Cressida J. Heyes shows in her analysis of *Extreme Makeover*,[2] makeover shows about plastic surgery "exploit fantasy narratives of radical transformation, and ... tell a sanitized fairy tale of identity becoming, in which the makeover enables the recipient to achieve longstanding personal goals presented as intrinsic to her own individual authenticity" (2007, 21). It will also be emphasised that these happy-ending bound shows are filled with tropes of fairytale inspiration. If "rarely do wonder tales end unhappily" (Zipes 2007, 4), neither do the contestants' stories in all the five seasons of *Let Me In*. The similarity between these shows and fairytales has also been discussed by media studies researchers, such as Jack Z. Bratich (2007), for whom "the closest cultural form to RTV [reality television] is actually the fairytale. With its emphasis on metamorphosis and transformation, RTV takes on the cultural function of the archaic fairy or wonder tale" (7). Consequently, the surgical change at the hands of the surgeons as representatives of the scientific objectivism can be interpreted as lending the fairytale transformation more power through the scientific rationality and objectivity of medical knowledge, an inherent and almost mythologised characteristic of the social sciences' discourse around medicine.

As in a fairytale, the participants of *Let Me In* are helped in their transformation by various agents. It is important to note here that the name of the show is a Chinese/English pun that comes from the Chinese characters for beautiful 美 (sounds like "me") and person 人 (sounds like "in"). While the metamorphosis staff includes surgeons, dentists, stylists and make-up artists, surgeons play the most important role. They are the active agents of metamorphosis, the creators of beauty, the "fairy godmothers" helping Cinderella-like women to metaphorically shed their meager background clothes, or the Frog Prince its skin, and to achieve beauty while overcoming their social standing. The fairytale metaphors I am using are embedded in the show's narratives and are most striking in the nicknames given to contestants. Grossly accentuating their defects, and even sometimes pathologising their appearance, the nicknames range from "Jaws" to "Frankenstein," "The Abandoned Wife," "The Son-like Daughter," or "The Half-faced Bride-to-be." These examples are taken from the website of ID Hospital, the clinic that sponsors the show and whose doctors perform the surgeries. In regard to how these representations of the participants' "ugliness" are visually supported through montage, the close-ups from the Before section of the show raise them to almost grotesque proportions. In her analysis of cosmetic surgery reality TV shows, Meredith Jones argues that participants' experiences of "almost magical transformations" are sometimes "the stuff of fairy tales and horror stories" and that this medium "has more in common with these older narratives than we might first think, sharing with them themes of rebirth, transition, hardship, endurance, and eventually reward and fulfillment" (Jones 2008, 517). The surgeons as agents of metamorphosis intervene to medically evaluate the contestants' features and to erase their physical defects in order to create a body beautiful. The surgeons' successful intervention is confirmed once again by the medium. In the After section, during the climactic Reveal, the same contestants are received in awe by the audience and presenters. Their looks will be compared to that of "modern princesses," celebrities and (Barbie) dolls: "as beautiful as a celebrity," "just like a star," and "more beautiful than a star" are recurrent evaluations of the surgically enhanced participants.

If fairytale-inspired depictions of patients' bodies have made their way to clinics' websites, showing how linguistically permeable medical knowledge can be, in the all-encompassing medium of the makeover shows, the surgeons' expert knowledge becomes even more permeable to the narrative structures of common knowledge. This linguistic and narrative permeability is simultaneous as can be seen in the fact that surgeons borrow expressions that also carry narrative meaning like "First Lady Facelift," "Bambi eye surgery," "V-line surgery," or "Customized Barbie Line Rhinoplasty" (ID hospital id 2017a, 2017b, 2017c). That such expressions can be found more often on the websites of plastic surgery clinics and tend to replace medical terms is of tantamount importance. Of obvious "modern" fairytale inspiration, they might serve the purpose of "humanising" sterile medical terms for the clinics' possible clientele. If we move outside the realm of reality TV, in the past two to three decades, researchers like Jones (2009) and Haiken (1997) have found that the dynamic between surgeon and patient has also been changing, altering the former's strong authority due to the need to conform to the consumer needs of the patient. Cosmetic surgery is one of the medical specialties that are found at the intersection with the consumer society dynamic and one of the most subordinated to it. It is a medical industry that also reflects the move of medicine from necessary health intervention to elective medical treatments that conform to business-like marketing strategies. In order to make the surgical change appealing, the doctors also need to adapt their medical vocabulary and to adopt popular narratives that capture patients' hopes of transformation. And what Korean woman would not want to become as beautiful and prestigious as a First Lady, or have a Barbie-like innocent beauty? The dynamic, of Foucauldian inspiration, that Armstrong, among others, has described is even more relevant in the context of a consumer society: in the relationship between doctor and patient, doctors are also evaluated and need to conform to the patient's hopes and needs: "the subject of knowledge became the object of knowledge," and "visibility was effectively reversed. For nearly two centuries, the eye of medicine had surveyed and fashioned the patient; now the naked form of the doctor was revealed to a penetrating gaze" (Armstrong 2002, 3).

Having mentioned visibility and the relationship between doctor and patient as subjects and objects of medical knowledge and their changing dynamic, it is necessary at this point to introduce some conceptual background. In this visual medium, the way participants and audience are taught to see as a medical expert will be referred to as the "surgical gaze." I have chosen to use this phrase instead of the more generic "medical gaze" as it is more appropriate for this particular field of analysis. In the makeover shows, the surgeons are the key representatives of medicine. As we will see, the surgeons as medical actors bring their own specificities and are different creatures than the clinicians that, for example, were found in Foucault's *Birth of the Clinic* (1963), the cardinal work for conceptualising the medical gaze and the evolution of modern medical knowledge. I will therefore use the surgical gaze concept in a manner similar to the more recent research of Sue Tait, for whom "viewers of surgical television are trained to survey the other with a surgeon's gaze, the ability to position one outside of, or speak back to surgical culture is increasingly confounded" (2007, 119). Through their expert authority, the surgeons' gaze is imposed on the contestants and the audience. Foucault's influence is, however, undisputed in regard to the link between what is seen and how it is communicated. For him, the birth of modern medicine towards the end of the eighteenth century is based on an important discontinuity, in the clinic-anatomical medicine dynamic,

> the relation between the visible and invisible – which is necessary to all concrete knowledge – changed its structure, revealing through gaze and language what had previously been below and beyond their domain. A new alliance was forged between words and things, enabling one to see and to say.
>
> (Foucault 2003, xiii)

From the middle of the twentieth century, as Armstrong points out, there has been a move towards patients' social narratives and subjectivities penetrating medical knowledge. Patients began to have a voice that was symptomatic of their "social milieu," of "their idiosyncratic self, their feelings, and their own experiences of the world," and

> patients' words, as they described their symptoms, were no longer a vicarious gaze to the silent pathology within the body but the precise technique by which the new space of disease could be established; illness was being transformed from what was visible to what was heard.
>
> (Armstrong 2002, 68, 65)

However, doctors still maintain a strong authority over patients and, sometimes, as Kaw shows in her research on the medicalisation of racial features for Asian-American women, they are perpetuating normative racial and gender ideologies that make women "mutilate" their bodies (1993, 75). Although Kaw's findings can be debated, we can follow Armstrong in acknowledging that patients are

> the constructs of medicine; their self-perceptions are themselves medically contaminated and – the parallel would be with Pygmalion – they can be

studied only as they have been rendered visible (which is as much as to say invisible) by the "medical gaze."

(Armstrong 2002, 2)

It can be concluded that "medical gaze," or, in the makeover shows analysis, the "surgical gaze," is representative of the power of doctors' authority over patients, but we should also take note of an ongoing dynamic that makes medical knowledge and its agents permeable to the patients' desire and to common knowledge on various levels.

It has been indicated that the integration of patients' subjectivities and their social background into the discussion about bodily enhancement can impact the discourse about medical knowledge. This becomes even more visible in the context of the makeover shows, as the medium's strict Before and After narrative arc inextricably links the Before to the suffering caused by the participants' physical appearance, and the After to the happiness achieved through surgical change. Both moments are tied together by surgical metamorphosis and carry deeper social implications. As the majority of the participants are from working-class backgrounds and cannot afford the surgeries, the suffering caused by their supposed physical defects is also due to their exclusion from the consumer market of plastic surgeries in South Korea. As Joanna Elfving-Hwang argues, the show deliberately "positions the contestants within the 'cosmetic underclass' (*miyong hawui kyegŭp*) of those who are considered unable to succeed because of their appearance and lack of means to fix their perceived flaws" (Elfving-Hwang 2009, 3). Consequently, the After section restores social justice. In a country where there is a conceptual and linguistic delimitation between "marriage cosmetic surgery" and "employment cosmetic surgery" solely in regard to the goal to be achieved surgically (for example, to attract a marriage partner or to secure a job), beauty is considered essential for succeeding in life (Holliday and Elfving-Hwang 2012, 74). Therefore, we can follow Alexander Edmonds in his analysis of the Brazilian plastic surgery phenomenon and conceptualise beauty as a social right, "where rights are re-interpreted as access to goods and the antidote to social exclusion is imagined as market participation" (2007, 371). That these shows' transformations ultimately create "subjects adequate to new economic and social conditions" is an aspect also captured by Jack Z. Bratich (2007, 7). The stories of their social background and their socio-economic suffering legitimate the need of medical intervention. As Schleifer and Vannatta show, this is not a modern development: "there has always been a close link between narrative and medicine – the oldest and among the most revered narratives in the Western culture are the ancient Greek tragedies that focused, like medicine, on human suffering" (2013, 258).

Before proceeding to analysing the way contestants' transformation stories are told and visually organised around the strict Before and After structure of the shows, it is important to highlight how the mix of magical and real-life elements, embedded with medical knowledge, can affect and determine viewers' preferences for plastic surgery. A North-American quantitative, survey-based study examined the perceptions of cosmetic surgery patients about these shows and whether these perceptions influence their decision making (Crockett, Pruzinsky, and Persing 2007). The authors, although warning that a causal relationship cannot be postulated based on the methodology used, found that

> there seems to be a significant association between viewing intensity of plastic surgery reality television shows and how patients perceive their own knowledge about plastic surgery, the similarity of these shows to real life, and the influence that these shows exert on patient decision making to seek consultation.
>
> (Crockett, Pruzinsky, and Persing 2007, 323)

Though no such studies have been found for South Korea, it can be argued that these media products do not have only an entertainment function; they also spread medical knowledge, making the surgical interventions attainable and, using Sue Tait's concept, "domesticating" the practice among viewers (Tait 2007).

Let Me In: stories of transformation in a globalised Korean makeover show

The characteristics of the makeover shows that were highlighted previously are not specific to a certain culture. They are shared by the Korean *Let Me In*, the British *10 Years Younger*, and the American *Extreme Makeover* or *The Swan* (which draws its name from "The ugly duckling" fairytale), to name a few. All these makeover shows tap into a globalised format that has at its foundation the narrative of transformation through surgical metamorphosis. For Sue Tait, such TV shows have played a significant role in the "domestication" of plastic surgery and this process has been done in "increasingly globalised contexts" (2007, 119). It is important to note that even though the narrative of transformation is the common characteristic, the Korean makeover shows present important cultural differences, and the main one I will stress pertains exactly to this narrative of transformation.

Since most of the literature used in this chapter is European and North-American, it is important to note that Western fantasies of transformation, of success by and for oneself, of individual self-affirmation, or aligning the outer appearance with the inner self through surgery (Heyes 2007, Jones 2008) are not entirely applicable to South Korean plastic surgery subjects. As Bratich emphasises, the "powers of transformation" of American makeover shows rest upon the assumption that "the capacity for reinvention is part of the American mythos. From the Jeffersonian self-made citizen to melting-pot ideologies, the American character has been defined around the ability to alter oneself in accordance with changing contexts" (2007, 8). The narrative tropes of individuality such as "from rags to riches" or "the self-made man" do not adequately describe the *Let Me In* contestants' hopes of transformation, and this can be exemplified by the active participation of their families on the show. The fantasies of transformation through surgical metamorphosis in South Korea originate more from the pressures of a collectivistic, competitive society, where one needs to conform to the norm and pragmatically use one's body as a vehicle for success (Voinea 2017). In Elfving-Hwang's view, it is also about family and "filial piety," as she argues that "cosmetic surgery in Korean popular narratives relates more to 'doing' surgery for the sake of performing a certain social class or status" (Jones, 2012; Sanchez Taylor, 2012), than it does to "'becoming' more the image that one holds of one's 'inner self'" (Elfving-Hwang 2013, 2). As Bondebjerg stressed, we should therefore talk about these globalised media-culture products in a "glocalized" perspective:

> as a massive media trend reality TV belongs to the deregulated and globalized media-culture of the 90s and onwards. In many ways reality TV combines a global format with a very "glocalized" perspective.... The same global formats create very different programs and social reactions.
>
> (2002, 159)

The globalised media culture has successfully disseminated not only the format of the makeover show, but also its characteristic narrative tropes like Cinderella. However, with a brief look at the metamorphosis trope in South Korean folklore, it can be argued that it is not a Western addition, but something that it is traditionally found in Korean folk-tales, legends, or fairytales, and is linked to fantasies of upward social mobility, although often with tragic endings. The shape-shifting moments occur, like in the legend of the "Lovesick Snake," when a protagonist of low social standing falls in love with someone higher in the social hierarchy: "conflict involving social class is a major factor in the haunting of spirit, and shape-shifting serves as a means of an individual expression which is prohibited in reality" (National Folk Museum of Korea 2014, 172). From premodern times, Korean fairytales of metamorphosis have therefore carried deeper social implications of class struggle and fantasies of personal transformation.

In order to understand the collective fantasies of transformation in South Korea, it is necessary to outline how they are related to the plastic surgery phenomenon. To give a statistical background, South Korea was in fourth place regarding total surgical procedures performed internationally in 2015 (ISAPS 2016). Unfortunately, the 2016 data for South Korea in the International Society of Aesthetic Plastic Surgery (ISAPS) survey is not available as not enough plastic surgeons provided their numbers. Older surveys, however, seem to confirm that South Korea is in a leading position worldwide regarding the number of cosmetic surgeries per capita (Voinea 2017). What made plastic surgeries so popular in South Korea is a complex discussion and would need a short historical overview. A previous study suggested that young women's motivations for undergoing surgery are related to the modernisation process of South Korea and the deep societal transformations of its society (Voinea 2017). Starting with the colonial period, the body of young Koreans became the predilect site to show their desires to participate in the modernisation project (Yoo 2001). During the Korean War, the encounter with Western bodies and surgeons, such as David Ralph Millard, Jr., who wanted to "normalize" the "Oriental eye" (Haiken 1997, 201), opened the way for what would become the desire, albeit debatable, of Koreans to look more Caucasian. During South Korea's economic boom, as women's bodies have been transformed into "consumer bodies" (Kim 2003, 98), their physical features became a site of transformation and investment. Today, women's motivations to change their bodies surgically "are derived from a pragmatic, instrumentalist view of the body as a vehicle for success in life, with two main goals: professional and personal" (Voinea 2017).

Unraveling the Before and After of *Let Me In*: familial ties, femininity, and professional aspirations

The contestants of *Let Me In* are, in their vast majority, young women from working-class backgrounds, with diverse motivations for changing their bodies, and various perceived physical defects. The structure of Before and After shows them in their evolution from the humble presentation of suffering caused by their appearance and their lack of means to change it, to the great reveal where they come to embody middle-class beauty. As Elfving-Hwang claims, the surgeries are not only about "fixing flaws and erasing evidence of aging, but also to literally embody the markers of middle class consumerist success" (2013, 3). A middle-class beauty is also the ideal that Meredith Jones (2004) finds representative for the contemporary plastic surgery phenomenon that isolates bodies from each other and eliminates individuality. Furthermore, South Korean makeover shows also transform participants' bodies towards a strict, normative Korean specific standard of a body beautiful: an innocent look with "a small face, pointy chin, high nose, visible forehead, under eye bags" (Voinea 2017, 14).

The Before part of *Let Me In* consists of the stories of two contestants competing for the chance to be "let in" the show. The *mise-en-scène* of the contestants' confessions of suffering makes use of melodramatic lights, music and voiceover. The participants place themselves and are placed in a position of inferiority, with humiliating close ups of their physical defects, and images from their dysfunctional private lives. Both contestants share stories of isolation, humiliation, depression, sadness, abuse from strangers and even, sometimes, from family due to their physical appearance. After the dramatic presentation of their suffering, a group of medical experts analyses their physical features and, on the basis of the greater abnormality and consequent suffering, they choose the person who will be let in the show. As Sue Tait notes, "these consultations with the surgeon function to extend the surgeon's gaze into the culture" (2007, 126). The fact that not only physical but also social and emotional features are important in the surgeons' decision comes to confirm how narratives are integrated in the medical evaluation and decision making. I will concentrate on three such narrative threads and how they pertain to Korean women's hopes of transformation, of overcoming their social background: familial ties; femininity; and professional aspirations. The Before part is the section of the show that allocates most space for such narratives.

Ji Hyun's story is that of strong "filial piety." She is verbally and even physically abused by her father for carrying the facial features of her mother, who left her family many years before. Ji Hyun admits that she wants "to erase my mother's vestige from my face" and by the end of the show she is "reborn as a beloved daughter" (ID Hospital Korea Plastic Surgery 2016a). Using Elfving-Hwang's analytical frame of the makeover show, this is a telling example of how plastic surgery embodies "filial piety." Without contesting her father's abuse, the daughter is willing to subject herself to surgery in order to restore the injustice inflicted upon their family by her mother. It could be argued that the scene of the father's abuse had been staged, but this is of lesser importance than the fact that the producers decided to include this narrative arc in the show. In the economy of *Let Me In*, showing "filial piety" by erasing an undesired genetic heritage is more important than the suffering caused by the father.

The abuse of Ji Hyun is an exceptional scenario, as most testimonials of friends and family come to support the contestants' plight and offer solidarity. In the collectivistic society of South Korea, a family member's suffering extends to the entire family. A protagonist of an episode, nicknamed "The Mask," begged the *Let Me In* staff on her knees for the chance to participate in the makeover show, as did her father on her behalf (StoryonTV 2014). Her successful metamorphosis was, in the end, welcomed with tearful eyes by her supportive mother. In another case, incapable of offering their son financial support, parents sent a letter themselves to the producers requesting help. Isolated from the rest of the world due to weight loss that left him with excess skin and temperamental problems, the first male participant of the show, Park Jin-Bae had a fairytale-like metamorphosis. "Shedding his skin," he was surgically transformed "from country boy to celebrity" (Korean Plastic Surgery Experience 2014).

The families' lower-class backgrounds and scarce financial resources that do not allow the surgical metamorphosis impact not only the children's present, but also their futures and hopes of a fulfilled life. As discussed previously, participating in the makeover show is presented as a way to restore social justice. The "Singer who can't sing" is a young woman whose musical talent and possible career was stopped due to abnormal jaw joint growth. Her mother's testimony is filled with remorse for their economic situation. She admits that she was even accused of not being able to offer her daughter the chance to have surgery, therefore not fulfilling her duty as a mother and provider: "If I had money I would've done it for her, but the financial situation was not so good. And everyone asked why I am not helping her to do the surgery" (ID Hospital Korea Plastic Surgery 2016b).

The role of the families on the show is not only relevant to the background of the participants, but also indicative of the intricate stories of transformation in South Korea, where it is not only about self-transformation and individual becoming, but about the family's identity and social position. Families are essential parts of children's past and future. As Elfving-Hwang shows, contestants' parents are shown to apologize to their children for passing on "faulty" genes to their daughters (*pumo-rŭl jal mot manass ŏ*), and also for lacking the funds to "fix" these "faults" through surgery (again enforcing the idea of the existence of a "cosmetic underclass" of those who cannot afford to fix their flaws).

(2013, 4)

For many women coming from this "cosmetic underclass" the main goal for altering their bodies is to succeed professionally. The surgical metamorphosis is therefore put in the service of a professional evolution. One participant who was preparing to start a career has admitted that the need for physical improvement is necessary in the competitive environment: "people my age are looking for a job and I really feel that having a soft image is important for finding a job since it is so competitive these days" (ID Hospital Korea Plastic Surgery 2014a). While looking for a job, another contestant was herself trying to improve her looks by modifying the pictures on her CV. Unfortunately, during job interviews this temporary alteration came apart and was frowned upon by her potential employers (StoryonTV 2014).

The previous testimony also brings to light another aspect, that a "soft image" is a key attribute for a feminine appearance. The participant nicknamed the "Singer who can't sing" received similar remarks prior to the surgery: "before she looked strong willed, now she is lovely" (ID Hospital Korea Plastic Surgery 2016b). Medical intervention therefore also comes to confirm the binary categories of femininity and masculinity. Surgeons include in their medical evaluations remarks pertaining to these categories, and this can be seen as another example of how medical knowledge is permeable to common knowledge and its cultural categories. A participant who was given the nickname "The son-like daughter" (ID Hospital id 2017d) is a relevant example of how, through surgical metamorphosis and with the help of medical experts, gender binaries are reinforced. Another young contestant's face was evaluated by a surgeon as "having a rough shape, a masculine physiognomy that needs to be corrected urgently" (ID Hospital Korea Plastic Surgery 2014b).

The mothers who come to regain their femininity and their young appearance are also typical cases of metamorphosis in makeover shows, what Jones calls "mommy makeover" (2008). "The Flat-Chested Mother" was a young mother who admitted that she "was not a woman anymore" and surgery "will bring her life back." With the help of the surgeons who did a "bikini breast augmentation surgery," they corrected her "male figure" and through this surgical "miracle" she was "born again" (ID Hospital Korea Plastic Surgery 2013). It is important here to stress the linguistic choice of the surgeon for the name of the medical intervention and the fact that all this contributed to reinforcing gender categories, and the examples are numerous.

My focus has mostly been on the Before section of the makeover shows and on presenting key narratives found in participants' stories. In unraveling the structure of the makeover show it is also important to briefly describe the middle section, as it is the segment where the candidates are most passive. They are presented in the sterile environments of the medical world; shots of medical equipment, X-ray, and bandages dominate this section of the show. The surgical gaze reigns over the participants' transformation. Left in the care of nurses, with no mirrors around and their faces wrapped in bandages, they are deprived of their own reflection. They are completely removed from their day-to-day lives, and are immersed in the medical universe fabricated on the set.

Although in real life this is the longest (around two to three months) and most difficult part of a participant's surgical metamorphosis, in the temporality of the makeover shows it gets similar or even less air-time than the Before and After sections. Here, the timeline gets twisted as in a fairytale, where days can be as long as years and years can pass in seconds. This is reminiscent of Bakhtin's theory of the chronotope, where "hours are dragged out, days are compressed into moments, it becomes possible to bewitch time itself" (Bakhtin 1981, 154). In the space of makeover shows, however, time and space are dictated by the show's producers and the surgeons, while the audience is purposely bewitched through the staged presentation of participants' time and space altered stories.

At this point, it is important to mention the main traits of the After section, the climactic part of the show, which could be said is the one most in the realm of fairytale, the part in which the fantastic metamorphosis is revealed. Makeover shows, more than other types of reality TV, leave no space for unexpected twists; the contestants are bound for a happy ending, visually constructed around the great reveal. Jones and Elfving-Hwang have associated the moment of the reveal to a rebirth and we saw the same metaphor in contestants' testimonies. This is the most dramatic part of the show; the presenters and the audience are in awe, there are loud, vocal expressions of wonder, and even expressions of disbelief at the extent of the transformation. The contestants are compared to modern princesses, celebrities, dolls. The metamorphosis is so dramatic that some contestants find it hard to recognise themselves; during one show, a presenter dramatically pinches a contestant to show she is not dreaming (ID Hospital Korea Plastic Surgery 2016b).

The After part is the section in which the surgeons, through their post-surgical evaluations, come to confirm the surgical metamorphosis; their medical vocabulary becomes most reflective of the permeability to common terminology. In the examples that follow we encounter once more the gender categories previously discussed. A surgeon evaluates his intervention on a young male participant as follows: "I created a straighter [jaw] line for a more masculine, cool, celebrity like look" (Korean Makeover TV Show, 2014). In the case of a female participant, the surgeon concluded that the orthognathic and jaw reduction surgeries gave the patient "a warmer image, a cuter appearance" and her nose was also modified for a "more feminine appearance" (ID Hospital Korea Plastic Surgery, 2014b).

In several cases, the After part extends into real life. The producers offer glimpses of participants' evolution to confirm the successful transformation of their lives and further emphasise the causal link between appearance and success. The aforementioned male participant is presented on a date, which was set up by a former contestant, one of the most popular participants of *Let Me In*, who has admitted being successful in finding a partner after the surgery (Korean Makeover TV Show, 2014).

During the Before, After, and especially the middle section of the show, medical knowledge becomes permeable to common knowledge on a narrative, linguistic and visual level. In this media universe, filled with narratives of trans-formation and fairytale-like metamorphosis, the participants are almost passive subjects, subordinated to the Before and After structure. Their human agency is put in the hands of the surgeons as creators of beauty and consequently of a better future. They are taught how to see surgically, to speak the medical jargon, and to integrate medical evaluations of their bodies into their narrative of trans-formation. As Tait, following Belling, has indicated, we witness "the creation of 'expert' patients via reality television depicting medical operations. Similarly, surgical make-over shows offer a pedagogy which equips the viewer for the sur-geon's office" (Tait 2007, 126). In this highly visual medium, it is the surgical gaze which dominates. However, medicine and its agents are not infallible to the marked narrative medium and this is where the patient-contestants restore some of their agency, although not intentionally, but mediated by the show's structure. The medical gaze borrows the pervasive fairytale tropes. If at times "ugliness" is medicalised through the use of medical equipment and scientific measurements, a reverse dynamic also takes place: in this visual medium, close-ups of patients' features, X-rays, medical tests are arranged to tell a story, to depict in a grot-esque manner the subjects' need of metamorphosis.

Conclusion

In the narrative arc of the show, the surgeon becomes more than just a scientist; he becomes the creator of beauty and the agent of transformation. His role is to causally link physical appearance to success and legitimate the surgical meta-morphosis in a person's story of transformation. Sometimes his intervention is as direct as, for instance, offering a job to a freshly made-over participant (Korean Plastic Surgery Experience 2013). Furthermore, the surgeons them-selves become active participants of the show. While disseminating medical knowledge, they are also borrowing common knowledge terminology and nar-rative structures. As participants, the doctors are tapping into the narrative of success. The successful metamorphosis of the patients also becomes their per-sonal and professional success. One surgeon, evaluating his patient's transforma-tion, said that "She looks so beautiful after the surgery. I feel very good that her natural beauty came to life after the surgery," while another stated that "After I saw her, I said to myself I did a very good job with the surgery" (ID Hospital Korea Plastic Surgery 2014). Describing the surgeries as "miracles" is a frequent occurrence on the shows, and so is comparing doctors to "God." In the case of a transgender female participant, the surgeons' work was depicted as an "unbe-lievable miracle," a presenter even exclaiming "Can I say you are all god-like doctors?" (View Plastic Surgery 2014). Associating plastic surgeons with the Pygmalion myth, with miracle makers, creators, or having God-like abilities, is not a new thing in the social history of plastic surgery, or, indeed, of medicine more broadly, and has been analysed by several researchers in this field. To name only one, Kathy Davis (2003) discusses at length the Pygmalion myth and how male plastic surgeons modify and control women's bodies. Although an aspect not tackled in this chapter, on the makeover shows, as well as in the plastic surgery industry, the surgeons are in their vast majority men, while the subjects are women. I have chosen not to pursue a gender studies direction in this chapter; however, it must be noted that feminist studies are a rich source of inspiration for the plastic surgery subject.

The makeover TV shows' plastic surgeon is a strange creature. He is a creator of beauty and a conveyor of success to his patients; he is an active agent in the surgical metamorphosis and contestants' stories of transformation; he disseminates medical knowledge and teaches participants and the audience to see surgically. The contestant of *Let Me In* is *homo narrans* in search of fulfillment: she goes through the surgical metamorphosis to look for the fairytale happy ending; she tells stories of familial ties, of professional dreams, and is looking for her femininity. She is, most of the time, a passive participant subjected to the surgical gaze. However, through her stories of transformation, medical knowledge is also transformed. She is recovering her agency by disseminating common knowledge, fairytale tropes, and embedding narratives in the medical discourse. Patient-contestant and surgeon are both actors controlled by the medium; the makeover show's strict structure dictates the surgical metamorphism happy ending, directs and assigns roles, and ultimately controls what is seen and told.

Notes

1 A South Korean television programme broadcasted on channel Story-on, 2 December 2011–11 September 2015.
2 An American reality makeover television series broadcasted on ABC, December 2002–July 2007.

Reference list

Armstrong, David. 2002. *A New History of Identity. A Sociology of Medical Knowledge*. New York: Palgrave.
Bakhtin, Mikhail. 1981. "Form of Time and Chronotope in the Novel." *The Dialogic Imagination: Four Essays*. Austin: University of Texas Press.
Bondebjerg, I. 2002. "The Mediation of Everyday Life: Genre Discourse and Spectacle in Reality TV." In *Realism and "Reality" in Film and Media*, edited by A. Jerslev, 159–92. Copenhagen: Museum Tusculanum Press.
Bratich, Jack Z. 2007. "Programming Reality. Control Societies, New Subjects and the Powers of Transformation." In *Makeover Television. Realities Remodelled*, edited by Dana Heller, 6–23. London: I.B. Tauris.

Crockett, Richard J., Pruzinsky, Thomas, and Persing, John A. 2007. "The Influence of Plastic Surgery 'Reality TV' on Cosmetic Surgery Patient Expectations and Decision Making." *Plastic & Reconstructive Surgery*, 120.1: 316–24.

Davis, Kathy. 2003. *Dubious Equalities and Embodied Difference. Cultural Studies on Cosmetic Surgery*. Lanham, MD: Rowman and Littlefield.

Edmonds, Alexander. 2007. "The Poor Have the Right to Be Beautiful: Cosmetic Surgery in Neoliberal Brazil." *Journal of the Royal Anthropological Institute*, 13.2: 363–81.

Elfving-Hwang, Joanna. 2013. "Cosmetic Surgery and Embodying the Moral Self in South Korean Popular Makeover Culture." *The Asia-Pacific Journal*, 11.24: 1–11.

Fisher, Walter R. 1987. *Human Communication as Narration: Toward a Philosophy of Reason, Value, and Action*. Columbia: University of South Carolina Press.

Foucault, Michel. 2003. *Birth of the Clinic*. London: Routledge.

Haiken, Elizabeth. 1997. *Venus Envy: A History of Cosmetic Surgery*. Baltimore, MD: Johns Hopkins University Press.

Heyes, Cressida J. 2007. "Cosmetic Surgery and the Televisual Makeover." *Feminist Media Studies*, 7.1: 17–32.

Holliday, Ruth, and Elfving-Hwang, Joanna. 2012. "Gender, Globalization and Aesthetic Surgery in South Korea." *Body & Society*, 18.2: 58–81.

ID Hospital id. 2017a. "Bambi Eye Surgery." Accessed 20 April 2017. http://eng.idhospital.com/eye/bambi/.

ID Hospital id. 2017b. "Customized Barbie Line Rhinoplasty." Accessed 20 April 2017. http://eng.idhospital.com/nose/vavinose/.

ID Hospital id. 2017c. "First Lady Facelift." Accessed 20 April 2017. http://eng.idhospital.com/antiaging/facelift/.

ID Hospital id. 2017d. "Let Me In." Accessed 7 May 2017. http://eng.idhospital.com/letmeinbest/.

ID Hospital Korea Plastic Surgery. 2016a. "Let Me In Eng Sub | She Became Barbie! Face Contouring, Orthognathic Surgery, Pt. 1." Accessed 20 April 2017. www.youtube.com/watch?v=B5kqM1dAeEs.

ID Hospital Korea Plastic Surgery. 2016b. "Eng sub) ID Hospital: Let Me In 5, Korea Plastic Surgery Part 1." Accessed 20 May 2017. www.youtube.com/watch?v=OkS_fEARUpw.

ID Hospital Korea Plastic Surgery. 2014a. "Underbite Jaw Surgery – Before & After (Oral and Maxillofacial Surgery)." Accessed 10 January 2017. www.youtube.com/watch?v=QFF4jBBJh24&index=4&list=PLeZD3wSpSMdrQBOZgeUhlYv9meG2c6gOP.

ID Hospital Korea Plastic Surgery. 2014b. "Jawline Surgery and Orthodontic Surgery Before and After (2)." Accessed 10 January 2017. www.youtube.com/watch?v=ivplmgi_QHU&index=13&list=PLeZD3wSpSMdrQBOZgeUhlYv9meG2c6gOP.

ID Hospital Korea Plastic Surgery. 2013. [Id Hospital Review Korean Plastic Surgery] "Amazing makeover show, Let Me In Hospital." Accessed 7 May 2017. www.youtube.com/watch?v=9aeqAFuUa8Q&index=22&list=PLeZD3wSpSMdrQBOZgeUhlYv9meG2c6gOP.

International Society of Aesthetic Plastic Surgeons (ISAPS). 2016. "ISAPS International Survey on Aesthetic/Cosmetic. Procedures Performed in 2015." Accessed 15 March 2017. www.isaps.org/Media/Default/global-statistics/2016%20ISAPS%20Results.pdf.

Jones, Meredith. 2004. "Cosmetic Surgery and Postmodern Space." *Space & Culture*, 7.1: 90–101.

Jones, Meredith. 2008. "Media-bodies and Screen-births: Cosmetic Surgery Reality Television." *Continuum: Journal of Media & Cultural Studies*, 22.4: 515–24.

Jones, Meredith. 2009. "Pygmalion's Many Faces." In *Cosmetic Surgery. A Feminist Primer*, edited by Cressida J. Heyes and Meredith Jones, 171–91. Farnham: Ashgate.

Kaw, Eugenia. 1993. "Medicalization of Racial Features: Asian American Women and Cosmetic Surgery." *Medical Anthropological Quarterly*, 7.1: 74–89.

Kim, T. 2003. "Neo-Confucian Body Techniques: Women's Bodies in Korea's Consumer Society." *Body & Society*, 9.2: 97–113.

Korean Plastic Surgery Experience. 2013. "Chinese Girl Came to Korea for Facial Bone Contouring (Cheekbone Reduction + Jawline) Surgery!" Accessed 20 May 2017. www.youtube.com/watch?v=t0ig9LloC9U.

Korean Plastic Surgery Experience. 2014. "Eng Sub, Orthodontic Jaw Surgery Before and After, Man's Plastic Surgery Korea Review." Accessed 20 May 2017. www.youtube.com/watch?v=eZ3sqdOMWec.

Korean Plastic Surgery Experience. 2014. "(Men) Let Me In Korean TV Show Eng Sub." Accessed 20 May 2017. www.youtube.com/watch?v=Gd-bISK3lkc.

National Folk Museum of Korea. 2014. *Encyclopedia of Korean Folk Literature*. Seoul: The National Folk Museum of Korea.

Schleifer, Ronald and Vannatta, Jerry B. 2013. *The Chief Concern of Medicine. The Integration of the Medical Humanities and Narrative Knowledge into Medical Practices*. Ann Arbor: University of Michigan Press.

StoryonTV. 2014. "LET 美人 2 1회 자존감 바닥의 마스크女 vs 20대 할머니." Accessed 20 May 2017. www.youtube.com/watch?v=Xyu0HajSDK0&oref=https%3A%2F%2Fwww.youtube.com%2F&has_verified=1.

StoryonTV. 2014. LET 美人 2 7회 승무원이 꿈인 볼거리女 VS 교사가 꿈인 거대 점女 메이크오버 주인공은. Accessed 20 May 2017. www.youtube.com/watch?v=2fDVfEHM2Wo&oref=https%3A%2F%2F.

Tait, Sue. 2007. "Television and the Domestication of Cosmetic Surgery." *Feminist Media Studies*, 7.2: 119–35.

Tanner, Claire, Maher, Janemaree, and Fraser, Suzanne. 2013. *Vanity: 21st Century Selves*. Basingstoke: Palgrave Macmillan.

View Plastic Surgery. 2014. "[LET Beauty 4] Beauty Stories between LET Beauties and VIEW Medical Group – ep1." Accessed 20 May 2017. www.youtube.com/watch?v=12hhkupfFEE.

Voinea, Carmen. 2017. "Plastic Surgery Phenomenon among South Korean Women. The Instrumental Body in a Rite of Passage to the Normative *Innocent Glamour*." *Romanian Journal of Sociological Studies*, 1: 69–87.

Yoo, S.Y. 2001. "Embodiment of American Modernity in Colonial Korea." *Inter-Asia Cultural Studies*, 2.3: 423–41.

Zipes, Jack. 2007. *When Dreams Came True. Classical Fairy Tales and Their Tradition*. New York: Routledge.

12 "John-o is interested in cutting up whatever he finds at the limits of life"

Monstrous anatomies and the production of the human body in Alasdair Gray's *Poor Things* and Hilary Mantel's *The Giant, O'Brien*

Kathryn Bird

Towards the end of Hilary Mantel's *The Giant, O'Brien* (1999) – an imaginative account of the eighteenth-century surgeon-anatomist John Hunter's acquisition of the skeleton of Charles Byrne (or O'Brien), the so-called "Irish Giant" – Byrne's acquaintances approach Hunter's assistant, Howison, with a proposition. They suggest that if Hunter advances them the money to rent cellars across London to exhibit a variety of "freaks," he will soon have their unusual corpses for dissection – because "[t]he life of a freak is not long ... once it has been brought to London and been worked" (Mantel 1999, 184). Howison doubts that Hunter has the funds but considers taking up the proposition himself and selling the corpses to his employer; after all, he knows that

> John-o is interested in cutting up whatever he finds at the limits of life. He is interested in what distinguishes plants from animals, and animals from man. The latter distinction, Howison thinks, may need more than a scalpel to make it.
>
> (184–85)

The story of Hunter's acquisition of Byrne's skeleton in 1783 continues to resonate over 200 years later. Indeed, in March 2017, a petition was launched seeking to have the skeleton removed from display in the Hunterian Museum in the Royal College of Surgeons in London (where it still hangs) and buried at sea according to Byrne's apparent wishes. Byrne, who suffered from a "growth disorder" and stood at roughly seven and a half feet tall (Doyal and Muinzer 2011, 1), made a living exhibiting himself in London and apparently "lived and died in fear that the anatomists would get his prodigious body" and submit it "to the second death and desecration of dissection" (Youngquist 2003, 3–4). Thus far the Royal College of Surgeons has dismissed the petition, stating that the value of his remains in terms of "educational and research benefits" outweighs Byrne's "apparent request" to have his body buried at sea (Lonergan 2017). Byrne's skeleton has certainly yielded significant research benefits in studies of acromegaly and pituitary adenoma, yet such research only requires Byrne's remains (particularly his DNA, which has already been extracted) to be medically accessible, which at the very least provides little justification for continued display (Doyal and Muinzer 2011, 3). In fact, the originator of the petition to have Byrne's skeleton removed and buried compares its continued display to "some circus freak show" (Lornegan 2017).

This is not a new criticism of medicine's approach to "extraordinary bodies," which must always "negotiate a long tradition of 'the curious' in British culture" (Kennedy 2008, 79). This is particularly true of anatomy, whose "practices, objects, and representations have always been an intricate mixture of science and art, and a hybrid of medical instruction and popular entertainment" (van Dijck 2005, 43). The above response from the Royal College of Surgeons can be understood as another attempt to justify medicine's own historical and continued curiosity about extraordinary bodies and their revelatory potential. Indeed, as Rosemarie Garland Thomson observes, "the word *monster* – perhaps the earliest and most enduring name for the singular body – derives from the Latin *monstra*, meaning to warn, show, or sign, and which has given us the modern verb *demonstrate*"; hence, the exceptional or "abnormal" body is never "simply itself" but always "betokens something else, becomes revelatory, sustains narrative, exists socially in a realm of hyper-representation" (1996, 3).

One narrative which the "monstrous" body has been called upon to sustain is a biomedical narrative of what it means to be human, particularly where medicine's production of a norm of human embodiment is concerned. This chapter will examine the depiction in two twentieth-century British novels – Hilary Mantel's *The Giant, O'Brien* and Alasdair Gray's *Poor Things* (1992) – of medicine's historical investment in obtaining and anatomising exceptional bodies in its quest to produce a norm of human embodiment, and of how this investment intersects with the legal, political and social implications of possessing the status of being fully human – or, conversely, of occupying an ambiguous position in relation to this category. While Mantel turns to historical sources for her depiction of medicine's production of a norm of human embodiment by "cutting up whatever [it] finds at the limits of life" (1999, 184), Gray turns to a fictional tradition: *Poor Things* imagines what might have happened if Frankenstein's creature had created his own female companion. The greater part of the novel centres on the memoir of Victorian public health officer Archibald McCandless, who recounts the story of his wife, Bella Baxter, a "surgical fabrication" created by Godwin Bysshe Baxter (apparently also made "by the Frankenstein method"), who creates her by transplanting the brain of her dead unborn child into her drowned body and reanimating it (1992, 35; 274). This narrative of Bella's life is later refuted in a letter from McCandless's wife, now known as Victoria, who describes her husband's "sham-Gothic" narrative as a "cunning lie" (1992, 275). These two narratives are in turn framed by an editorial introduction and "Notes Critical and Historical"; additionally, scattered throughout the text are anatomical illustrations from another "Gray" – this time, from *Gray's Anatomy*.

The first section of this chapter examines the novels' evocation of the role of monstrous specimens in the history of anatomical constructions of the human body. Drawing on Giorgio Agamben's analysis of the "example," I consider how the use of such "abnormal bodies" foregrounds medicine's deeper struggles to demonstrate an exemplary form of human embodiment through morbid anatomy. Then, turning to Agamben's work on the "exception," the second section focuses on Mantel's and Gray's depictions of the intersection of medicine's production of a norm of human embodiment with the political, legal and social abandonment of those considered ambiguously human, with particular emphasis on the Anatomy Act and on the conflation of monstrosity with other experiences of social exclusion, including poverty. The final section draws on work from the critical medical humanities to explore Mantel's and Gray's emphasis on the entanglement of literary and biomedical imaginations of the human.

Monstrosity, medicine and the anatomical example of what it means to be human

Although it has become something of a critical commonplace to note that "the body as we know it is always a discursive construction" (Shildrick 2008, 32), this point does bear repeating when thinking about medicine's historical entanglement with monstrous bodies. As Katharine Young puts it, the body "is not given as the physiological substrate on which medical discourse is mounted; rather, it is invented and transformed by medical discourse" – in other words, medicine "fabricates a body" (1997, 1). A key area in which this fabrication takes place is anatomical dissection, which should be understood not simply as the "partition" of "organic integrity," but as "an act whereby something can also be constructed, or given a concrete presence" (Sawday 1995, 2). What is constructed through this process is not just any "body," but "a cultural norm of human embodiment" (Youngquist 2003, xi). Moreover, it is not necessarily "normal" bodies which make this production of human embodiment visible; instead, "monstrosities provide a material occasion ... for observing norms of embodiment in action" (Youngquist 2003, xxvii).

That both the normal and the abnormal body are discursive and interrelated productions is emphasised in *Poor Things* and *The Giant, O'Brien*. The most obvious manifestation of this in *Poor Things* lies in the novel's intertextual references to Bella and Baxter being created "by the Frankenstein method" (1992, 274). In his fabrication of Bella, Baxter succeeds in uniting "discarded" remains into a totality resembling a norm of human embodiment, such that, even for those who are aware of her origins, Bella's "most striking abnormality is her lack of it" (223). By contrast, Baxter's "progenitor" has produced in him a body at once "dwarfish" and yet also "ogreish" and possessed of a "monstrous bulk" (12, 44). Moreover, Baxter's body also lacks the normal boundaries associated with human embodiment. Because he has "little or no pancreas," Baxter must "make his digestive juices by hand, stirring them into his food before chewing and swallowing," a process which involves the use of his own "bodily wastes"

(72). Yet the novel also emphasises that even where extraordinary bodies such as "anacephalids, bicephalids, cyclops" are ostensibly born out of "nature" rather than being fabricated, it is medicine which produces and confirms their status as "unnatural"; indeed, such beings are declared unnatural precisely because they require medicine's "artificial help" to survive (33), which foregrounds the foundational presence of medicine's authority in the construction of supposedly self-evident divisions between "natural" and "unnatural" bodies.

In *The Giant, O'Brien*, Hunter's project of "cutting up whatever he finds at the limits of life" in order to decide what constitutes a norm of human embodiment (1999, 184–85) resonates with Agamben's emphasis on the role played by anatomical dissection (particularly "the solid grounds of comparative anatomy") in the functioning of "the anthropological machine of humanism," which governs decisions on what constitutes human life (2004, 25; 29). According to Agamben, the "division of life into vegetal and relational, organic and animal, animal and human" – the same question of "what distinguishes plants from animals, and animals from man" (1999, 185) that preoccupies Hunter in Mantel's novel – "passes first of all as a mobile border within living man." Decisions on the position of this "intimate caesura" enable "the very decision of what is human and what is not" (Agamben 2004, 15). However, the question of what constitutes "the truly human being" is never settled once and for all; instead, the category of the human is "only the place of a ceaselessly updated decision in which the caesurae and their rearticulation are always dislocated and displaced anew" (38). Given the etymological roots of *caesura* in "cutting," Agamben's conception of the production of human life is echoed in Mantel's depiction of Hunter's project of dividing human from non-human with his "scalpel" (Agamben 1999, 185).

Yet the role of monstrous bodies in decisively carving out a norm of human embodiment is complicated by their ambiguous relationship with the category of the "human." As Elizabeth Grosz points out, the "monster" or "freak" marks the threshold "not of humanity itself" – monsters, unlike nonhuman animals, are rarely perceived as belonging to a different species – but of "acceptable, tolerable, knowable humanity" (1996, 55). Monstrosities might "haunt the human" (Youngquist 2003, xi), but as with all hauntings, it is never clear whether they trouble ideas of what it means to be human from a position inside or outside of this category. In the history of medicine in early modernity, for example, monstrous bodies were dissected not as "mere curiosities" or to specifically explore manifestations of anatomical abnormality, but to provide "empirical evidence to sustain anatomical claims" concerning the norms of human anatomy (Moscoso 1998, 358). Moreover, this approach continues to hold sway in contemporary biomedical research; for example, William Viney observes how human twins – often depicted as "quasi-monstrous" or as an "exceptional phenomenon … in a state of monstrous proximity to the norm" – continue to be "utilised as examples, models, and 'equipmental figures'" in medical science to "investigate who and what we are" (Viney 2014, 48–49). In other words, medicine's production of a norm of human embodiment from modernity to the present day has been significantly built on evidence drawn from extraordinary bodies which have been used as examples to produce and demonstrate this norm.

Yet the presence of visibly unusual bodies in the anatomical fabrication of a norm of human embodiment also draws attention to anatomy's fundamental difficulties in finding any examples which are sufficiently "average" to succeed in "emphasis[ing] the body's representativeness rather than its uniqueness" (van Dijck 2005, 128). For instance, in her study of the "Visible Human Project" (VHP), which sought to produce an online repository of complete anatomical detail for a standard male and female body, Catherine Waldby observes that this project encountered "one of the central epistemological problems in anatomy generally: the problem of the norm and the ordering of the distinction normal/pathological" (2000, 18). In choosing an anatomical example to be representative of a norm of human embodiment, it was necessary for the VHP to choose a sample which would "exclude the possibility of any visible pathology, anything which might detract from the project's claim to present strictly healthy and normal anatomies" (Waldby 2000, 13). However, this anatomical fantasy of finding a standard body necessarily falters at what Margrit Shildrick describes as the "resistance of flesh to normativity" (2008, 42). Although "the fundamental socio-cultural belief in the fixity of corporeal boundaries" is "easily set aside in the case of the extraordinary body at the margins," the "normative body" also harbours "the ever-present threat of excessive proliferation, and of disintegration and decay," such that all bodies "are more or less unstable" (2008, 34; 32–33).

Medicine's difficulty in producing a representative example of a norm of human embodiment can be productively read in relation to Agamben's analysis of the concept of the "example" itself. For Agamben, both the example and the exception "constitute the two modes by which a set tries to found and maintain its own coherence" (1998, 21). What makes the "example" so intriguing is that it "is one singularity among others, which, however, stands for each of them and serves for all":

> On one hand, every example is treated in effect as a real particular case; but on the other, it remains understood that it cannot serve in its particularity. Neither particular nor universal, the example is a singular object that presents itself as such, that *shows* its singularity.
>
> (9–10)

For Agamben, this functioning of the example can be seen in the Greek term for "example:" "*para-deigma*, that which is shown alongside" (10). In other words, as Steven DeCaroli puts it, the example "is simultaneously a simple member of a set as well as the defining criteria of that set"; hence, because it provides "its own criteria of inclusion, the example remains ambiguously positioned alongside the class of which it is most representative, neither fully included in a class nor fully excluded from it" (2011, 145). As a result of this ambiguous position in relation to the set it paradoxically founds and represents, the example retains a persistent "singularity" that can never be separated from "its exemplarity"

(Agamben 2009, 31). It is through this persistent singularity that the example becomes capable of calling the criteria of belonging to a set "radically into question" (Agamben 1993, 10), such that the example simultaneously demonstrates and undoes the coherence of the category which it both founds and represents.

Like any example, then, the anatomical example that both founds and demonstrates the category of normal human embodiment always already exists "beside itself," as Agamben puts it (1993, 10), in an ambiguous relation to the human, which troubles the coherence of this category. Moreover, at a practical or material level, anatomical examples of a norm of human embodiment are particularly apt for demonstrating the persistent singularity of "exemplary being" itself. Whether the raw materials for medicine's fabrication of the human body are drawn from visibly extraordinary or ostensibly ordinary bodies, all anatomical examples retain "their organic materiality, their specific ties to individual bodies with their inescapable idiosyncrasies" and will thus "fail to be representative" (van Dijck 2005, 131). We might therefore construe all anatomical examples of a norm of human embodiment as "monstrous," both in the sense that flesh may always exhibit some singularity, some lack or excess that makes it deviate from an ideal or norm, and in the sense that such examples nevertheless *demonstrate*; like the body of a monster, the anatomical example of the human body is both singular and yet never "simply itself" because it also "betokens something else, becomes revelatory, sustains narrative" (Thomson 1996, 3). Hence, like monstrous bodies more generally, an anatomical example such as those used in the VHP can only ever ambiguously belong to the medical norm of the human body that it helps to found and sustain, and which it therefore also suspends and disrupts.

It is striking that in both *Poor Things* and *The Giant, O'Brien*, the surgeon-anatomists who attempt to fabricate human bodies are ultimately troubled not by any obvious monstrosity, but by the persistent singularity of ostensibly ordinary and anonymous bodies. In Mantel's novel, when John Hunter first comes to London to join his older brother at his anatomy school, he is asked "to dissect, to make preparations" of some arms in order "to serve the students with a feast for their eyes" (1999, 36). When John Hunter asks his brother who the arms belonged to, William Hunter's response – "'Whose?' The little query dripped with ice" – leads John to regret "bursting out like that … as if it should matter where limbs came from"; yet "he couldn't help wondering, speculating in his mind: making up a life to fit the possessor of the fibrous, drained muscle" (36–37). Here, what should be anonymous anatomical examples of human arms for instruction persist in their "historical and irreducibly singular" nature (DeCaroli 2001, 11), which disturbs the anatomist's attempts to reduce them to inert representative matter, "drained," in Mantel's words, of particularity. In *Poor Things*, Baxter's attempt to literally fabricate a "perfect" and anonymous female body using a "discarded body and discarded brain from our social midden" also struggles in the face of the persistent singularity of these raw materials (1992, 27; 34). Having transplanted the brain of Bella's unborn child into her body and reanimating her, instead of gaining "what men have hopelessly yearned for throughout the ages: the soul of an innocent, trusting, dependent child inside the opulent body of a radiantly lovely woman" (36), what Baxter ends up with is a strong-willed woman with a medical and legal history that constantly returns, rather like Frankenstein's own recalcitrant creature, to haunt him.

From example to exception: abandonment at the limits of life

That Baxter finds his materials for producing Bella "discarded" in the "social midden" (1992, 34) resonates with the typical sources of raw materials for anatomists, whose knowledge "relied on the bodies of those excluded from the social contract, ... those useless or dangerous beings at the margins of the human" (Waldby 2000, 53–54). Waldby's emphasis on "the margins of the human" is echoed by Mantel's focus in *The Giant, O'Brien* on anatomy's search for its materials "at the limits of life" in the bodies of "freaks" and "monsters" (1999, 184). Yet in Mantel's novel, Hunter appears less interested in what he can learn from the Giant's extraordinary body than he does in acquiring a trophy for his anatomical collection: he surveys his specimens and decides that he "will move that armadillo three feet to the left, and the giant bones will sway, suspended on their wires, boiled and clean" (1999, 127). As José van Dijck observes, the "primary appeal" of anatomical collections such as Hunter's "was their focus on the aberrant – especially the monstrous aspects of pathological cases, such as embryos with spina bifida and fetuses with hydrocephalus" (2005, 46). This display does, of course, have echoes of the freak show, but rather than presenting "pathological creatures and 'monsters' as objects of spectacle" – though this aspect of "titillation" undeniably persists in anatomical collections – their display rendered them part of "an authoritative medical culture" (46).

In Mantel's novel, Hunter's displays demonstrate the investment of this "authoritative medical culture" in delimiting the category of the human by focusing on ambiguously human figures, including preparations with "deformities and distortions" (1999, 63), and preparations drawn from nonhuman animals. For example, Hunter arranges his collection of skulls thus: "Croc. Dog. Macaque. A monkey is half-beast, half-man, he thinks.... Chimp. Savage. European Male" (103). With every preparation and display, Hunter attempts to "understand hierarchy" as it applies to living beings (135), ranging from fully human to nonhuman. Both *The Giant, O'Brien* and *Poor Things* are concerned with the implications of being classified at the bottom of this hierarchy, and hence with the dangers of occupying an ambiguous position in relation to the category of the human itself.

These dangers can be examined by turning to Agamben's later emphasis on the "exception," described as "the photographic negative or dark image of the example" (Meskin and Shapiro 2014, 425). As the other of "the two modes by which a set tries to found and maintain its own coherence," the exception "is situated in a symmetrical position with respect to the example, with which it forms a system" (Agamben 1998, 21). However, the "mechanism of exception" is opposite to that of the example: while the example is "excluded from the set insofar as it belongs to it, the exception is included in the normal case precisely because it does not belong to it" (1998, 21). Moreover, just as "belonging to a class can be shown only by an example – that is, outside the class itself – so non-belonging can be shown only at the center of the class, by an exception" (1998, 21). These "correlative concepts" of example and exception "come into play every time the very sense of the belonging and commonality of individuals is to be defined" (1998, 21–22).

Indeed, for Agamben, the exception is closely related to the "ban," the mechanism whereby certain beings are excepted from the rights and protection conferred by the laws of a community or nation, and are exposed to any form of violence. Again, the abandoned person retains an ambiguous relationship with the category or community from which they have been excluded; just as "non-belonging can only be shown at the center of the class, by an exception" (1998, 21), so it is also the case that "what has been banned is delivered over to its own separateness and, at the same time, consigned to the mercy of the one who abandons it – at once excluded and included, removed and at the same time captured" (110). It is striking that Agamben should use a "monstrous" figure to illustrate this relation of the ban: the werewolf, "a monstrous hybrid of human and animal" who "is precisely *neither man nor beast*, and who dwells paradoxically within both while belonging to neither" (105). Such figures appear in *The Giant, O'Brien*, in which the Giant passes through a ruined village in Ireland and glimpses "one of those hybrids that are sometimes seen to scuttle, keen and scrape in ruins … their human parts weeping, their animal nature truffling for dead flesh" (1999, 9). Once in England, he learns that such hybridity is risky – that the English "do not have werewolves. For them, you're either one thing or the other" (159).

While Agamben draws on folklore and myth, we might equally think of the more mundane "monsters" used in the history of medicine not simply as unexpected examples of human anatomy but as abandoned beings excepted from dominant ethical and legal conceptions of human life; as Javier Moscoso observes, monsters were popular choices for anatomists because they "were devoid of the same ethical and pragmatic issues that surrounded human dissections" (1998, 358). Yet this experience of abandonment applies more broadly to anatomists' sourcing of materials for dissection. For example, Margaret Lock and Vinh-Kim Nguyen emphasise how "the plundered bodies of the poor" (among others) were "effectively assigned to a 'state of exception'; their bodies were not due the respect given to the rest of society" (2010, 207). For Lock and Nguyen, this ability to consign certain bodies to a state of exception stems from the 1832 Anatomy Act of Britain, which gave surgeons the right for the first time to dissect the unclaimed bodies of the poor, and was instituted in response to the need to bring an end to practices of body-snatching by so-called "resurrectionists" – the very practices, in fact, which Mantel depicts Hunter engaging in, and against which the Giant's companions riot (1999, 98).

While Mantel's novel depicts the events leading up to the implementation of the Anatomy Act, Gray's novel is concerned with the later nineteenth-century period when it was in force. There are numerous references to the Act in *Poor Things*; for example, the corpse out of which Baxter constructs Bella is described as "advertised, but not claimed" (1992, xiv); and an editor's note to the novel states that McCandless later authored a "five-act play about the Burke and Hare murders" – involving two men who "took graverobbing to its logical conclusion" by murdering people and selling the corpses to anatomists (Marshall 1995, 4) – which treats the surgeon whom they supplied "more sympathetically than usual" (1992, 300). The Burke and Hare scandal also makes a subtle appearance in Baxter's revelation that his refinement of surgical techniques would enable him to "replace the diseased hearts of the rich with the healthy hearts of poorer folk, and make a lot of money," but he adds that "it would be unkind to lead millionaires into such temptation" (1992, 22). McCandless's response is telling in its failure to pick up on the nuances of Baxter's pronouncement: he tells Baxter that it would not be "murder" because the corpses they have access to "have died by accident or natural disease," and if Baxter can "use their undamaged organs and limbs to mend the bodies of others" he will be hailed as "a greater saviour than Pasteur or Lister" (1992, 23). What McCandless fails to realise is that Baxter's pronouncement implies not only the use of "spare parts" from the unclaimed bodies of the poor which the Anatomy Act legally provides for, but (*pace* Burke and Hare) the appropriation of living bodies and the "temptation" to murder them solely to provide these parts. Indeed, there are indications in *Poor Things* that the living bodies of the poor are already vulnerable to such legal and medical abandonment and violence: as Baxter observes, "public hospitals are places where doctors learn how to get money off the rich by practising on the poor," which is "why poor people dread and hate them" (1992, 17). As Clara Tuite points out, the unwholesome conditions in the public hospitals and workhouses led to early deaths, such that these institutions formed "an efficient central collection point for 'unclaimed' human refuse" (1998, 144).

In Mantel's novel, poverty is also shown to produce vulnerability before medical authority; for example, among the many "monstrous" bodies Hunter demands Howison should find for him, he also frequently requests "paupers" for his experiments (1999, 110). But in this novel, it is monstrosity in particular which mediates the fates of other categories of abandoned beings, both through the body of the Giant, and through those of the other "freaks" confined in the cellar with him as he dies, all of whom are marked for delivery to the anatomist. As Mantel puts it, "for the poor man and the giant there is the scrubbed wooden slab and the slop bucket, there is the cauldron and the boiling pot, and the dunghill for his lights" (1999, 205). In particular, Mantel's depiction of the ability of monstrous corpses to command a high price speaks to anatomy's role in "a whole economy of biovalue" (Waldby 2000, 51). Anatomy, Waldby points out, "involves finding a use-value for the corpse, calling it to account in order to produce a surplus of vivification for the living" (2000, 51–52). This "surplus of vivification" is

> produced through setting up certain kinds of hierarchies in which marginal forms of vitality – the foetal, the cadaverous and extracted tissue, as well as

the bodies and body parts of the socially marginal – are transformed into technologies to aid in the intensification of vitality for other living beings.

(2000, 19)

In Mantel's novel, the Giant's acquaintances recognise the possibilities of extracting the maximum value from the monstrous and marginal bodies they intend to display; hence, because they know that "the life of a freak is not long … once it has been brought to London and been worked" (1999, 184), they discover a course for getting even more money out of their "freaks" after their deaths by selling their bodies to Hunter.

Indeed, if these marginal bodies and anatomical preparations produce a "surplus of vivification" for those who belong to the category of the "fully human" (Waldby 2000, 51–52), it is less clear exactly how "vital" these marginal entities are themselves. Both novels point to the ways in which certain beings (whether monstrous or socially marginal, or both) are situated not just at the limits of the human but, as Mantel puts it, "at the limits of life" (1999, 184). In *The Giant, O'Brien*, the Giant is so horrified by Hunter's offer to buy his corpse while he is still living, that he says "I'll buy you while you're still breathing, I'll buy you now against the hour of your death" (191). This isolation of the "biovalue" of the Giant's corpse in his still-living body is akin to the treatment of the strange existence of the "freaks" in the cellars discussed above. In both cases, these marginal beings exist before the medical gaze in "a kind of suspended life" that fascinates Hunter, who wishes to experiment on "drowned persons" to see if he can revive them from a state of apparent death (96, 22). In *Poor Things*, this reanimation of the drowned is precisely what Baxter achieves, although he takes his discovery further through his ability to "arrest a body's life without ending it" (1992, 13). In other words, he can place bodies into a kind of living death, which enables him to perform organ transplants – perhaps (as he suggests to McCandless) using organs harvested from the bodies of the poor (22).

This imagery recalls what Des Fitzgerald and Felicity Callard have recently described as "the bioethically over-invested scene of the prone figure hooked up to a life support machine," which has become paradigmatic of "the most pressing sites of the biopolitical redistribution of bodily potencies" (2016, 42). While an over-investment in this "scene" does attest to what DeCaroli describes as the potentially "normative" force of such "exemplary objects" (2001, 10), the image of the comatose patient as a paradigm of the vulnerability of ambiguously human beings does retain a useful analogical relationship with other scenes of the "biopolitical redistribution of bodily potencies" – including, in Mantel's and Gray's novels, some of the broader questions around issues such as welfare provision that Fitzgerald and Callard rightly suggest are equally deserving of attention (2016, 42). Indeed, both novels were published in a period in which Fred Botting argues Britain was "still reeling from the effects of Thatcherism," and he suggests that Gray's emphasis on the "suffering, socialism and the filth of Victorian modernity" provides a stark commentary on "the dismantling of the Welfare State" (2008, 129–30). Similarly, Elizabeth Klaver argues that in *The Giant,*

O'Brien Mantel "deploys the act of human dissection as a means to tropologize a brutal class and colonial system" (2005, 21) – one whose effects are still evident in the "ontological insecurity" suffered by the victims of the global organ and tissue trade, who exist "in a world that values their bodies more dead than alive, and as a reservoir of spare parts" (Scheper-Hughes 2002, 32). This contemporary experience of "ontological insecurity" finds an apt parallel in the bodies of the poor and the "freaks" in Gray's and Mantel's novel who are shunted to "the limits of life" where they can be cut up with impunity.

Conclusion: biomedical and literary entanglements

In *Poor Things*, Victoria McCandless (known as "Bella" in her husband's narrative) leaves a letter for her descendants damning her husband's "sham-gothic" account of her life, not only because she claims it is untrue – by her own account, she was born in a Manchester slum, not on a surgeon-anatomist's table, and Baxter was never "a monster whose appearance made babies scream" – but also because she fears that his gothicised version of her life will divert attention from the real horror of the material conditions into which she was born (1992, 259). The "morbid Victorian fantas[ies]" he has "filched from" involve and encourage a form of "useless over-ornamentation" which glosses over "the stunted lives of children, woman and men," and she laments that she has "no time to go through every page separating fact from fiction" (1992, 274–75). Interestingly, Victoria's "review" of her husband's account has a curious resonance with a review of *The Giant, O'Brien* in the *BMJ*, which accuses Mantel of "stretch[ing] the limits of literary licence ... to suit her own peculiarly unpleasant agenda," which apparently includes an over-emphasis on the victimisation of the colonial subjects and an utterly "fanciful" portrayal of Byrne and the Hunters. "Coming from an experienced author," the reviewer concludes, "this book has to be classed as an unusually disappointing potboiler depending, it would seem, on the outlandish and the macabre to attract a readership" (Cohen 1998, 1533). What is also striking about this review – besides its rather prudish attitude to historical fiction – is its source: the reviewer is Bertram Cohen, who at the time was the chairman of the board of trustees at the Hunterian collection in the Royal College of Surgeons – the very place where Charles Byrne's skeleton still hangs.

Perhaps Cohen would have done well to pay attention to Mantel's choice of epigraph for the novel, an extract from George MacBeth's "The Cleaver Garden":

> But then
> All crib from skulls and bones who push the pen.
> Readers crave bodies. We're the resurrection men.
> (Mantel 1999)

Besides emphasising the fictionality of her account, Mantel's choice of epigraph also hints at a much deeper relationship between fictional and medical imaginations of human life and death. Mantel depicts Hunter both decrying those medical men whose work displays "too much imagination ... unbuttressed by results," and yet also worrying that he, "a man bound to fact and observation," might "embroider the tale" (86, 132). Mantel's portrayal of Hunter's attitude to his anatomical specimens is certainly suggestive of this capacity for embroidery. While walking through his collection at night, he imagines that he sees "in the shadows" the "creeping of a polydactyl hand across marble ... or perhaps the ripple of flesh and fluid, as conjoined twins elbow for space in their bottle" (103); moreover, as I noted earlier, Hunter cannot resist the temptation of imaginatively resurrecting the singular life behind the "drained" flesh of an anonymous anatomical preparation (37). In *Poor Things*, Gray similarly has the medically trained McCandless insist that "the imagination is, like the appendix, inherited from a primitive epoch," and "in modern scientific industrial nations" is "mainly a source of disease" which he had "prided" himself on lacking – yet he discovers that it "had only lain dormant" in him (1992, 55), and Gray's fictitious "editor's notes" state that McCandless later "devoted himself to literature," including (according to his wife) that of a "gothic" and "morbid" variety (1992, 55; vi; 274–75).

What both Mantel and Gray emphasise in their depiction of (sometimes reluctantly) imaginative medical men is what Waldby describes as the "biomedical imaginary," which "refers to the speculative, propositional fabric of medical thought, the generally disavowed dream work performed by biomedical theory and innovation" (2000, 136). Waldby argues that alongside its "properly scientific ... deductive strategies and empirical epistemologies," medicine also derives its "impetus from the fictitious, the connotative, and from desire" (2000, 136–37). Moreover, this imaginary dimension of medicine is "hopelessly enmeshed in a gothic cultural imaginary around life, death, reanimation, and the status of the corpse" (2000, 18). Given their focus on medicine's fascination with the monstrous, perhaps traces of the gothic or macabre are an unavoidable feature of Mantel's and Gray's novels, but they also serve to illuminate the imaginative aspects of medicine, not least in its approach to constructing a norm of human embodiment and, by extension, of the value of particular lives at the limits or margins of this category.

In this respect, Mantel's and Gray's literary depictions of medicine's production of the human foregrounds the very "entanglement" that is so central to the field of critical medical humanities. "Entanglement" describes the "creative boundary-crossing" between the various scientific and humanities disciplines which make up the field of medical humanities – a form of boundary-crossing "in and through which new possibilities can emerge" (Whitehead and Woods 2016, 8). As I have argued in this chapter, *Poor Things* and *The Giant, O'Brien* consistently emphasise the most damaging aspects of biomedicine's conception of human life and its collusion with the biopolitical hierarchies according to which lives are either fostered or abandoned. Yet both novels also provide sympathetic ground for the emphasis in critical medical humanities on the "need to displace, if not significantly reimagine, how medical humanities has tended to figure the 'human,'" which exists in conjunction with the need to displace a model in which empathic or caring humanism is positioned as ready to tame the clinical coldness of the biomedical – or in which the inventiveness of the "human spirit" is imagined as ready to combat the deadening and reductive effects of scientific rationalism.

(Fitzgerald and Callard 2016, 43)

Not only do both novels trouble any clear distinctions between the literary and biomedical imaginaries of human embodiment and life, they also refute the depiction of an "empathic or caring humanism" as a straightforward means of combating the most negative effects of biomedicine's production and repro-duction of hierarchies of human and nonhuman life. Hunter's moments of sym-pathy with his anatomical subjects – "who move him to tears" (1999, 97) – do not prevent him from acts of cruelty in deciding the boundaries of human life; nor does Baxter's humanistic view of medicine as a "kindly art" prevent his exploitation of the remains he finds "discarded" on the "social midden heap" (1992, 223; 34). To return to the quotation with which I began this chapter, con-cerning Hunter's desire to produce the human by "cutting up whatever he finds at the limits of life," his assistant Howison's reflection that the division of "animals from man ... may need more than a scalpel to make it" (Mantel 1999, 185) is certainly apt; but both Mantel's and Gray's novels are clear that if an exploration of the nature of human embodiment and life takes "more than a scalpel," it also takes more than a pen.

Reference list

Agamben, Giorgio. 1993. *The Coming Community*. Translated by Michael Hardt. Minne-apolis and London: University of Minnesota Press.

Agamben, Giorgio. 1998. *Homo Sacer: Sovereign Power and Bare Life*. Translated by Daniel Heller-Roazen. Stanford, CA: Stanford University Press.

Agamben, Giorgio. 2004. *The Open: Man and Animal*. Translated by Kevin Attell. Stan-ford, CA: Stanford University Press.

Agamben, Giorgio. 2009. *The Signature of All Things: On Method*. Translated by Luca D'Isanto with Kevin Attell. New York: Zone Books.

Botting, Fred. 2008. *Gothic Romanced: Consumption, Gender and Technology in Con-temporary Fictions*. London and New York: Routledge.

Cohen, Bertram. 1998. "*The Giant, O'Brien*, Hilary Mantel." *BMJ* 317: 1533.

DeCaroli, Steven. 2001. "Visibility and History: Giorgio Agamben and the Exemplary." *Philosophy Today* 45: 9–17.

DeCaroli, Steven. 2011. "Paradigm/Example." In *The Agamben Dictionary*, edited by Alex Murray and Jessica Whyte, 144–47. Edinburgh: Edinburgh University Press.

Doyal, Len and Thomas Muinzer. 2011. "Should the Skeleton of the 'Irish Giant' Be Buried at Sea?" *BMJ* 342: 1–5.

Fitzgerald, Des and Felicity Callard. 2016. "Entangling the Medical Humanities." In *The Edinburgh Companion to the Critical Medical Humanities*, edited by Anne Whitehead and Angela Woods, 35–49. Edinburgh: Edinburgh University Press.

Gray, Alasdair. 1992. *Poor Things*. London: Bloomsbury.

Grosz, Elizabeth. 1996. "Intolerable Ambiguity: Freaks as/at the Limit." In *Freakery: Cultural Spectacles of the Extraordinary Body*, edited by Rosemarie Garland Thomson, 55–67. New York and London: New York University Press.

Kennedy, Megan. 2008. "'Poor Hoo Loo': Sentiment, Stoicism, and the Grotesque in British Imperial Medicine." In *Victorian Freaks: The Social Context of Freakery in Britain*, edited by Marlene Tromp, 79–113. Columbus: The Ohio State University Press.

Klaver, Elizabeth. 2005. *Sites of Autopsy in Contemporary Culture*. Albany: State University of New York Press.

Lock, Margaret and Vinh-Kim Nguyen. 2010. *An Anthropology of Biomedicine*. Malden, MA and Oxford: Wiley-Blackwell.

Lonergan, Aidan. 2017. "A Dying Wish – Battle on to Release Irish Giant's Skeleton from British Museum for Sea Burial." *The Irish Post*, 15 March. Accessed 4 June 2017. http://irishpost.co.uk/a-dying-wish-battle-on-to-return-irishs-giant-skeleton-from-british-museum-for-burial-in-ireland/.

Mantel, Hilary. 1999. *The Giant, O'Brien*. London: Fourth Estate.

Marshall, Tim. 1995. *Murdering to Dissect: Grave-robbing, Frankenstein, and the Anatomy Literature*. Manchester and New York: Manchester University Press.

Meskin, Jacob and Harvey Shapiro. 2014. "'To Give an Example is a Complex Act': Agamben's Pedagogy of the Paradigm." *Educational Philosophy and Theory* 46: 421–40.

Moscoso, Javier. 1998. "Monsters as Evidence: The Use of the Abnormal Body during the Early Eighteenth Century." *Journal of the History of Biology* 31: 355–82.

Sawday, Jonathan. 1995. *The Body Emblazoned: Dissection and the Human Body in Renaissance Culture*. London and New York: Routledge.

Scheper-Hughes, Nancy. 2002. "Commodity Fetishism in Organs Trafficking." In *Commodifying Bodies*, edited by Nancy Scheper-Hughes and Loïc Wacquant, 31–62. London: Sage.

Shildrick, Margrit. 2008. "Corporeal Cuts: Surgery and the Psycho-social." *Body and Society* 14: 31–46.

Thomson, Rosemarie Garland. 1996. "Introduction: From Wonder to Error – A Genealogy of Freak Discourse in Modernity." In *Freakery: Cultural Spectacles of the Extraordinary Body*, edited by Rosemarie Garland Thomson, 1–19. New York and London: New York University Press.

Tuite, Clara. 1998. "Frankenstein's Monster and Malthus' 'Jaundiced Eye': Population, Body Politics, and the Monstrous Sublime." *Eighteenth-Century Life* 22: 141–55.

van Dijck, José. 2005. *The Transparent Body: A Cultural Analysis of Medical Imaging*. Seattle and London: University of Washington Press.

Viney, William. 2014. "Curious Twins." *Critical Quarterly* 56: 47–58.

Waldby, Catherine. 2000. *The Visible Human Project: Informatic Bodies and Posthuman Medicine*. London and New York: Routledge.

Whitehead, Anne and Angela Woods. 2016. "Introduction." In *The Edinburgh Companion to the Critical Medical Humanities*, edited by Anne Whitehead and Angela Woods, 1–31. Edinburgh: Edinburgh University Press.

Young, Katharine. 1997. *Presence in the Flesh: The Body in Medicine*. Cambridge, MA: Harvard University Press.

Youngquist, Paul. 2003. *Monstrosities: Bodies and British Romanticism*. Minneapolis and London: University of Minnesota Press.

13 In Lady Delacour's shadow

Women patients and breast cancer in short fiction

April Patrick

The study in himself and others of the human understanding, its modes and laws as objective realities, and his gaining that power over mental action in himself and other, which alone comes from knowledge at first-hand, is one which every physician should not only begin in youth, but continue all his life long.

(John Brown 1858, xi)

In Maria Edgeworth's 1801 novel *Belinda*, Lady Delacour receives a sharp blow to the breast, which she fears has caused a cancerous tumor to form. Her desire for secrecy allows a doctor to manipulate her and use treatments that worsen her condition. Through the support of a friend's kindness, she eventually changes doctors and makes a full recovery. This seemingly miraculous cure occurs not because of the new doctor's excellent treatment, but because she never had breast cancer at all. While many nineteenth-century patients faced the risks of mistreatment and quackery, such a recovery from breast cancer does not reflect the vast majority of women's experiences in the period. Expanding the study from this popular representation to more realistic portrayals of illness raises the questions: how does the human condition enter into literary representations of illness, and how does fiction engage in medical discourse and debates? Or put more simply, how does medicine affect literature, and how does literature affect medicine?

This chapter explores possible answers to those questions through analysis of two much more realistic portrayals of breast cancer in the nineteenth century, presented in physician John Brown's "Rab and His Friends" (1858) and Katharine Tynan's "Willie" (1898). In these short stories, both authors draw on actual experiences observing breast cancer to represent the realities of the illness, treatment for it, and the likelihood of recurrence and death. Additionally, both texts engage in contemporary medical discourse through their representations of doctors that resist the institutionalisation of medicine in their compassion for the patients and of the ways social class affects a patient's treatment.

Brown first published "Rab and his Friends" in his 1858 *Horæ Subsecivæ*, a volume of essays on a wide variety of topics. In the story, Brown reflects several times on the perceived callousness of the doctors, an issue of the day with the increasing institutionalisation of medicine through the establishment of the British Medical Association in 1856 and passage of the Medical Act of 1858. Tynan's story, originally published in *The Speaker*, engages in a discussion about public health and class that appeared on the periodical's pages in the preceding year. Additionally, the issue of class and the treatment of both characters in hospitals reflect larger concerns about healthcare for the poor. By engaging in these issues, the two short stories demonstrate the ways fictional representations of illness both respond to and shape medical discourse.

Over the course of the nineteenth century, literary realism shaped fictional portrayals of all aspects of life, including health and medical treatment, as the realistic Dr. Lydgate in George Eliot's *Middlemarch* (1871) and Harriet Martineau's nonfiction account of her *Life in the Sickroom* (1844) replaced the romantic and miraculous recovery of Lady Delacour. Realism highlights the powerful influence nonfiction had over fiction and the connection that developed between the seemingly distinct genres. For example, Jason Tougaw argues that the medical case history and the novel

> share subject matter – suffering protagonists – but more significantly, they appeal to readers by appearing to engage in, but ultimately also providing a respite from, the classification, system making, and categorization that the science, moral philosophy, and education of the period stressed.
>
> (Tougaw 2006, 2)

By simultaneously engaging with and digressing from scientific discourse, writers of medical fiction and nonfiction face a "unique rhetorical dilemma" in seeking to combine fidelity to medical realism with "humane sympathy for suffering patients on the other" (2). Such a conflict between the medicalised body and the human being is, of course, one that today's field of medical humanities seeks to bridge.

In the nineteenth century, some doctors feared the connection between humanity and medical practice was slipping out of their grasp. As John Brown's words in the epigraph above indicate, he believed the study of the humanities critical to the work of the doctor, and he wrestled with how to reconcile the increasing institutionalisation of the medical field with his beliefs about the effect of medical compassion. In the "Preface" to *Horæ Subsecivæ* Brown concludes that the study of humanity was an essential complement to the study of the medicine, that one must study the human being in order to treat the human body.

In the same year that Brown's collection appeared, the Medical Act of 1858 legally recognised a distinct occupation for qualified medical practitioners and "set up a general medical council with powers to monitor standards of professional training, to register qualified practitioners, and to de-register practitioners found guilty of criminal acts or of 'infamous conduct in any professional respect'" (Roberts 2009, 37). Though this Act provided the foundation for the British medical profession, it "can be seen as the culmination of [a] conflict ...

between the members and supporters of 'traditional professional groups,' the apothecaries, physicians, surgeons and their professional associations, and those other individuals who aspired to the status of medical practitioner" (Carrier and Kendall 2016, 10). While supporters of the Act hoped it would reduce the prevalence of commerce-driven quackery, others worried about "losing that sense of 'gentlemanly' responsibility for management of the patient as an individual and instead seeing each case as material for scientific observation and experiment" (Roberts 2009, 54). This concern was amplified by differences in the views of the patients and medical professionals:

> From the lay, or patient's perspective, a complex set of cultural interactions, both secular and religious, had begun to transform attitudes to the meaning and management of suffering: in a romantically adjusted age pain became more culturally disturbing, and empathy with the sufferer more culturally admirable. Yet, from the perspective of general practitioner campaigners for medical reform over the same period, reform more often than not meant asserting one's credentials as a "man of science" – a dedicated observer of the regularities and pathological irregularities of nature – rather than as a comforter with an individual knowledge of the patient.
>
> (55)

Some medical professionals themselves, including Brown, also worried about impacts of the regulation of medicine on the doctor-patient relationship. Though he was a fellow of the Royal College of Physicians of Edinburgh, Brown's comments on the profession in *Horæ Subsecivæ* indicate his continued belief

> that a cheerful face, and step, and neckcloth, and button-hole, and an occasional hearty and kindly joke, a power of executing and setting agoing a good laugh, are stock in our trade not to be despised. The merry heart does good like a medicine.
>
> (1858, xxvii)

Indeed, for Brown and many other physicians, the institutionalisation of medicine in the Victorian period created a tension between professionalism and humanity, between doctor and patient.

Though Brown does not explicitly mention the move towards the Medical Act in *Horæ Subsecivæ*, the volume as a whole promotes his conservative views on the practice of medicine and the importance of the relationship between the family physician and his patients. This belief is abundantly clear in "Rab and His Friends," which was inspired by Brown's experience apprenticing under famed surgeon James Syme, who pioneered the use of the operating theatre as a place for educating future doctors. Brown first prepared the account for a speech in his hometown of Biggar and later revised that speech into the story.[1] In the Preface to an illustrated edition of *Rab and His Friends* published in 1862, Brown explains how his uncle invited him to speak and his concern over what he should say:

I had an odd sort of desire to say something to these strong-brained primitive people of my youth, who were boys and girls when I left them. I could think of nothing to give them. At last I said to myself, "I'll tell them Ailie's story."

(Quoted in Brown and Forrest 1907, 117)

He describes a sense of urgency in the need to tell the story of Ailie Noble, the breast cancer patient, James her husband, and their dog Rab, saying,

it came on me at intervals almost painfully, as if demanding to be told, as if I heard Rab whining at the door to get in or out ... or as if James was entreating me on his deathbed to tell all the world what his Ailie was.

(117)

This desire to share a patient's story with an understanding of her and her family's perspective rather than presenting it through the style of the medical case study emphasises Brown's position on the importance of medical professionals in literary culture.

"Rab and His Friends" tells a story from 1830, when the narrator is "a medical student, and clerk at Minto House Hospital" and sees James Noble and his mastiff Rab weekly (299). As the narrator leaves the hospital one day, James explains that his wife is ill: "Maister John, this is the mistress; she's got a trouble in her breest – some kind o' an income we're thinkin'" (300).[2] Brown examines Ailie's breast and observes,

there it was, that had once been so soft, so shapely, so white, so gracious and bountiful ... hard as a stone, a centre of horrid pain, making that pale face, with its grey, lucid, reasonable eyes, and its sweet resolved mouth, express the full measure of suffering overcome.

(302)

In this brief description of Ailie's condition, Brown compares the diseased breast with its former healthy and beautiful appearance and laments the effect of the illness on the patient herself, noting how her face indicates Ailie's pain and concern. These details indicate Brown's view of Ailie as a patient, focusing not only on her malady but also on her human response to illness, and foreshadow his approach to treating her as a contrast to that of his mentor and his fellow medical students. This initial examination of Ailie's breast builds upon Brown's introduction of James, Ailie, and Rab, including James's occupation as a carrier, detailed descriptions of the appearance of all three, and his weekly interactions with James and Rab. The details included indicate the personal relationship between Brown and his patient, introduce Brown's emphasis on humanity in the doctor/patient relationship, and demonstrate the working-class status of the family.

The verbose presentation of this initial examination, including dialogue between Brown and James and an observation of Rab's presence, directly contrasts with Syme's examination and diagnosis the next day. As Brown explains, "Next day, my master, the surgeon, examined Ailie. There was no doubt it must kill her, and soon. It could be removed – it might never return – it would give her speedy relief – she should have it done" (304). The short phrases of the surgeon's diagnosis, while not an actual quote, demonstrate the clipped language the surgeon uses in his interaction with Ailie and James. The recorded dialogue between the two parties is reduced to just two words: "Ailie … said, 'When?' 'Tomorrow,' said the kind surgeon – a man of few words" (304). While Brown's own rapport with the Nobles directly contrasts with Syme's approach, his narration of the scene avoids any judgement of Syme by dismissing the seemingly curt behaviour as a personality trait and by describing Syme as kind. To support this portrayal of Syme, Brown describes him as Ailie's "friend the surgeon" at the start of the surgery on the following day.

Similarly, Brown describes the reaction of the medical students entering the operating theatre, "eager to secure good places" and chatting about the case. While initially they may seem insensitive, Brown contextualises their response:

> Don't think them heartless; they are neither better nor worse than you or I: they get over their professional horrors, and into their proper work; and in them pity – as an *emotion*, ending in itself or at best in tears and a long drawn breath, lessens, while pity as a *motive*, is quickened, and gains power and purpose. It is well for poor human nature that it is so.
>
> (305)

Interestingly, through this description, Brown distinguishes himself from the other medical students and from the standard views of medical professionals, aligning himself instead with his audience. His theorising about the place of pity in medicine acknowledges concerns about the institutionalisation of the field and the ways that medical professionals can retain their humanity in treating patients.

Brown continues the story by describing how Ailie's beauty quieted the excited students as soon as she walked in, confirming his own response to Ailie's appearance in his initial examination just a few days before. Throughout the surgery, Ailie "was still and silent" (306) in spite of the operation being performed without anesthesia. As the surgery ends, Brown describes Ailie's behaviour: "she is dressed, steps gently and decently down from the table, looks for James; then, turning to the surgeon and the students, she curtsies, – and in a low, clear voice, begs their pardon if she has behaved ill" (307). This part of the account emphasises the patient's response following the surgery over the operation itself, highlighting Brown's focus on the humanity of the patient. Her behaviour inspires a deeply human response from those observing the surgery, as Brown explains, "The students – all of us – wept like children" (307). Here, instead of separating himself from the other medical students as he did before, Brown reconnects with them in their human response to Ailie's bravery. What he formerly described as a valuable form of medically distant pity dissolves into the emotional pity that doctors often seek to overcome.

In the days that follow, Ailie recovers in the hospital with regular visits from the other medical students, who "came in quiet and anxious, and surrounded her bed. [Ailie] said she liked to see their young, honest faces" (308). By including Ailie's response to the medical students, Brown gives the patient a voice in the medical narrative and develops her deeply human responses into an ironic maternal care for her medical providers. The shift in the medical students' behaviour from loudly entering the operating theatre to quietly approaching a recovering patient's bedside indicates the continued effect of Ailie's humanity during the operation and the emotion of pity they felt for her. Additionally, when they arrived at the operating theatre before, the patient was not yet in the room; here, they enter into a relatively private space where the patient is already present. Syme's response also indicates his feelings towards Ailie as he "dressed her, and spoke to her in his short kind way, pitying her through his eyes" (308). This description continues the portrayal of Syme's seeming short manner of speaking as kind and adds, for the first time, pity. Brown does not evaluate the nature of Syme's pity – as emotion or motive – but based on his extensive experience as a surgeon, this pity seems different from the emotion that led the medical students to tears immediately following the operation.

Even with a combination of her husband's loving care and attention from a medical team, Ailie contracts an infection shortly after the surgery, which was common before Lister's 1867 publication of *Antiseptic Principle of the Practice of Surgery* and the subsequent adoption of antiseptic surgical practices. The dog Rab's presence in the operating room is a key indicator that Syme likely did not follow any sort of antiseptic procedures. After a few days of steady recovery, though, Brown explains, "my patient had a sudden and long shivering" and observes "her eyes were too bright, her cheek coloured; she was restless, and ashamed of being so; the balance was lost; the mischief had begun" (308–09). Even in detailing the symptoms that indicate Ailie's infection, Brown includes Ailie's feelings about the change in her condition, indicating that her reaction is as important as his evaluation of her and highlighting her human response as her health worsens. This is the only point in the story where Brown uses the possessive to identify Ailie as his patient rather than Syme's, and after this change in Ailie's condition, no other medical professionals are mentioned again in the story. Once Ailie is clearly expected to die from the infection, Syme and the medical students seemingly abandon the case and focus on others. Brown, on the other hand, joins James and Rab in caring for Ailie as she dies and writes in explicit detail of her final days. Though only four days pass between the first signs of infection and Ailie's death, Brown dedicates as many pages of the story to her decline as he does to the other six days of her diagnosis, surgery and initial recovery.

Brown describes the many ways he and James attempt to comfort Ailie as her condition worsens. In the midst of these more general observations, Brown describes a specific moment in the night before she dies when Ailie deliriously gathers a gown lying on the bed to her breast as if nursing an infant:

> She held it as a woman holds her sucking child; opening out her night-gown impatiently, and holding it close, and brooding over it, and murmuring foolish little words, as over one whom his mother comforteth, and who sucks and is satisfied. It was pitiful and strange to see her wasted dying look, keen and yet vague, – her immense love.... And then she rocked backward and forward, as if to make it sleep, hushing it, and wasting on it her infinite fondness.
>
> (311)

In this scene, Ailie behaves like an amputee with phantom pains in the lost limb, but instead, "the pain in the breast, telling its urgent story to a bewildered, ruined brain, was misread and mistaken; it suggested to her the uneasiness of a breast full of milk" (311–12). The heartbreaking scene becomes even more so with James's explanation that Ailie is seeking to nurse their child that had died 40 years before. The narration of this scene in explicit detail, rather than another of the moments when the men sang songs and recited Psalms with Ailie, heightens the sentimentality of the story and emphasises Ailie's humanity through acknowledgement of her life before she became a patient. Considering his audience of medical professionals and lay people, Brown seems to challenge them to maintain a medically distant pity and not dissolve into "pity as an *emotion* ending ... in tears and a long drawn breath" (305).

If the detail of Ailie's decline and the image of "Ailie's hand, which James had held, ... hanging down ... soaked with his tears" then licked carefully by Rab (312–13) does not produce such a response, Brown concludes the story with the deaths of James and Rab in short succession. Not long after burying Ailie, James catches a fever because of "his want of sleep, his exhaustion, and his misery" and he dies (316). Upon Brown's queries about Rab shortly after James's death, he learns that Rab, too, had died after refusing to obey his new master, behaviour described almost in terms of suicidal desire as Rab acts in a way that forces the new master to kill him. And so the story ends with all three gone within a few weeks. Brown follows the family's story beyond the loss of his patient, presenting a deep human compassion not required of doctors who may know nothing of their patients' families after death or discharge.

In addition to the professionalisation of medicine, the social position of James and Ailie influences their response to her treatment. Brown describes James as "the Howgate carrier" (301), indicating that James transported goods with his horse and cart, a career that certainly impacted their ability to pay for medical treatment. As Mary Wilson Carpenter (2010) explains, hospitals through much of the nineteenth century were places for the poor that seemed more like prisons in terms of the food and care provided. James's insistence on nursing Ailie in her recovery suggests a sense of discomfort with the level of care provided beyond the surgeon's visits. Additionally, doctors treated patients "as cases from which medical students could learn" (29), which explains the behaviour of the medical students in the operating theatre as part of the motivating, rather than emotional, pity needed in practicing medicine and the fact that Syme and the students disappear once Ailie's case becomes hopeless.

From the start of the story, the couple's social class shapes their access to treatment. Since they would be unable to pay for a private physician, the Nobles must rely on an institution like Syme's Edinburgh Surgical Hospital for Ailie to receive treatment, where he examined "patients who are desirous of admission, and also those treated as out-patients" in the operating theatre each day (Paterson 1874, 43). This did not guarantee treatment, however; as Anne Digby explains, "voluntary hospitals found that local demand outstripped their resources so that poor patients were turned away without treatment" (1994, 44). Indeed, Syme's "Sixth Report of the Edinburgh Surgical Hospital, from August 1830 to February 1831" notes that in this six-month period – the same period when Ailie was treated – "925 patients … applied for relief, and 149 [were] admitted into the house" (1831, 233). Since the challenges of receiving treatment were commonly known, James directly approaches Brown, likely the only person in the medical community he knew, as he leaves the hospital and directly asks Brown to look at Ailie's diseased breast. This appeal to Brown seems the couple's only hope for treating Ailie's breast cancer. Thus, Ailie's public mastectomy in the operating theatre and her recovery, or lack thereof, at the hospital rather than her home are both results of her social class.

Brown's description of Ailie's mastectomy and death just 10 days later demonstrates the reality of breast cancer for many patients in the nineteenth century. The style of the story brings important information about medical treatment for breast cancer and the risk of death following a mastectomy to an audience that was unlikely to be reading the medical literature of the period. The portrayal of a woman from the working class facing breast cancer makes the story even more significant because few, if any, narratives of breast cancer by or about nineteenth-century working-class women exist. Brown's role as a physician and writer of medical essays expands the audience from the general public reading his book of miscellaneous essays to include other doctors who could learn from his account about the psychological trauma for a patient and her family as she undergoes a mastectomy.[3] The details of her emotional response and that of the medical professionals treating her remind readers about the human responses of both doctors and patients in the face of illness and death. The dual audience of such a text, including both general public and medical professionals, makes the story particularly important as a narrative of breast cancer.

The issues related to social class and medical treatment continued to intensify throughout the century. Concerns about the institutionalisation of medicine that, for Brown, was depersonalising the doctor-patient relationship were compounded by the need to treat the rising number of poor and working class that often lived and worked in unsanitary conditions. Not only did poor patients have to worry about whether hospitals would treat their cases, they also had to worry about diseases that resulted from their living conditions. The combination of the realities facing breast cancer patients and the issues of disease in working class communities appears in another short story 40 years after Brown published "Rab and his Friends." Katharine Tynan's "Willie" tells the story of a poor mother with breast cancer living in a community struck by diphtheria. The protagonist's poverty shapes both her response to and treatment for breast cancer, as it also leads to her family's tragic experience with contagious diseases.

The intersection of social class and the spread of disease developed throughout the century, with the cholera epidemic of 1831, mid-century fiction representing the poor living and working in unsanitary conditions, and public health measures of the 1860s, including the Contagious Diseases Acts in 1864, 1867, and 1869. By the 1890s, this debate centred on the outbreaks of diphtheria that had spread from rural communities and reached London. While diphtheria was a clinical diagnosis as early as the 1850s and the diphtheria bacillus was discovered by 1884, understanding of its causes and thus the ways it spread "was a source of confusion and argument within the English medical profession" for another decade (Hardy 1993, 84–85). Even though this proved that defective drainage and contaminated milk did not cause diphtheria, the general public and many medical professionals still suspected a connection between the living conditions of the poor and outbreaks of diphtheria.

An evolving understanding of the disease is evident in the coverage of it in periodicals of the 1890s. *The Speaker*, a politically liberal intellectual weekly founded in 1890 that included sections of general interest and well-known contributors in the arts, addressed the topic a number of times. In 1891, the periodical reported outbreaks of diphtheria and other diseases at St. Bartholomew's Hospital, suggesting a connection with either a recently reopened ward previously closed because of contamination or "grave charges ... about the general sanitation of the hospital – charges of defective drainage and of offensive smells" ("Misfortune" 1891, 215–16). In presenting the 1894 research that suggested the effectiveness of an anti-toxin in treating diphtheria, H.E. Roscoe explains the crisis the disease presented:

> for amongst all the diseases known to medical science there is none more infectious than diphtheria, and none so dangerous or so fatal to children of school age and under. It is a fact no less alarming than true that diphtheria is spreading by leaps and bounds; in rural districts its ravages are even more serious than in our crowded towns.... In some cases the young children of a village have been literally swept away as by the plague.
>
> (1894, 708–09)

Roscoe notes that around "three thousand children died [in 1893] in London alone from diphtheria," so the larger spread in the rural villages is particularly concerning (1894, 708). In a report on "The Health of London" three years later, this number remained steady, with statistics from 1895 indicating diphtheria specifically caused "2,292 deaths among some eleven thousand sufferers" and suggesting that the large number "was due entirely to the mortality among children under five years old" (1897, 452). Regardless of the causes of diphtheria, the fact that it spread quickly among groups of young children playing together meant that the children of the poor were often more susceptible to the disease.

In the midst of these discussions about diphtheria and public health, the 18 June 1898 issue of *The Speaker* included Katharine Tynan's short story "Willie," which combines these larger issues with the effects of breast cancer. Just as "Rab and His Friends" engaged with the major medical debates around the profession-alisation of medicine while representing the realities of breast cancer, "Willie" responds to the concerns about diphtheria as it also presents another complica-tion in treatment for breast cancer leading to the patient's inevitable death. The story centres on issues of social class, illness and medical treatment in the final years of the nineteenth century while also highlighting the human awareness essential to the doctor/patient relationship evident in Brown's work. The titular Willie is the seven-year-old son of Judy Carroll, described as the "poorest of the poor" because her husband Terrence drowned while she was pregnant with Willie (761). The family's poverty is evident in the fact that Willie is the only boy "still in petticoats, which consorted oddly with his very masculine little personality" (761). As Willie suffers insults from the other children, Judy hopes to get enough fabric to make him "the finest trousers in the place" (762). The Carroll family's poverty is remarkable in that it stands out among a town described from the opening of the story as "very poor" (761).

After the brief background information on the town and the story's primary characters, the remainder focuses on Judy's and Willie's illnesses and inter-actions with medical professionals. Judy's ailment begins first, as she has "pain in her breast, sharper than an arrow" and sees Dr. Sharp a week or two later (762). Dr. Sharp, the closest medical professional based in a larger town eight miles away, only visited the "very poor" village of Oyster Creek (761) periodic-ally to provide vaccinations in the hopes of keeping the residents as healthy as possible. His treatment of these patients appears to be charity work and is done primarily out of a deeply human concern for the community. Dr. Sharp examines Judy's "white breast disfigured by an eruption" and diagnoses breast cancer, which will need surgery, explaining, "You'll have to go to the hospital. This thing has roots and will have to be taken away." Like Ailie, Judy's class dictates her treatment at a hospital, away from her home and her son, a fact that worries her nearly as much as the diagnosis. Before she speaks, Judy's response appears through her behaviour, as she "trembled all over, and her eyes were like the eyes of a bird that has been shot." This description simultaneously emphasises Judy's humanity through the emotion of her response and removes it through a compar-ison to a wounded animal. Judy's first words to the doctor actually concern her son rather than her own condition: "'But Willie, doctor,' she said helplessly sitting down in the chair he had placed for her. 'What is to become of Willie?'" (762). Because of her rural location and position as a widow, Judy must travel to a town large enough to have a hospital for the operation and leave Willie in Oyster Creek, relying on other families in the village to care for him in her absence. The overwhelming sense of charity here – in both the doctor's appearance in the village and the support from Judy's neighbours – powerfully highlights the human side of medical treatment, making the patient vulnerable and the doctor generous.

Judy's concerns about the mastectomy extend beyond Willie's care for a few weeks, as she recognises the likelihood that the cancer will still kill her. She confides in the doctor, "if only I'd last till Willie was a man; I'd feel he was all right then for me to go from him" (762). The narration of Judy's thoughts indicates that she is aware of the realities facing her in being treated for the cancer. In the immediate aftermath of the diagnosis, "the terror of women [overtook] her, and she knew what it meant; for even in Oyster Creek women had died of cancer." After Judy asks the doctor several times about the chances that the operation will cure her, Dr. Sharp reluctantly assures her, "we'll do our best for you," as the text confirms, "he spoke with a confidence he was far from feeling." This response, in spite of his understanding of the situation, makes both the doctor and patient appear more human. As a medical professional, Dr. Sharp was expected to be direct and honest in presenting the realities of Judy's illness, but his humanity and his belief in the humanity of his patient leads him to soften the reality without making false promises. Judy, too, knew the likelihood that her cancer would return because "she knew other women to be cut for the cancer, and it had always come back" (762). While Dr. Sharp and Judy determine that a mastectomy is the best treatment for her, both clearly understand the grim reality that few women were cured of breast cancer for the long term.

Though the surgery is successful and she returns to Willie after a few weeks, Judy's poverty shapes her experience in recovery, making her unable to work. She refuses public welfare and is supported through the kindness of neighbours to survive the winter (761–62). In her fear of the surgery and refusal to receive public assistance, Judy's poverty and pride shape her response. As the hope of spring returns, however, Judy discovers that "the cancer [had] started in the other breast." Instead of consulting the doctor, she hides it by "wrapping her little shawl across the breast that was eaten as by vultures" (762). This graphic description illustrates both the reality of how breast cancer could appear and how likely it was to return or spread even after a mastectomy. As in the moment of her diagnosis, the recurrence of the cancer highlights Judy's humanity through her fear of illness while simultaneously dehumanising her in the description of her breast, with the attack of vultures suggesting her body is already dead.

After dedicating over two-thirds of the story to the introduction and Judy's illness, the story turns to Willie's illness when he comes home one evening with a headache, sore throat and fever. When he does not improve with traditional remedies overnight, Judy visits a neighbour where she learns that other children of the village have similar symptoms. Once the first child dies, the villagers "sen[t] a boy running for his life the eight miles to town to fetch the doctor," and though "Dr. Sharp came with all speed, [he] found Oyster Creek full of dead and dying children." With a diagnosis of "diphtheria of a virulent type," the doctor calls in other medical professionals and tries to treat as many children as he can (762). By the time he reaches Judy's cabin, though, Willie has been lying on Judy's lap dead for two hours. When she asks what killed all of the children,

Dr. Sharp replies, "It's something you never heard of, my poor Judy.... It's the diphtheria, though God knows how it ever got here, and not a drain within miles of you" (763). This suggests that Dr. Sharp continues to believe that the illness spread through unsanitary conditions, a view disproven in the years before. As a rural doctor serving a poor community, he lacks the most current medical knowledge to treat the village. Addressing the grieving mother as "my poor Judy," Dr. Sharp's explanation recalls Brown's feelings about Ailie. Not only does the doctor use a possessive "my" to indicate his connection to her as a person and a patient, but the use of "poor" shows a sense of pity for her.

The story concludes with a paragraph of reflection from the narrator:

> The doctors and nurses came too late, and Oyster Creek was swept almost clear of children. When I have gone there since and have seen the quiet women, and the few children playing on the beach, I have always recalled Willie, a big boy in his petticoats, riotously leading his madcap little crowd.
>
> (763)

As the story returns to its titular focus on Willie with the image of his poverty apparent in his apparel, the larger message seems to be about the diphtheria outbreak and its effects on a poor, rural village, as a fictional response to the discussions about public health and diphtheria on the pages of *The Speaker* in the 1890s. The inclusion of Judy's illness, however, complicates this, particularly because less than a third of the story actually includes the outbreak and its aftermath. Rather than being simply a story about the effects of one type of disease, which was still often dismissed as a result of unsanitary conditions, "Willie" addresses the larger issues at the intersection social class and medical treatment at the end of the nineteenth century, including both patients' mistrust of medical institutions and lower quality of medical treatment. The relationship between doctor and patient in the tragic story emphasises the value of humanity for both parties in facing illnesses they did not fully understand.

Judy's decision to endure the treatment is explicitly connected to both her son and her social class: "Like all her class, she had a deep horror of an operation, but since it promised at least a respite, she endured what they feel to be the degradation of being cut and maimed, for Willie's sake" (762). This reference to her class dismisses Judy's valid concerns about undergoing surgery, implying that the poor may lack the education or knowledge to understand the benefits of such an operation and only find the surgery degrading in some way. The narrator separates himself from this working-class misconception with the word *they*, noting this fear is not one shared by those of the narrator's class. Working-class fears of surgery, however, were still common in the 1890s primarily due to decades of Poor Laws and public health practices that bred mistrust of medical treatment.[4] This feeling is evident among the villagers when Dr. Sharp visits Oyster Creek in order to vaccinate the children, whose "matrons ... came unwillingly, hugging their yet unhurt babies to their breasts" (762). Logie Barrow (2002) explains the many reasons for resistance to compulsory vaccination through the Poor Law Guardians, including that "parents ... objected to what they saw as the confusing and unfair workings of the state machinery of compulsion" and because of issues with "the public vaccination facilities set up to provide for the poor" (206). Parents of the lower class viewed these public health stations "as dangerous to their children and demeaning to themselves" (220). Such suspicions demonstrate the larger mistrust that Judy and the other villagers have of medical treatments, including both the compulsory vaccinations and going away to a hospital for surgery.

Perhaps one of the reasons Judy is willing to endure the operation is Dr. Sharp's willingness to develop a human relationship with her. His kindness to Judy is evident from the beginning but is unique enough to warrant an explanation as to why he treated a woman patient in this way: "His young wife had died before the honeymoon was old, and he was compassionate to women" (762). Including the doctor's own background, something unnecessary to the plot, demonstrates the shared human experience of loss that motivates his kindness in treating female patients. Twice when speaking with Judy, he addresses her as "my poor Judy," first in his diagnosis and call for the mastectomy and then in his explanation of the diphtheria that killed her beloved son. Even his assurances of her recovery, which the narrator notes conflict with the doctor's fears, seem driven by compassion and kindness. Dr. Sharp resembles Brown in his conversation with Judy, and this demeanour seems to be somewhat exceptional when compared to Syme's clipped speech in "Rab and His Friends" and influences Judy's decision to accept treatment.

Just as Brown based "Rab and His Friends" on his knowledge of breast cancer as a medical student, so too does "Willie" draw on Tynan's experience with breast cancer through the illnesses of two of her literary mentors in the decade prior to the story's publication.[5] First, Ellen O'Leary died in 1889 after enduring a mastectomy while gripping a crucifix after she refused anesthetics and facing a recurrence of the disease. Then, Christina Rossetti died in 1894 when her breast cancer returned two years after her mastectomy. The addition of breast cancer to a text that in its title and its context seems to have initially focused on diphtheria and public health demonstrates Tynan's own, though secondary, experience with the illness and recognition of the harsh realities for women facing breast cancer at the end of the nineteenth century. Tynan uses a topic of current public interest for her audience to introduce a narrative that was largely suppressed in nineteenth-century fiction. "Willie" and the issue of diphtheria in children also provided Tynan with an important basis (the affective appeal of a child) for talking about women undergoing medical examinations during which they disrobed and revealed that the symbols of maternal generosity and female beauty were also sites of disease and suffering. The short story fits into *The Speaker*'s mission well by making the topic of diphtheria of interest to general readers, while presenting the issues of class and illness in the politically charged context of the periodical.

The inclusion of real experiences with breast cancer certainly separates "Willie" and "Rab and His Friends" from the representation of Lady Delacour's cancer scare in *Belinda*. Not only do Ailie and Judy endure mastectomies, but they also eventually die because of their breast cancer. By incorporating the realities of illness into their stories, Brown and Tynan represent the humanity of the patient through fiction. The patients experience all of the fear that comes with cancer, including worries before the diagnosis, about the operations they endure, and about the complications or recurrence that cause their deaths. They bare cancerous breasts for the doctors, showing bodies ravaged by disease. They submit to treatments in hospitals away from home without much expectation of a positive result. In many ways, the women's social classes shape their realities in facing illness, as the stories represent the human experience of many nineteenth-century patients.

Perhaps the larger distinction between these two stories and *Belinda*, however, is in the way that they reflect contemporary medical debates. While *Belinda* acknowledges the dangers of quackery, it only does so through the fictional representation of a doctor taking advantage of Lady Delacour. In their texts, however, Brown and Tynan explicitly engage in the medical discourse around medical professionalisation, the relationships between doctors and patients, the impact of social class on medical treatment, and policies around public health. The stories show the effects of these debates in the lives of the patients, as the narration addresses the issues directly. The interaction between medicine and literature in these texts demonstrates the myriad ways each shapes the other in representing the human condition.

Notes

1 Brown describes the differences in the two versions of the stories and his own troubles with public speaking:

> I was at Biggar the other day, and some of good folks told me, with a grave smile peculiar to that region, that when Rab came to them in print he was so good that they wouldn't believe he was the same Rab I had delivered in the school-room – a testimony to my vocal powers of impressing the multitude somewhat conclusive.
> (Quoted in Brown and Forrest 1907, 117)

2 Erin O'Connor explains the nineteenth-century use of the term *income* for a tumor or growth and discusses the complicated associations between this definition and the more common monetary meaning (2009, 60).

3 Brown explains this purpose for his stories in the preface to *Horæ Subsecivæ* along with the importance of returning to the days when physicians were also involved in literary culture (1858, xi–xii).

4 Elizabeth Hurren's "Poor Law versus Public Health: Diphtheria, Sanitary Reform, and the 'Crusade' against Outdoor Relief, 1870–1900" and Logie Barrow's "In the Beginning was the Lymph: The Hollowing of Stational Vaccination in England and Wales, 1840–98" provide valuable overviews of these topics and the reasons members of the working class distrusted institutionalised medicine.

5 Tynan memorialised both women in essays for the periodical press including "A Fenian's Sister" about O'Leary for *The Speaker* and "Some Reminiscences of Christina Rossetti" for *The Bookman*.

Reference list

Barrow, Logie. 2002. "In the Beginning was the Lymph: The Hollowing of Stational Vaccination in England and Wales, 1840–98." In *Medicine, Health and the Public Sphere in Britain, 1600–2000*, edited by Steve Sturdy, 205–23. London: Routledge.

Brown, John. 1858. *Horæ Subsecivæ: Locke and Sydenham with Other Occasional Papers*, Edinburgh: Thomas Constable.

[Brown, John], and D.W. Forrest, ed. 1907. *Letters of Dr. John Brown, With Letters from Ruskin, Thackeray, and Others*. London: Adam and Charles Black.

Carrier, John and Ian Kendall. 2016. *Health and the National Health Service*, 2nd edn. Milton Park and New York: Routledge.

Digby, Anne. 1994. *Making a Medical Living: Doctors and Patients in the English Market for Medicine, 1720–1911*. Cambridge: Cambridge University Press.

Hardy, Anne. 1993. *The Epidemic Streets: Infectious Diseases and the Rise of Preventive Medicine 1856–1900*. Oxford: Clarendon Press.

Hurren, Elizabeth. 2005. "Poor Law versus Public Health: Diphtheria, Sanitary Reform, and the 'Crusade' against Outdoor Relief, 1870–1900." *Social History of Medicine* 18.3: 399–418.

"The Health of London." 1897. *The Speaker*, 24 April: 451–52.

Kent, Christopher. 2009. "The Speaker." In *Dictionary of Nineteenth Century Journalism*, edited by Laurel Brake and Marysa Demoor, 587. Gent: Academia Press.

"Misfortune or Mismanagement at St. Bartholomew's?" 1891. *The Speaker*, 21 February: 215–16.

O'Connor, Erin. 2000. *Raw Material: Producing Pathology in Victorian Culture*. Durham, NC: Duke University Press.

Paterson, Robert. 1874. *Memorials of the Life of James Syme*. Edinburgh: Edmonston and Douglas.

Roberts, Michael J.D. 2009. "The Politics of Professionalization: MPs, Medical Men, and the 1858 Medical Act" *Medical History* 53.1: 37–56.

Roscoe, H.E. 1894. "Diphtheria and Its Cure." 29 December: 708–09.

Syme, James. 1831. "Sixth Report of the Edinburgh Surgical Hospital, from August 1830 to February 1831." *Edinburgh Medical and Surgical Journal* 35.107: 233–58.

Tougaw, Jason Daniel. 2006. *Strange Cases: The Medical Case History and the British Novel*. New York: Routledge.

Tynan, Katharine. 1894. "A Fenian's Sister." *The Speaker*, 19 May: 554–56.

Tynan, Katharine. 1895. "Some Reminiscences of Christina Rossetti." *The Bookman*, February: 141–42.

Tynan, Katharine. 1898. "Willie." *The Speaker*, 18 June: 761–63.

Wilson Carpenter, Mary. 2010. *Health, Medicine, and Society in Victorian England*. Santa Barbara, CA: Praeger.

14 "My lawful wife and mistress"

A physician's perspective

Uzo Dibia

> Medicine is my lawful wife and literature is my mistress. When I get tired of one I spend the night with the other. Though it's disorderly, it's not dull, and besides neither loses anything from my infidelity.
>
> (Letter from Anton Chekhov to A.S. Suvorin, 11 September 1888)

Russian-born physician, playwright and author Anton Chekhov (1860–1904) demonstrated both in his practice of medicine and through his writing a deep understanding of his patients and their ailments. In his letter to A.S. Suvorin, in which he describes medicine as his wife and literature as his mistress, he suggests that neither suffered from his infidelity: "when I get tired of one, I spend the night with the other" (Chekhov 2004), as if medicine and literature were oblivious of each other's existence; that one would satisfy where the other fell short. Yet such a reading of Chekhov's meaning gives a false impression of the relationship he saw between the two. Indeed, rather than unrelated, distinct entities that never cross paths, Chekhov understood the ways in which medicine and literature speak to each other. His literary characters reveal an author whose knowledge of people transcended the superficial, reaching right through to the core of their individuality, assembling, disassembling and restructuring their essence, hence rendering a clearer, truer picture of the reality they may inadvertently conceal. In much the same way, he was known to care for the whole being of his patients:

> [Chekhov] did everything with attention and a manifest love of what he was doing especially towards the patients who passed through his hands. He listened quietly to them, never raising his voice however tired he was and even if the patient was talking about things quite irrelevant to the illness. The mental state of the patient interested him particularly. As well as traditional medicines, he attached great significance to the effect the doctor had on the psyche of the patient, and on his way of life.
>
> (Hart 1997, 1243)

Medicine has come a long way from its humble beginnings to the marvels of science and technology we now see. Yet somewhere between the demystification of precepts and the accretion of facts, the science and art of medicine have drifted away from each other. It appears that physicians treat the ailing body, but have forgotten about the human being. Lip service is paid to "holistic medicine" but compassion and empathy seem to elude this definition. Medicine has become a victim of the growing divide between technological advancement and the human side of care.

If our knowledge of medicine is much greater than it has ever been, and yet our understanding of the patient's plight seems ever more remote and distant, then we must address this anomaly. Doctors are taught to present facts in a bland manner, to "get rid of adverbs and adjectives, pictures, first person, and just let the science sing" (Brook 2010, 2528). We have let the science sing but the song we hear lacks rhythm, cadence and imagination: factual, yes, but not deeply engaging; concise, but not punctilious enough to evoke deeper ruminations over what illness means to the individual, his immediate family and society as a whole. This sense of detachment that one is taught in medical school all but desensitises and dehumanises doctors towards patients. A sense of duty trumps an avowal of empathy, "a stance that compromises our capacity to directly respond to the human dimension of the clinical encounter" (Oyebode 2010, 243).

The art of taking a patient's history, followed by a clinical examination, are time-honoured crafts of medical enquiry. Here, details of symptoms are given credence, as important signs are discovered during a physical examination, followed by laboratory tests, which are adjuncts to making an accurate diagnosis. These observations and accompanying tests reveal the obvious; that is, the physical condition of the patient and the complications of disease. What is sometimes overlooked is usually subtler – how the disease impacts the patient and his wider world, or the diurnal pressure physicians face in an attempt to do the best for patients. In the face of all this, our response as physicians should still be on diagnostic accuracy without compromising empathy, or disregard for our own wellbeing.

I argue that literature can lead us back to the tenets of empathy, patience, and understanding of ourselves, whether as patients or as healers. A greater understanding of humans – of what it means to be human – may be found in the arts and not the sciences. Through focusing on works by Anton Chekhov, Franz Kafka, T.S. Eliot and Alexander Solzhenitsyn, I will examine the ways in which literature informs the practice of medicine, as well as how we can use our literary past to enrich our experience of a better medical future. Literature creates an aesthetic distance – a detachment from the subject being studied – and in doing so, it allows a narrative to be engaged with more deeply, therefore facilitating reflection and empathy (Cupchik 2002; Koopman and Hakemulder 2015). Furthermore, it provides "a place in which to test emotions and experiences without the consequences of a real encounter" (Wellbery 2000), leading to personal and intellectual enrichment. The works I have chosen deliberately engage, directly and indirectly, with medical precepts and practice, providing paradigms that relate to the often simple, sometimes complex, relationship between the doctor and patient. Chekov, for example, portrays figures suffering from illness and their doctors with an insight that suggests his first-hand experience of what they felt, indicating a translation of ideas between his writing and his practice as a physician. His convictions regarding empathy and the art of listening to one's patients are made clear throughout his writing, yet the most crucial question that hovers over Chekov's perspective remains: is it necessary for the doctor to keep his or her humanity in check in order to treat patients in a professional manner?

"A Doctor's Visit" (1898): spot diagnoses and empathy

Korolyov, the eponymous doctor in Chekhov's tale, is a physician from Moscow, who travels to the country to attend to a wealthy heiress, Lizanka, living with her mother, Madame Lyalikov, whose factory she will inherit. When Korolyov visits her, Lizanka has apparently been ill for a long time, suffering violent palpitations of the heart, and has seen various other doctors who have given her various medications to little effect. On meeting Lizanka, Korolyov is easily able to diagnose her anxiety, but unable to unravel to its genesis. Lizanka tells him: "I have palpitations of the heart.... It was so awful all night.... I almost died of fright!" (Chekhov 2003, 175). After examining her, Korolyov responds:

> The heart is all right ... it's all going on satisfactorily; everything is in good order. Your nerves must have been playing pranks a little, but that's so common. The attack is over now; one must suppose; lie down and go to sleep.
>
> (176)

Korolyov's dismissal of Lizanka's initial complaint as something trivial is redolent of the anxious patient who always presents to the emergency room, even though he or she has presented multiple times and nothing wrong is ever found. More importantly, this is nineteenth-century Eurasia, where primitive ideas about women and their illnesses still held sway. The disproportionate representation of morbidity among women seems to suggest that the "sick role" seemed more culturally acceptable for them (Nathanson 1975): malingering, or pretense, on the part of women was more acceptable to the nineteenth-century paternalistic world. If this indeed was Korolyov's initial purview, we can then understand why his initial reaction appears dismissive and nonchalant.

However, Korolyov's "spot diagnosis" – an unconscious recognition of a particular non-verbal pattern, auditory or visual (Heneghan *et al.* 2009) – and use of heuristics (that is, short-cuts or memory aides as used by doctors the world over) remain familiar to many in medicine and have their uses. Yet heuristics potentially lead to cognitive biases, which can result in diagnostic errors. They make assumptions about a patient's condition that, while not entirely wrong, are grossly incomplete. Korolyov initially regards Lizanka's symptoms as nothing more than "nerves," and would have left but for the entreaties of Lizanka's mother. Doctors, especially more senior and experienced ones, do resort to short-cuts and heuristics to diagnose quickly and manage patients, but inappropriate selectivity has consequences (Minué *et al.* 2014).

A spot diagnosis should always be followed by a formal enquiry into the nature of the problem, and the attendant signs and symptoms need to be explored thoroughly. Revisiting a patient's presentation by going back to the history of the signs and symptoms may reveal important facts missed or overlooked during the first encounter. It is Korolyov's willingness to dwell for a time in Lizanka's situation – to walk in her shoes – that enables him to understand her anxiety as a symptom of other concerns. That night, his senses are overwhelmed by the nature of life at Madame Lyalikov's home and its proximity to the factory she owns. Existence there is full of drudgery and monotony – the sounding of the bell punctuating each hour that passes; the loud refrain from frogs and gales in their nighttime tryst; the trains and carriages in their slow revelry: all was repetitive, gloomy and dull. His preconception of factories is confirmed:

> He always thought how quiet and peaceable it was outside (factories), but within there was always sure to be impenetrable ignorance and dull egoism on the side of the owners, wearisome, unhealthy toil on the side of the work-people, squabbling, vermin, vodka.
>
> (Chekhov 2003, 174)

His views here echo those of a young Friedrich Engels observing the precarious working conditions of factory workers in Manchester, the city itself described as a place of "filth, ruin and uninhabitableness." Yet Korolyov's example is a privileged young woman, so the question arises whether her anxiety is the product of, or a reaction to, the plight of the working-class people who work for her mother. Lizanka's is a different kind of imprisonment. Her anxiety can be read as a reaction to being sheltered from experiential existence – not being able to explore the world beyond her country manor.

Deliberately connecting Lizanka's condition to factory life, Korolyov's impression is written in terms of an incurable disease:

> As a doctor accustomed to judging correctly of chronic complaints, the radical cause of which also was incomprehensible and incurable, he looked upon factories as something baffling, the cause of which was obscure and not removable, and all the improvements in the life of the factory hands he looked upon not as superfluous, but as comparable with the treatment of incurable illness.
>
> (Chekhov 2003, 178)

Chronic diseases often have no cure. Some live with them, managing flares as they present. Others pursue endless investigations and tests in the hope of finding a cure that may not exist. Not all symptoms readily lend themselves to a firm diagnosis and it appears that Korolyov is powerless to do much in this situation. He knows Lizanka has tried various medicines and concoctions but has never been cured. The constant siege of her senses, by both known and strange stimuli, manifests as a morbid anxiety. Categorising diagnoses into physical, emotional or unknown causes opens the door to consider alternative diagnoses when physicians cannot ascertain a condition's cause (Breen and Greenberg 2010). Korolyov thinks Lizanka's problem may be emotional, or at least an emotional response to a yet undiagnosed problem. He suspects her external milieu lends itself to a perturbation of the senses: the never-ending noise of peasants working during the day; the palpable silence that consumes the night. And in that silence, the sentience of the factory's soul burns in the flames that it generates, a constant reminder of its *raison d'être*: to serve its mistress and nothing else. This inveterate thought of her place in society is now the same knot that ties her to an existence where she seems to not have much volition. Korolyov posits that her position of wealth and privilege unsettles her:

"You in the position of a factory owner and wealthy heiress are dissatisfied; you don't believe in your right to it; and here now you can't sleep. That, of course, is better than if you were satisfied, slept soundly, and thought everything was satisfactory. Your sleeplessness does you credit; in any case, it is a good sign."

(Chekhov 2003, 182)

Lizanka never acknowledges this as the issue, and it is only by listening to her again that Korolyov begins to understand the way she earlier expresses the nature of her plight:

"I am lonely. I have a mother I love, but, all the same, I am lonely. That's how it happens to be. Lonely people read a great deal, but say little and hear little. Life for them is mysterious; they are mystics and often see the devil where he is not. Lermontov's Tamara was lonely and she saw the devil."

(181)

Korolyov's preconceived notions about Lizanka are, to a degree, overturned after this declaration. While he initially saw her as a rich, spoilt heiress, what he sees now is an only child with an overbearing mother who sees the need to shelter her daughter from every potential harm. Listening to Lizanka, more attentive to the details of her immediate environment and surroundings, Korolyov earns her trust and empathises with her. It is this, the physician's ability to sit back and listen, this empathetic bond created between patient and doctor that leads her to trust him implicitly, this shared recognition of each other's humanity that leads to a better and more fruitful doctor-patient relationship.

"A Country Doctor" (1916): duty and vulnerability

German-Jewish writer Franz Kafka (1883–1924), well known for maintaining a healthy cynicism towards religion, extended that same courtesy to the medical profession. His short story "A Country Doctor" elucidates the moral dilemma doctors sometimes face, torn between a sense of duty and an instinct for self-preservation; trying to ensure order in the midst of chaos; attempting to make sense out of disorder, to find meaning when none exists. Which is more important, to attend to the patient or your own needs first? Should the patient's problems supersede all others, even your own? Should a doctor, when faced with this moral dilemma, negate his responsibility to family, friends and loved ones, even if they, too, are faced with their own problems?

In this story, an old doctor has to go out to tend to a sick patient 10 miles away. His horse died the night before; it is an unforgiving Russian winter, and he has sent his servant girl out to borrow a horse from any of the villagers, to no avail. A groomsman appears, who kindly lends him horses but tries to take advantage of the servant girl, as the doctor departs. The doctor, it seems, sacrifices his servant girl's safety, by leaving her to attend to a patient, miles away. He wrestles with the decision he has made, to leave her to an uncertain fate, because when duty calls, he must obey. Even when he arrives at his destination, there is some ambivalence, anger even. Is there some affection deeper than would be expected between master and servant, or something less complicated but sincere, humane? Why doesn't the doctor make an effort to stay back? Why does the groomsman want to defile the doctor's maid?

Even though the doctor decides to go to the patient's, he still questions whether he made the right decision:

> I had to sacrifice Rosa as well, that lovely girl who has been living with me for a year, most of the time stupidly overlooked by me – that loss is simply too great, and I must work hard to shrink it in my own head so as not to take it out on this family here, which with the best will in the world is not going to restore Rosa to me.
>
> (Kafka 2008, 188)

Here he laments his inability to have negotiated the circumstances of his predicament, even with its obvious paradoxes: he scarcely notices his maid, who has lived with him all year long, yet now he acknowledges her beauty; that he is going to save a life yet must rationalise why that life is more important than that of his maid, who is about to be defiled; he must remain self-possessed despite an urge to lash out at the family who sought his help at such an inauspicious time. Perhaps it is not his failing as a doctor as such, but as a man, that preoccupies him. It is this inability to "anticipate and control the bewildering flow of experience" (Guth 1965, 427) that he laments and broods about, to the point of despair, yet a sense of duty prevails: "I am employed by the parish, and do my duty to the point where it is almost too much for one man. Though badly paid, but I am generous and helpful to the poor" (Kafka 2008, 188).

A survey of doctors at different levels of training in the United Kingdom found that the absence of a work-life balance was not uncommon, with high expectations of service provision yet little support for the providers (Woolf *et al.* 2016). One doctor even commented, "you can't be a person and a doctor," emphasising how the demands of the job lead to a negation of other aspects of one's life, even when the remuneration is incommensurate. Kafka's doctor, and all doctors, then, see medicine as a calling, not dissimilar to the religious calling of priesthood. The larger society's perceptions of disease and healing seemed to be shaped by this tenet of faith, and Kafka's doctor, at a point, mocks the town's people who have elevated him to the status of a priest:

> That's the way people are in this parish. Always demanding the impossible from the doctor. They have lost their old faith; the priest sits around at home, ripping up his altar garments one after another; but the doctor is expected to perform miracles with his delicate surgeon's hand.
>
> (Kafka 2008, 189)

While he derides the apostasy of the villagers, he also seems to find himself partly culpable for this perception they have of him, this ability to "achieve everything." The high expectations of him from the villagers stand in stark contrast to what he believes he will be able to achieve for the dying patient. The patient, even in his delirium, is able to see the doctor's ambivalence towards this visit, accusing him of "taking up room on his deathbed," an indictment of the doctor's attention, and, ultimately, commitment. The doctor acknowledges his inattention but is also quick to point out that he, just like his patient, has other concerns, worries, doubts, fears. He says: "Believe me, it's not easy for me either" (Kafka 2008, 190).

When faced with such personal challenges, how does the physician cope? When does the healer become the patient, looking for some healing of his own? Do physicians recognise the need to seek help during personal crises, as these may adversely affect their work, or do they hide under the casuistry of self-assuredness, telling themselves and their patients, that everything is okay when it isn't? More likely than not, doctors fail to attend to their own problems. Burnout is common (Halliday *et al.* 2016); depression, and even suicide, is higher among physicians when compared to the general population, much of this stemming from the pressures of balancing expectations at work with life outside of it (Merlo 2016). There is a wide chasm between one's ability to heal as a physician, and the acknowledgement of one's shortcomings, especially in moments of deep personal anguish. This "conspiracy of silence" is a lack of acknowledgement of the physician's need to respond to their own physical and mental stressors, prior to dealing with patients, that will likely compromise patient care (Merlo 2016). Doctors must recognise that they are as imperfect and flawed as the people who seek their help; doctors must recognise that they are human. It is this recognition of their vulnerabilities that will make for a deeper appreciation of what they do to, and for, their patients.

Cancer Ward (1968): trash and trauma

Cancer Ward is Alexander Solzhenitsyn's semi-autobiographical account of the fate of prisoners under Stalin, seen through the eyes of patients in a cancer unit.

The theme of dispossession runs through the accounts of Oleg Kostoglotov, who has stomach cancer, Dyoma, a young socially conscious youth who has a lower limb amputation, and Anya, a gymnast and Dyoma's lover, who undergoes a mastectomy for breast cancer. Oleg fears loss of his libido as a result of the treatment he is receiving; Dyoma contemplates life without a limb; and Asya questions her womanhood without what she feels is its very essence – her sexuality, immanent in how she feels she will be looked upon (or not) by others, with the loss of a breast. To refer to these characters as "just patients" would be incomplete; like the word "specimen," it suggests an "otherness," an object of scientific enquiry, the word "patients" evokes pity, rather than an attempt to understand what they actually are – humans who have lost something precious.

Oleg's account begins after several injections of Sinestrol, an oestrogen-containing drug. While cancer chemotherapy agents were limited in those days, and hence some experimental drugs may have been tried, being a prisoner of the state, Oleg fears that this was another form of humiliation, a chemical castration. While the motivation is unclear in the text, what is not in doubt is the drug's side effects in men, which may include feminisation and a loss of male sexual urges. Oleg contemplates whether its effects, over time, add up. He addresses his concerns to Lev Leonidovich, a surgeon with whom he is acquainted:

> "They're giving me a course of hormone therapy by reason of … intramuscular Sinestrol injections, in doses of…" (Kostoglotov took pride in his ability to talk to doctors in their language, with full precision. It was the basis of his claim that they should talk to him with complete frankness). "What interests me is this: is the effect of the hormone therapy cumulative or not."
>
> (411)

The doctor's reply does not satisfy him. Oleg was insistent on knowing his fate:

> "It's very important for me to understand," said Kostoglotov. He looked and talked as if he was threatening the other. "After this treatment will I lose the ability to … well, I mean, as far as women are concerned? Or will it just be for a limited period? Will the injected hormones leave my body or will they stay forever? Or perhaps the therapy can be reversed for a while by cross-injections?"
>
> (411)

Lev Leodinovich's response to this is to state how the pursuit of women is a distraction from one's goals: "Listen to me," he said, "do you really think women are the flower of life? You know, you can get fed up with them after a while … All they do is stop you achieving anything serious" (412).

The doctor fails to understand, or rather ignores, the pertinence of the question put to him. For Oleg Kostoglotov, there seems to be no point in living, if one cannot perform one's sexual duties. Not far removed from procreation, yet the knowledge that these thoughts and desires can be pursued to fruition, to rise in the moment of crisis, is a thought that plagues Oleg, that makes him question his self-worth. There is a long-held perception that a "real man" is a virile, sexually motivated man (Reed 2014), and Leodinovich's attempt to make Oleg focus on other things beside a loss of libido, though well-intentioned, is apathetic at best, and displays a lack of empathy at worst. It does raise the question of what it is that makes us feel more alive, more human; sexual desire and its consummation represent one spectrum of that ideal.

Dyoma's narrative begins a week after he has had a lower limb amputated, most likely due to bone cancer. His phantom limb experience challenges the physical loss: "The operation was receding into the past, but his leg stayed with him, torturing him as if it hadn't been removed. He could feel each toe separately" (417). What was more severe, the amputation itself or the constant reminder of his missing appendage? French doctor Ambrose Pare's work on phantom limbs focused on understanding its origins. It leaves its victims often in pain, sometimes depressed but always constantly reminded of the absence of that limb. Avoidance is not an uncommon phenomenon, but it has the potential to aggravate the phantom pain. Embracing the finality of the dismemberment may have been bearable for Dyoma but for the "phantom sensation," a constant reminder of what he now has to learn to do without. His way of coping with loss seems to be focusing on when he will be discharged from the hospital, and the things he would love to do; a way of distraction that may make living with his amputation a bit more bearable (Trevelyan, Turner and Robinson 2016). Self-reliance and fierce independence sometimes mask an underlying poor coping mechanism, which may give rise to further phantom pain, and grief months and even years after the amputation (Maguire and Parkes 1998). As physicians, we must remind ourselves that psychological scars are often refractory to physical therapies, medications and one-off hospital visits. Knowing that we care by devoting the time and energy to these, makes patients more human to us, and us, more humane, to patients.

Asya, a beautiful, young gymnast who comes to visit Dyoma while he contemplates a limbless future, is distraught, angry and terrified. Lumps had been found in her right breast, and now the surgeons were going to perform a mastectomy: "'they are going to cu-c-cut it off…!' She cried and she cried. And then she started to groan, 'O-o-oh!'" (423). It is not just the loss of a mere body part that troubles her – it is the loss of a breast, a symbol of her womanhood. The preservation of its entirety is of utmost concern to her, even though its integrity has been compromised by cancer. The same way she had pleaded with Dyoma earlier to preserve his diseased leg, she now faced a similar tragedy, or worse in her opinion. Even now, Dyoma's entreaties to her to calm down, to listen to reason, and focus on her inner qualities as the bases of future expressions of love and romance, rather than dwell on her cancerous breast, is redolent of Lev Leodinovich's attempts to downplay the joys of sexual love. He tells her: "You know how people get married … They have the same sort of opinions … the same sort of characters" (423–24). To this, Asya retorts:

"What sort of a fool loves a girl for her character?" She started up angrily, like a horse rearing. She pulled her hand away, and Dyoma saw her face for the first time – wet, flushed, blotched, miserable and angry. "Who wants a girl with one breast? Who wants a girl like that? When she's seventeen!" She shouted the words at him. It was his fault.

(424)

Asya conflates physical desire and physical appearances; one is dependent on the other. Her desirability is a function of how she looks, and she shudders at the thought of how her femininity will be perceived once she is dismembered. For Asya, the breast had not yet served its purpose and now it was going to cut off, excised and thrown away like a piece of rubbish. This need to be loved, admired and sought after, through the cultural objectification of the female form, informs her perception of herself, and her reaction to her impending mastectomy. While not perverse in itself, this type of thinking may not necessarily lead to happiness (Ramsey *et al.* 2017). Asya believes she will be judged by her looks, her disproportionate body, her imperfection, her forgotten breast. Asya's head is full of thoughts of undesirability, fear of negotiating the present, adjusting to a new normal, and uncertainties about future breast cancer recurrence. These could inevitably lead to depression and negative ideas about oneself. The notion that the breast is unworthy, hence its disposal, becomes the realisation of the unworthiness of the body as a whole (Arroyo and López 2011). She pleads with Dyoma:

"You'll remember? ... You'll remember, won't you? You'll remember it was there, and what it was like?" ... When she did not take it away, he returned to its rosy glow again and again, softly kissing the breast. He did what her future child would never be able to do. No one came in, and so he kissed and kissed the marvel hanging over him. Today it was a marvel. Tomorrow it would be in the bin.

(425)

A surgeon's blade may take away a cancerous growth, or cut out a gangrenous limb, but will never address the feelings of inadequacy it produces on the patient. Healing should commence long before the surgical knife intervenes; it is the doctor's duty to pay attention to the details of a patient's hopes, doubts and fears, in the acceptance of personal loss, before and after it actually occurs. In this way, the patient's grief is given life, addressed more humanely and managed more appropriately.

"Eyes that Last I Saw in Tears" (1919): reflections on death

Most of T.S. Eliot's (1888–1965) work takes on a sombre, reflective tone. His poem "Eyes that Last I Saw in Tears" draws on this sombre tradition, leading down the paths of remembrance and remorse that doctors may experience when patients die: "I see the eyes but not the tears / This is my affliction" (Eliot 2011, ll. 5–6). The poet's last encounter with the deceased was not a pleasant one. Earth is described as "death's other kingdom" (l. 3), a biblical reference to life as a kind of death, and the final resurrection, when the Christ returns, as the beginning of a new life. If we substitute the doctor for the poet, we can engage more deeply with this regret. The doctor is human, and his last encounter with the patient was not a pleasant one. It may be that the patient was about to die, and perhaps a failure to recognise, say, metastatic cancer, or administration of the wrong drug, has led to the patient's eventual demise.

There has been much recent focus on medical mistakes, the vilification of medical personnel, the "Swiss cheese effect" of breaks in protocols that inevitably led to deaths or egregious harm to patients, but little literature on the effect of these mishaps on the lives of those accused of causing them. An article in the *Student British Medical Journal* recounts several stories from now senior medical officers, who talk about mistakes they have made in their careers. One of those stories, by Elisabeth Paice, a rheumatologist, and former deanery director of the London deanery, is particularly telling. She saw a patient with a condition called dermatomyositis, something usually associated with cancer, and had requested tests to screen for cancer and a chest x-ray. Everything else had come back with no evidence of cancer, but she ultimately forgot to check the chest x-ray. It was a few months later, while reviewing the patient's notes, she was able to retrieve the x-ray, and much to her dismay, the chest x-ray showed a tumour. She recounts:

> It was months before I noticed that the x ray report was not in the notes and opened the envelope to look at the film. The film showed an obvious tumour, duly identified by the radiologist whose report was still in the envelope. I had to tell the woman that she had cancer, that I would have to refer her to a cancer specialist, and that the delay in doing so was my fault. She died not long after because of an allergic reaction to her first dose of chemotherapy.
>
> ("Medical Mistakes" 2012, n.p.)

One can only imagine the guilt and regret that Dr Plaice felt in this case. Having confronted the patient, and told her about her, the doctor's, error, she promptly referred to an oncologist, but the patient succumbed to the treatment. If the chest x-ray had not been missed in the first place, would the tumour have been confined and amenable to surgical treatment without the need for chemotherapy? In accepting culpability for her errors, and hence vulnerability, the physician here becomes at once more accessible, more flawed, more human. That she has now put checks in place so that such mistakes never occur again is beside the point. We are able to see the human behind the doctor's mask, behind the façade that positional power erects and keeps all others away; we see how disappointed she is at her mistake, we feel the unease that gnaws away at her thoughts, knowing that her error may have cost someone their life. Perhaps after the grieving, one can, like Eliot, re-imagine the deceased again, this time without the tears, calmer and more peaceful, serene and self-assured: "The eyes outlast a little while / A little while outlast the tears" (Eliot 2011, ll. 12–13). Doctors' mistakes are well documented and, though checks and safe-guards may help alleviate the risk of harm to patients, the ones that do occur in many cases still represent changeable circumstances, and they are the ones that seem to haunt those who feel culpable for much longer (Roese and Summerville 2005). Reflection on one's practice goes far beyond thinking about mistakes and how they have, or could have, affected patients. It calls for wilful assertion to be more punctilious, to attempt to understand what went wrong, and in the future to prevent, or at least mitigate, those circumstances that may compromise the care of patients. This practice has become more widespread, with some hospitals providing regular sessions where doctors can debrief, and talk about their mistakes and near-misses, in a non-judgemental environment, where the origins of these mishaps can be traced. Support needs to be offered, not only to the direct victims of the misfortune, but the doctors as well – the silent, forgotten victims whose mistakes are always fodder for the sensationalism of tabloids. Unless both victims are attended to, real healing can never occur. This is what the reading of Eliot's poem reminds us who wait in "death's other kingdom:" physicians live with the regret of not having saved one life, but a hope that others may be yet be saved.

Conclusion

Empathy, engagement (with people), ambivalence, doubt and regret are all human qualities, inherent traits that affect us all, and make us more human. As a physician, one is expected to be more empathetic, to care more, to engage more with patients, and at the same time one is expected not to show ambivalence, fear or regard for oneself, as doing so would make doctors seem less competent and less in control of the situation. Should the physician respond to patients as themselves – vulnerable, sometimes timid, human – rather than put up an act of what a physician should be like (Weiner and Auster 2007)? The old models of caring for patients that focus on detachment need to be re-evaluated. While medical texts will always be about the anatomical and physiological departures from the norm, we can perhaps lean towards literature for psychological guidance on the nature of humans and how we interact with them. The medical curriculum itself is saturated with the scientific, giving little or no room to the psychosocial aspects of medicine. Diseases are studied, and the ever-growing cache of drug treatments is sought. We, as doctors, are taught, through systematic scientific enquiry, how to approach illness and disease, with technological solutions given emphasis; yet more complex diseases may call for more innovative and often expensive solutions that may or may not improve the disease outcome. In this morass of scientific discovery, the patient has been reduced to a symptom, not a human being. If the most fundamental aspect of being a doctor, that is caring, is lost, then the essence of treatment in itself is defeated. If the medical curriculum cannot address this issue, perhaps we should seek help outside the bounds of the medical narrative, and within the solace of the fictional and imaginative world of literature.

Not everyone is convinced by the use of literature as an adjunct to understanding people and being more empathetic towards patients. The use of narratives to inform practice has been seen as being disingenuous and pretentious:

> Doctors should – and generally do – treat their patients with courtesy, dignity, and kindness. It is inevitable that they sometimes fall short in this regard and fail to show grace under the intense pressure of modern practice. The narrative medicine imperative to express an empathy which the doctor may or may not feel cheapens, undermines, and coarsens the relationship between patient and doctor. Older, more stoically inclined patients in particular may find this form of engagement with their doctor vulgar, embarrassing, and intrusive.
>
> (O'Mahony 2013, 615)

There are many varied and distinct aspects of medicine, and one may argue that not all these lend themselves easily to literary discourse. Surgeons focus on the precision of excision, the physicians on the potency of their pills, while psychiatrists linger in the land of the mind and its afflictions. But it is not about the medical specialties per se. The need to care for, and understand the plight of, patients, transcends speciality or area of expertise. It is a broader discourse, one that encompasses the individual patient, his/her current condition, and how that affects their wider social and psychological environment. It is for this reason that detachment will not do. If we can draw parallels between the characters we read about and our patients, perhaps we can learn better approaches towards communicative behaviour, and arm ourselves with the knowledge and understanding of how to care for them.

Reflecting on Chekhov's statement now, I do not see medicine and literature as the twin faces of Janus, with literature as a relic of our distant past, not concerned or connected with how medicine, the future, is to be shaped. Rather, I see literature acting as the proverbial lighthouse, guiding lost doctors from the rocky shores of detachment and overreliance on technology. Literature will lead us back safely to where everything begins – an understanding of ourselves as human beings.

Reference list

Arroyo, José Manuel García and María Luisa Domínguez López. 2011. "Psychological Problems Derived from Mastectomy: A Qualitative Study." *International Journal of Surgical Oncology*, 2011: 1–8.

Brook, Robert H. 2010. "A Physician = Emotion + Passion + Science." *JAMA*, 304.22: 2528.

Chekhov, Anton Pavlovich. 2004. *Letters of Anton Chekhov*, trans. Constance Garnett. Project Gutenberg.

Cupchik, Gerald C. 2002. "The Evolution of Psychical Distance as an Aesthetic Concept." *Culture & Psychology*, 8.2: 155–87.

Eliot, T.S. 2011. *The Complete Poems and Plays of T.S. Eliot*. London: Faber & Faber.

Guth, Hans P. 1965. "Symbol and Contextual Restraint: Kafka's 'Country Doctor.'" *PMLA: Publications of the Modern Language Association of America*, 80.4: 427–31.

Halliday, L., A. Walker, S. Vig, J. Hines and J. Brecknell. 2016. "The Relationship between Grit and Burnout: How Do Surgical Trainees Compare to Other Doctors?" *International Journal of Surgery*, 36: 36.

Hart, J.T. 1997. "Doctor Chekhov: A Study in Literature & Medicine, by John Coope." *BMJ*, 315.7117: 1243–43.

Heneghan, C., P. Glasziou, M. Thompson, P. Rose, J. Balla, D. Lasserson, C. Scott and R. Perera. 2009. "Diagnostic Strategies Used in Primary Care." *BMJ*, 338.7701: 1003.

Koopman, Eva and Frank Hakemulder. 2015. "Effects of Literature on Empathy and Self-Reflection: A Theoretical-Empirical Framework." *Journal of Literary Theory*, 9.1: 79–111.

Maguire, Peter and Colin Murray Parkes. 1998. "Coping with Loss: Surgery and Loss of Body Parts." *BMJ*, 316.7137: 1086.

"Medical Mistakes." 2012. *Student BMJ*, 20.

Merlo, Lisa J. 2016. "Healing Physicians." *JAMA*, 316.23: 2489–90.

Minué, Sergio, Clara Bermúdez-Tamayo, Alberto Fernández, José Martín-Martín, Vivian Benítez, Miguel Melguizo, Araceli Caro, María Orgaz, Miguel Prados, José Díaz and Rafael Montoro. 2014. "Identification of Factors Associated with Diagnostic Error in Primary Care." *BMC Family Practice*, 15.1: 92.

Nathanson, Constance A. 1975. "Illness and the Feminine Role: A Theoretical Review." *Social Science and Medicine*, 9.2: 57–62.

O'Mahony, Seamus. 2013. "Against Narrative Medicine." *Perspectives in Biology and Medicine*, 56.4: 611.

Oyebode, Femi. 2010. "The Medical Humanities: Literature and Medicine." *Clinical Medicine, Journal of the Royal College of Physicians of London*, 10.3: 242–44.

Ramsey, Laura R., Justin A. Marotta and Tiffany Hoyt. 2017. "Sexualized, Objectified, but Not Satisfied: Enjoying Sexualization Relates to Lower Relationship Satisfaction through Perceived Partner-objectification." *Journal of Social and Personal Relationships*, 34.2: 258–78.

Reed, Eva E. 2014. "Man Up: Young Men's Lived Experiences and Reflections on Counseling." *Journal of Counseling and Development*, 92.4: 428–37.

Roese, Neal J. and Amy Summerville. 2005. "What We Regret Most … and Why. (Author Abstract)." *Personality & Social Psychology Bulletin*, 31.9: 1273.

Trevelyan, Esmé G., Warren A. Turner, and Nicola Robinson. 2016. "Perceptions of Phantom Limb Pain in Lower Limb Amputees and its Effect on Quality of Life: A Qualitative Study." *British Journal of Pain*, 10.2: 70–77.

Weiner, Saul J. and Simon Auster. 2007. "From Empathy to Caring: Defining the Ideal Approach to a Healing Relationship." *The Yale Journal of Biology and Medicine*, 80.3: 123–30.

Wellbery, C. 2000. "Do Literature and the Arts Make Us Better Doctors?" *Family Medicine*, 32.6: 376.

15 A humanistic perspective on the healing power of language at the end of life

Restoration of the self through words and silence[1]

Andrea Rodríguez-Prat and Xavier Escribano

In the 1960s a new way of treating patients at the end of life began to emerge, one that focused not just on the physical but also on psychological, social, existential and experiential aspects of illness (Clark 2002). The philosophy of palliative care, championed by Cicely Saunders (1965), also helped promote a more holistic approach that challenged the widespread idea that little could be done for the terminally ill patient. Thus, even in situations where no cure was available, attention began to be paid to ways of managing the person's symptoms and of addressing aspects such as depression, fear of what the future might hold, anxiety, and a loss of dignity and meaning in life (MiL[2]). The aim of this was to overturn a situation that, since its beginning in Parisian hospitals, had become more generalised in medicine. As stated by Saulius Geniusas: "the history of clinical medicine has been a history of the decline of dialogue and the upsurge of the technically mediated 'discourses on tissue'" (2016, 162).

More recently within this framework, good communication has come to be seen as an important component of end-of-life care (Abdul-Razzak *et al.* 2016; Evans *et al.* 2012; Garner *et al.* 2011; Generous and Keeley 2017; Murray, McDonald and Atkin 2015; Norton *et al.* 2013; Parry, Land and Seymour 2014; Sinuff *et al.* 2015), and various studies have concluded that communication is a crucial factor in helping these individuals come to terms with their illness, to make decisions and to maintain quality of life (Bernacki and Block 2014; Sleeman 2013). This new perspective contributed to the understanding of the human being through a holistic look that set out a foundation of medicine focused on the person.

In one of the first studies of psychotherapy with terminally ill patients, Zuehlke and Watkins (1977) cited earlier research (cf. Eissler 1955), suggesting that some clinicians avoided telling patients their diagnosis for fear of provoking psychological disturbances. Several decades later, the situation does not seem to have changed significantly. While the UK leads the way in Europe in terms of the percentage of patients who are informed of their diagnosis (94.6 per cent) and prognosis (91.8 per cent) (Vassilas and Donaldson 1998), rates in other European countries range between as low as 25 per cent and 50 per cent (Centeno and Núñez Olarte 1998). There is also evidence of a lack of training in communication skills for health professionals, leading many of them to be wary of addressing issues related to the end of life (Bolt *et al.* 2016; Ciemins, Brant, Kersten, Mullette and Dickerson 2015).[3] For example, some authors note that while doctors are invariably taught the technical skills they need to treat illness and maintain health, they rarely receive training on how to communicate with advanced patients and their relatives (Balaban 2000; Granek *et al.* 2013; Jackson *et al.* 2008; McCormick and Conley 1995; Moir *et al.* 2015; Quyen *et al.* 2008). In 1998, the American Society of Clinical Oncology surveyed over 6,000 oncologists about the training they had received on communicating with terminally ill patients and found that over half reported using trial and error as a source of learning about end-of-life care (cited in Jackson *et al.* 2008). In short, the thesis that is supported in this work is that adequate communication between doctors and patients is an essential aspect – and not merely an accessory – of humanising healthcare. The need for appropriate communication is even more relevant at the end of life, where the opportune use of language and silence come to constitute the only instruments for the recuperation of the sense of humanity that serious illness can distort.

If, as we have seen, communication should be regarded as an integral part of care and the healing process, and in the end-of-life context as a crucial factor in enabling patients to accept their illness and experience a "good death," why do so many studies find patient-physician communication to be poor? Why is there such reluctance to speak openly about death and dying? In contemplating these questions, one also needs to ask whether communication is a skill implicit to medical science or, on the contrary, a kind of supplementary tool whose use implies certain skills that doctors are not necessarily required to have.

The relationship between patient and physician has not always been characterised by a lack of communication. Indeed, for centuries language occupied a central role in the healing process. The heroes of the Homeric epics, for example, are healed through the uttering of magical formulae (Laín Entralgo 2001). Likewise, the writings of Plato contain numerous references to body and soul as an inseparable duality, such that any attempt to treat the body's ills must also take the soul into account:

> Zalmoxis … says that as you ought not to attempt to cure eyes without head, or head without body, so you should not treat body without soul; and this was the reason why most maladies evaded the physicians of Greece – that they neglected the whole, on which they ought to spend their pains, for if this were out of order it was impossible for the part to be in order.
>
> (*Charmides*, [156d–157a])

In keeping with this classical tradition we would argue that effective communication between physician and patient should be regarded as a therapeutic resource. It is "only through dialogue [that] the patient and the physician [can] overcome the ontological gap that separates them" (Geniusas 2016, 163), that is, the gap between the lived experience of illness and the objectifying gaze of medicine.

Socio-anthropological barriers to end-of-life communication

In recent decades, Western societies have witnessed a profound change in terms of how pain, suffering, illness, death and dying are conceived (Ariès 1975; Ariès 1981; Gorer 1955; Illich 1976). In this section, we will discuss three key aspects that can help in understanding why health professionals often avoid talking about the end of life: technological and medical control of illness; the contemporary experience of pain; and the denial of death. The social representation of suffering, death and dying is closely linked to technological advances in clinical care and to what is known as medicalisation (Clark 2002; Illich 1976; van Wijngaarden, Leget and Goossensen 2016), defined as "the process by which 'non-medical' problems become understood and treated as 'medical' problems" (Conrad 2008, 5). The spectacular development of the technique and the consequent growing prestige of the medical profession produced a transformation in the understanding of death: it went from being a part of life to being an illness that should be treated (Ariès 1975). In this reshaping of the experience of illness, control shifted from patients to doctors, and even to the patient's relatives, who often took on the mantle of decision making, including over whether or not the patient should be informed of his or her diagnosis. As the process of medicalisation became more widespread, death came to be seen as an illness to be treated (Callahan 1989), and by some as a problem that would one day be solved by technology (Morin 1994).

This belief in the eventual triumph of technology has fostered a society in which people are reluctant to accept and speak about pain and death (Illich 1976). Unsurprisingly, therefore, studies that have examined communication in the end-of-life context have noted how difficult it can be to engage in conversation about death and dying (Balaban 2000). The potential impact of this silence should not be underestimated because, as noted earlier, patients facing the end of life, and especially those receiving palliative care, can benefit from a clinical approach that takes into account the psychological, social and existential aspects of their situation. However, research suggests that many health professionals struggle to connect with patients and understand their concerns in this regard (Bolt *et al.* 2016; Ciemins, Brant, Kersten, Mullette and Dickerson 2015; McCormick and Conley 1995). Consequently, Trice and Prigerson (2009) conclude that much of the time that doctors spend with patients is dedicated to discussing technical or medical aspects with them, and also that doctors often fail to pick up on the information that most matters to the patient and find it difficult to assess fully the patient's needs and symptoms. As we will address, a purely technical approach to illness limits the content of doctor-patient conversations and overlooks aspects that are crucial for adequate end-of-life care.

Just as technological advancement has enabled the avoidance of death, the widespread availability and use of anaesthesia in Western societies have meant that people are less exposed to physical pain. Indeed, the effective relief of pain is now the goal of specialist clinics and physicians, of researchers and the pharmaceutical industry, and of organisations such as the International Association for the Study of Pain. It is important to note, however, that these developments in the field of pain relief, guided by the aforementioned technological paradigm, were accompanied by the introduction into the public imagination of a mechanistic and Cartesian view of the body (Walter 1994). This in turn led to a reductionist view of pain which accounts, in two ways, for how pain is experienced today. First, once pain or suffering became seen as a purely organic phenomenon, it was no longer recognised as an inevitable part of personal human experience that might have deeper meaning or as something of which a person might make a virtue (Illich 1976; Le Breton 1999). From the reductionist point of view, pain was simply an unpleasant sensory experience (Merskey and Bogduk 2012) that should be treated pharmacologically. This biomedical viewpoint is, however, incapable of understanding the experience of patients at the end of life, which encompasses not only physical pain but also psychological and existential distress. Nevertheless, the fact that pain could now be treated, coupled with the development of the welfare society and the establishment of new standards for health and quality of life has meant that people today generally expect to be given pain relief much sooner and regard pain as generally unnecessary. This resistance to pain is reflected in studies that have examined the wish to hasten death among patients with advanced disease, who often say they would prefer to die rather than experience unbearable suffering (Rodríguez-Prat *et al.* 2017). These studies suggest that suffering is the most distressing aspect for patients, and the cause of their greatest fears. This illustrates how, in a context characterised by trust in technology, it is easy to create the illusion that every kind of pain or suffering – and even death – has a cause that can be tackled by medical science.

The term "forbidden death" was coined by Ariès (1975) to refer to how, in contemporary society, death has been relegated to the anonymous setting of hospitals, becoming a phenomenon that no longer has a place in the collective imagination, and about which people do not wish to speak (Baudrillard 1993). Death, rather than sex, is now the great taboo (Gorer 1955). Whereas prior to the middle of the twentieth century, people made time for funeral and grieving rites, death today has become an event about which it is better not to think and which, as far as possible, should not disrupt everyday life. These social changes in relation to death have also affected the ability of doctors to speak about it. Health professionals today are often reluctant to accept that an illness may be incurable, and together with patients and their relatives they may feel frustrated by and reject the reality of death.

Doctors' own beliefs and fears can also influence how they approach issues related to the end of life. For instance, equating the absence of a cure with failure, a focus on cure that potentially leads to overtreatment, a feeling of being unable to live up to patients' expectations or starting from a different series of premises to those held by the patient are all potential obstacles to good communication (Granek *et al.* 2013; Sleeman 2013; Trice and Prigerson 2009). Some studies have found that even when patients have an incurable disease, health professionals often fail to acknowledge that they will likely die as a result

(Anderson, Kools and Lyndon 2013). For example, Granek noted that "because oncologists were focused on curing patients, they continued to offer more interventions and treatments instead of having a conversation about end-of-life care" (2013, e131). Sleeman (2013) likewise points out that these barriers to communication derive from the idea that death is a failure of medicine rather than an inevitable part of life.

Psychotherapeutic interventions at the end of life

Depression, anxiety, despair, demoralisation, a loss of dignity and of MiL, and even a wish to hasten death are all relatively common phenomena among patients with advanced disease (Chochinov *et al.* 2002; Kissane, Clarke and Street 2001; Monforte-Royo *et al.* 2011). There are numerous reports of psychological interventions that seek to address these aspects, and studies of their effectiveness suggest that psychotherapy (etymologically, "treatment of the soul") can lead to improvements not only in the aforementioned aspects but also in terms of "reduced suffering, physiological indicators, treatment retention, enhanced interactions with other people, work performance, and other indexes of recovery" (Norcross and Lambert 2010, 1). Research into the efficacy of psychotherapeutic interventions has often focused on analysing how their proposed mechanism of action and the context in which they are applied may interact to produce certain outcomes (3) – and depending on the outcomes being sought, the clinician may choose among various models that focus on different clinical needs and which make use of different conceptual frameworks. Our aim in this section is to draw attention to some of the key therapeutic elements in the doctor-patient relationship, and we will do so through reference to the findings of a systematic review and realist synthesis of MiL interventions that was carried out recently by our research group (Guerrero-Torrelles *et al.* 2017). These findings will then serve as the basis for a more in-depth discussion of the relationship and communication between doctor and patient from the perspective of Laín Entralgo's work on the healing power of language. Pedro Laín Entralgo (1908–2001) was a Spanish physician, philosopher and historian who made a profound intellectual contribution to medical history and anthropology. One sees reflected in his extensive writings the interdisciplinary training that led him to address various topics of medical interest from a humanistic perspective, and it is this which makes his work particularly relevant.

In the field of psychotherapy, reference is often made to the dichotomy between a medical-scientific model, based on treatment methods and randomised control trials, and a relational-contextual model, based on the therapeutic relationship and process-outcome studies (Norcross and Lambert 2011, 3). Here, following Norcross,[4] we adopt an integrative (rather than dualist) perspective which recognises that both approaches can make a useful contribution to the healing process, even though our focus is primarily the relational-contextual model.

In 2017 our research group published a review of the literature in which we identified 12 studies describing psychotherapeutic interventions whose aim was to improve MiL among advanced patients. The analysis and synthesis of studies was carried out according to the criteria proposed by the RAMESES project, which enables complex interventions to be analysed in terms of their context, mechanisms and outcomes. In this chapter we will focus solely on those aspects of the therapy relationship that were shown to contribute to the healing process; greater detail regarding the effective elements of each of the interventions (including the conceptual framework and the setting in which they were applied) can be found in the original article (Guerrero-Torrelles *et al.* 2017). In the following we will briefly discuss the notions of context and mechanisms, and then, having introduced the work of Laín Entralgo, we will compare the outcomes reported in the MiL studies with the concepts developed by this Spanish physician.

Our review of MiL interventions concluded that the interpersonal encounter between therapist and patient was the key element. This encounter occurs within the context of an ongoing therapeutic conversation that enables the patient to begin reflecting on his/her life, connecting past, present and future and redefining his/her identity and relationship to others by considering what it is that gives meaning to life. Some authors (Henry *et al.* 2010; Zuehlke and Watkins 1975) argue that a crucial element of this encounter is the therapist's capacity for patience; that is, the ability to give patients time to develop the sense of security and trust they need in order to begin speaking about significant aspects of their life. A common core feature of the studies included in our review was a dynamic conversation between patient and therapist, and it was this narrative aspect of the interventions which enabled patients to share with the therapist key elements of their life story. In this regard, the authors of the interventions indicated that reflection, self-exploration, acknowledgement, self-awareness and acceptance were key elements in the process of identifying MiL. Other important and related tasks included enabling patients to explore concepts and sources of meaning, to discuss life priorities and goal changes that give meaning to their life, to review the impact and meaning of their diagnosis, to explore past significant life events and successful ways of coping, to re-evaluate events as positive, to place their life in a historical and personal context, to achieve gratitude for a life lived, to prepare and organise farewell gatherings with significant others, to leave an inter-generational legacy or spiritual will, and to resolve past conflicts and achieve forgiveness.

Before looking more closely at the work of Laín Entralgo, it will be useful to consider three premises regarding illness and human nature that are implicit within many of the studies reviewed. The first is that the healing power of language has to do with understanding illness from the perspective of both body and soul. While there is a tendency nowadays to reduce illness to an organic dysfunction and to offer treatment accordingly, if we are to understand the meaning of illness for a given individual and to appreciate the enormous impact that an incurable disease can have on a person's sense of identity, then we need to engage with the whole person: with the self that feels itself fragmented by illness. Language, as a bearer of meaning and reasons, is able to capture the existential aspect of illness. The patient who reflects, who looks inward and gains awareness of his/her situation and of what matters most in life, may be better able to bear the suffering produced by the apparent meaninglessness of existence, by the sense that one's identity and dignity have been lost.

The second premise which emerges is that a person's illness may come to be acknowledged more fully through dialogue. If "diagnosis" is understood as the ability to discern or recognise, then the task of diagnosing is not exclusive to the physician but, rather, must involve both physician and patient working together in the search for truth. The diagnostic process might therefore be regarded as a kind of maieutics, in which the physician questions the patient in order to draw out the important information that lies within.

The third and final premise is that illness and, ultimately, death are part of life. Indeed, one of the guiding principles of palliative care and of a more multi-dimensional approach to patients with advanced disease is that these individuals should not simply be left to die but, rather, are deserving of dignified care to the very end. From this perspective, and contrary to the attitude that denies illness and death a place in life, or to the utilitarian view that regards persons at the end of life as no longer dignified, it becomes possible to accept the end as a final opportunity for personal growth, as a moment that can be lived in true accordance with one's beliefs and values, and where a deep connection can be re-established with oneself and with others.

The healing power of language in the writings of Laín Entralgo

As early as the 1960s, Laín Entralgo began to express concern about the increasing artificiality and distance of the doctor-patient relationship. His belief that both diagnosis and treatment had come to rely too heavily on technology, and that the medical consultation had become depersonalised and bureaucratic, led him to reflect on the structure of the doctor-patient relationship and to examine "what this relationship once was, is and should be" (Laín Entralgo 1969, 10). In his view, one of the key structural elements of this relationship was communication, which he defined as the principal techniques that the physician must employ when seeking to capture the objective and subjective reality of the patient, namely observation, touch and the use of both words and silence (Laín Entralgo 1969, 160). However, as Entralgo himself notes, one must also ask how relevant communication is to the bond between doctor and patient: "Is the spoken word an essential aspect, or is medicine a technical discipline in which what is said is only of secondary importance?" (1964, 4).

To give context to the origin of the use of the word for healing purposes, it was Plato who first set out a rational argument for the use of words in the treatment of certain diseases. He also stated that the word can be seen to be "the very expression of humanity" (Laín Entralgo 1964, 7). As noted earlier, if we are to view illness as more than a physio-pathological condition, then the biographical dimension must be seen as a key element in the healing process and thus, by expressing through words the humanity, can emerge this personal dimension. Therefore, argues Laín Entralgo, it is necessary to develop a narrative in which patients, through words, are able to express the meaning they ascribe to their illness, since its origin, development and manifestation (symptoms) are inseparable from their personal biography. Hence, physician and patient must join forces to interpret imaginatively the illness and to establish links between the diagnosis and lived experience.

In contrast, medicine has also been described as *muta ars*, a silent art. For example, in Virgil's *Aeneid* we learn that the doctor Iapyx "preferred to know the potencies of herbs, and the practice of healing, and to ply this quiet art, resigning fame" (XX, 396–97). Similarly, four centuries later, Vegetius wrote that "animals and men must not be treated with vain words but with the sure art of medicine" (quoted in Szasz 1988, 12). And even in Plato's *Laws*, we find the following description of how the slave-doctors work:

> None of these doctors gives any explanation of the particular disease of any particular slave – or listens to one; all they do is prescribe the treatment they see fit, on the basis of trial and error – but with all the arrogance of a tyrant, as if they had exact knowledge.
>
> (Laín Entralgo 1964, 4)

Laín Entralgo argues that this view of medicine is founded on a false premise, namely that the physician may, solely through his powers of observation, understand what is troubling the patient without needing to hear from the patient himself.

According to Laín Entralgo, a conversation between doctor and patient always has two simultaneous facets, diagnostic (anamnesis) and therapeutic (psychotherapy) (1969). Although the different functions of language are concurrent within a medical consultation, as we will see in the next section, Laín Entralgo nonetheless distinguishes between four of them. The vocative function has to do with how words simultaneously call out to and invite the attention of the listener. Then there is the informative function, which reflects how the uttered word both communicates and lifts a weight from the speaker (catharsis). Third, there is the nominative function, which refers to how the process of naming one's experience can bring some sense of order and recognition to reality (clarification). Finally, the self-affirming function has to do with consolidating and affirming one's own discourse: "Whoever speaks to another, affirms himself in the process" (Laín Entralgo 1969, 180).

Laín Entralgo goes on to argue that these functions must be located within a series of "moments," which may be synchronic. Thus, all the functions would have what he calls a "cognitive moment," in which the word serves as a means of acquiring knowledge. Alongside this there would be an "operative moment" in which treatment is administered, and here the encounter between doctor and patient would become a healing relationship. In the "affective moment," the clinical conversation between patient and doctor leads to the establishment of "friendship" or "transference." And finally, there is an "ethical/religious moment," defined by the cultural assumptions of both parties.

Just as the spoken word has its functions, so too may silence be informative and revealing, a way of communicating something meaningful. On the one hand, a negative form of silence may occur when patients or health professionals do not speak because they do not know how – or do not wish – to communicate a certain piece of information or some aspect of themselves. However, there is also a positive form of silence that points towards the transcendence of human existence. For authors such as Heidegger, silence is an essential possibility of speaking:

> In talking with one another the person who is silent can "let something be understood," that is, he can develop an understanding more authentically than the person who never runs out of words.... But to keep silent does not mean to be mute.... And the person who is by nature accustomed to speak little is no better able to show that he can be silent and keep silent. He who never says anything is also unable to keep silent at a given moment. Authentic silence is possible only in genuine discourse ... Then reticence makes manifest and puts down "idle talk." As a mode of discourse, reticence articulates the intelligibility of Dasein so primordially that it gives rise to a genuine potentiality for hearing and to a being-with-one-another that is transparent.
>
> (2000, 183–84)

This is a silence which recognises that some things are ineffable, and that sometimes what has been said or heard can only begin to be understood by remaining silent. In the field of palliative care, the experience of illness, suffering, the finiteness of humanity and death can foster this meaningful silence. Indeed, once we experience and acknowledge our limits as human beings, silence, as a form of communication, may be regarded as our final narrative resource, one that leads to a kind of "interpersonal communion" (Quevedo 2003, 55) between patient and doctor and which enables an understanding of the former's predicament.

Applications of dialogical medicine

Returning to the aforementioned analysis of MiL interventions, it is possible to see how their reported outcomes illustrate the positive impact of what we will refer to here as "dialogical medicine." More specifically, some of the main features of the interventions that were shown to promote wellbeing and a change of attitude among patients with advanced disease involved enhancing their self-understanding through the clarification of life views, the exploration and acknowledgement of suffering and illness, and helping them to accept and find new meaning in life.

These aspects are consistent with the functions of language described by Laín Entralgo, for whom an awareness of the therapeutic power of words may foster dialogue between patient and physician. Thus, if we apply his framework to the studies of MiL interventions we can see how the spoken word served the four functions he describes: vocative (inviting the other's attention); informative (catharsis); nominative (clarification); and self-affirmation. Through their encounter with the therapist, the advanced patients who took part in these studies were able to reflect upon and clarify their life situation, and through the greater awareness they obtained could then begin to name their experience. By informing another person of their predicament they felt understood and accompanied (the invited other who listens), and in the process some of the weight of their experience was lifted from them (catharsis). In the clinical context, some authors have suggested that persons at the end of life often need to resolve certain conflicts or seek forgiveness before they die (Alon 2010). The cathartic function of the spoken word, therefore, would not merely imply the sharing of one's experience, which is often done privately, but may also involve a more public reparation of past mistakes or damaged relationships.

Turning to another concept used by Laín Entralgo, an awareness of different "moments" in the conversation with patients is also important for health professionals as it may enable them to understand how they themselves, through their attitudes and behaviour, are an instrument for healing not just the body but also – as Plato suggested – the soul. In a context of medicalised health care, it is easy to forget that the art of healing requires not simply technical knowledge but also the capacity to interpret and understand the lived experience of the patient, the biographical dimension that is crucial to the diagnostic process.

Finally, it is worth remembering that silence may be the manifestation of a profound interpersonal encounter rather than of a lack of communication. Silence is a problem if the patient is not involved or engaged (in which case one might speak of a conspiracy of silence), but it can acquire a healing quality when it derives – as in the studies of MiL interventions – from acknowledgement and understanding. Indeed, silence is an important part of medical communication:

> The physician must know how to remain silent. By remaining silent in the presence of the patient, but listening attentively and with an attitude of benevolence, the physician comes to know and heals, because it is only through silence that one fully discovers the meaning of what has been said and heard, and – above all – because nothing brings greater relief to the speaker than the realisation that his words are being gathered in the lap of silence made available by the listener.
>
> (Quevedo 2003, 56)

Conclusion

Many people with advanced disease experience great physical, psychological and existential suffering and feel that they have lost their sense of identity, dignity or MiL. If we are to help them regain or maintain these aspects, we need to recognise that both the spoken word (*logos*: reason, motive, signification and meaning) and silence are crucial elements of the encounter between doctor and patient. The work of thinkers such as Laín Entralgo, who was deeply concerned about the dehumanisation of medicine, can help us to situate clinical practice within a long tradition of philosophical reflection on the art of healing, and in doing so we may come to reimagine the human being as someone defined by – and capable of being healed by – words. The medical consultation, thus conceived, may have a transforming effect not only on the ill person but also on the physician who is turned to by the patient, the patient who expresses in words his inner experience and who remains silent about all that is ineffable in life.

Notes

1 The authors would like to thank Alan Nance for his contribution to translating and editing the manuscript. We are grateful for the funding received from Recercaixa 2015 and WeCare Chair: End-of-life care at the Universitat Internacional de Catalunya and ALTIMA.
2 The Viennese psychiatrist Viktor Frankl was the first to consider meaning in life (MiL) as a clinical variable. Although this concept has been considered from various perspectives (psychological, spiritual, etc.) it can be assumed that MiL has a cognitive component (ideas, beliefs) and a volitional component (the fulfilment of useful activities).
3 In the biomedical field there has been an exponential growth in the number of publications claiming that communication promotes not only individual patient wellbeing but also the quality of the relationship that patients have with health professionals and others in their immediate social environment.
4 John C. Norcross is a key figure in this field as he undertook "to investigate the association between elements of the therapy relationship and treatment effectiveness" (2010, 1). His research was supported by the American Psychological Association's Division of Psychotherapy and Division of Clinical Psychology and gave rise to 20 meta-analyses on this topic.

Reference list

Abdul-Razzak, Amane, Diana Sherifali, John You, Jessica Simon and Kevin Brazil. 2016. "'Talk to Me': A Mixed Methods Study on Preferred Physician Behaviours during End-of-Life Communication from the Patient Perspective." *Health Expectations* 19.4: 883–96.

Alon, Shirly. 2010. "Tradition, Heritage and Spirituality. Researching the Meaning of Life: Finding New Sources of Hope." *Asian Pacific Journal of Cancer Prevention* 11: 75–78.

Anderson, Wendy G., Susan Kools and Audrey Lyndon. 2013. "Dancing Around Death: Hospitalist-Patient Communication about Serious Illness." *Quality Health Research* 23.1: 1–13.

Ariès, Philippe. 1975. *Western Attitudes towards Death: From the Middle Ages to the Present.* Baltimore, MD: Johns Hopkins University Press.

Ariès, Philippe. 1981. *The Hour of Our Death.* New York: Vintage.

Balaban, Richard B. 2000. "A Physician's Guide to Talking about End-of-Life Care." *Journal of General Internal Medicine* 15.3: 195–200.

Baudrillard, Jean. 1993. *Symbolic Exchange and Death.* London and Thousand Oaks, CA: Sage.

Bernacki, Rachelle E. and Susan D. Block. 2014. "Communication about Serious Illness Care Goals." *JAMA Internal Medicine* 174.12.

Bolt, Eva Elizabeth, H. Roeline Willemijn Pasman, Dick Willems, Bregje Dorien Onwuteaka-Philipsen, S. Hales, C. Zimmermann and G. Rodin. 2016. "Appropriate and Inappropriate Care in the Last Phase of Life: An Explorative Study among Patients and Relatives." *BMC Health Services Research* 16.1: 655.

Callahan, Daniel. 1989. "Can We Return Death to Disease?" *The Hastings Center Report* 19.1: 4–6.

Casell, E.J. 1982. "The Nature of Suffering and the Goals of Medicine." *New England Journal of Medicine* 306.11: 639–45.

Centeno, Carlos and J.M. Núñez Olarte. 1998. "Studies about the Communication of the Diagnosis of Cancer in Spain." *Medicina Clínica* 110.19: 744–50.

Chochinov, Harvey Max, Thomas Hack, Susan McClement, Linda Kristjanson and Mike Harlos. 2002. "Dignity in the Terminally Ill: A Developing Empirical Model." *Social Science and Medicine* 54.3: 433–43.

Chochinov, Harvey Max, Thomas Hack, Thomas Hassard, Linda J Kristjanson, Susan McClement and Mike Harlos. 2004. "Dignity and Psychotherapeutic Considerations in End-of-Life Care." *Journal of Palliative Care* 20.3: 134–42.

Ciemins, Elizabeth L., Jeannine Brant, Diane Kersten, Elizabeth Mullette and Dustin Dickerson. 2015. "A Qualitative Analysis of Patient and Family Perspectives of Palliative Care." *Journal of Palliative Medicine* 18.3: 282–85.

Clark, David. 2002. "Between Hope and Acceptance: The Medicalisation of Dying." *BMJ* 13.324: 905–07.

Conrad, Peter. 2008. *The Medicalization of Society: On the Transformation of Human Conditions into Treatable Disorders*. Baltimore, MD: Johns Hopkins University Press.

Eissler, K. 1955. *The Psychiatrist and the Dying Patient*. New York: International Universities Press.

Evans, N., H.R. Pasman, S.A. Payne, J. Seymour, S. Pleschberger, R. Deschepper and B.D. Onwuteaka-Philipsen. 2012. "Older Patients' Attitudes towards and Experiences of Patient-Physician End-of-Life Communication: A Secondary Analysis of Interviews from British, Dutch and Belgian Patients." *BMC Palliat Care* 11.1: 24.

Gadamer, Hans-Georg. 1992. *The Enigma of Health. The Art of Healing in a Scientific Age*. Stanford, CA: Stanford University Press.

Garner, Kimberly K., Archie A. Henager, Jo Ann E. Kirchner and Dennis H. Sullivan. 2011. "The Elephant in the Room: Facilitating Communication at the End of Life." *Family Medicine* 43.4: 277–78.

Generous, Mark A. and Maureen Keeley. 2017. "Wished for and Avoided Conversations with Terminally Ill Individuals during Final Conversations." *Death Studies* 41.3: 1–29.

Geniusas, Saulius. 2016. "Phenomenology of Chronic Pain: De-Personalization and Re-Personalization." In *Meanings of Pain*, edited by Simon van Rysewyck, 147–64. Cham: Springer International Publisher.

Gorer, Geoffrey. 1955. "The Pornography of Death." *Encounter* 5.4: 49–52.

Granek, Leeat, Monika K. Krzyzanowska, Richard Tozer and Paolo Mazzotta. 2013. "Oncologists' Strategies and Barriers to Effective Communication about the End of Life." *Journal of Oncology Practice. American Society of Clinical Oncology* 9.4: e129–35.

Guerrero-Torrelles, Mariona, Cristina Monforte-Royo, Andrea Rodríguez-Prat, Josep Porta-Sales and Albert Balaguer. 2017. "Understanding Meaning in Life Interventions in Advanced Illness Patients: A Systematic Review and Realist Synthesis." *Palliative Medicine*. doi: 10.1177/0269216316685235.

Heidegger, Martin. 2000. *El Ser Y El Tiempo* [*Being and Time*]. Madrid: Fondo de Cultura Económica.

Henry, Melissa, S., Robin Cohen, Virginia Lee, Philippe Sauthier, Diane Provencher, Pierre Drouin and Philippe Gauthier. 2010. "The Meaning-Making Intervention (MMi) Appears to Increase Meaning in Life in Advanced Ovarian Cancer: A Randomized Controlled Pilot Study." *Psycho-Oncology* 19.12: 1340–47.

Illich, Ivan. 1976. *Medical Nemesis: The Expropriation of Health*. London: Alder and Boyars.

Jackson, Vicki A., Jennifer Mack, Robin Matsuyama, Mathew D. Lakoma, Amy M. Sullivan, Robert M. Arnold, Jane C. Weeks and Susan D. Block. 2008. "A Qualitative Study of Oncologists' Approaches to End-of-Life Care." *Journal of Palliative Medicine* 11.6: 893–906.

Kissane, D.W., D.M. Clarke and A.F. Street. 2001. "Demoralization Syndrome: A Relevant Psychiatric Diagnosis for Palliative Care." *Journal of Palliative Care* 17.1: 12–21.

Laín Entralgo, Pedro. 1964. "El Silencio Y La Palabra Del Médico." *Medicina e Historia* 3: 1–14.

Laín Entralgo, Pedro. 1969. *El Médico Y El Enfermo*. Madrid: Ediciones Guadarrama.

Laín Entralgo, Pedro. 2001. "La Racionalización Platónica Del Ensalmo Y La Invención de La Psicoterapia Verbal." *Revista Frenia* 1: 107–29.

Laín Entralgo, Pedro. 2005. *La Curación Por La Palabra En La Antigüedad Clásica*, 2nd edn. Barcelona: Anthropos.

Le Breton, David. 1999. *Antropología Del Dolor* [*Anthropology of Pain*], 1st edn. Barcelona: Seix Barral.

Leder, Drew. 1992. "A Tale of Two Bodies: The Cartesian Corpse and the Lived Body." In *The Body in Medical Thought and Practice*, edited Drew Leder. Dordrecht: Springer Science & Business Media.

McCormick, T.R. and B.J. Conley. 1995. "Patients' Perspectives on Dying and on the Care of Dying Patients." *The Western Journal of Medicine* 163.3: 236–43.

Merskey, H. and N. Bogduk. 2012. "IASP Taxonomy." *IASP Task Force on Taxonomy*. www.iasp-pain.org/Taxonomy (accessed 25 May 2017).

Moir, Cheryl, Renee Roberts, Kim Martz, Judith Perry and Laura J. Tivis. 2015. "Communicating with Patients and Their Families about Palliative and End-of-Life Care: Comfort and Educational Needs of Nurses." *International Journal of Palliative Nursing* 21.3: 109–12.

Monforte-Royo, Cristina, Christian Villavicencio-Chávez, Joaquín Tomás-Sábado and Albert Balaguer. 2011. "The Wish to Hasten Death: A Review of Clinical Studies." *Psycho-Oncology* 20.8: 795–804.

Morin, Edgar. 1994. *El Hombre Y La Muerte* [*Humanity and Death*], 6th edn. Barcelona: Kairós.

Morris, David. 1993. *The Culture of Pain*. Berkeley: University of California Press.

Murray, Craig D., Claire McDonald and Heather Atkin. 2015. "The Communication Experiences of Patients with Palliative Care Needs: A Systematic Review and Meta-Synthesis of Qualitative Findings." *Palliative & Supportive Care* 13.2: 369–83.

Nancy, Jean-Luc. 2002. *L'Intrus*. East Lansing: Michigan State University Press.

Norcross, John C. and Michael J. Lambert. 2010. "Evidence-Based Therapy Relationships." In *Evidence-Based Therapy Relationships*, edited by John C. Norcross, 1–4.

Norcross, John C. and Michael J. Lambert. 2011. "Evidence-Based Therapy Relationships." In *Psychotherapy Relationships That Work: Evidence-Based Responsiveness*, edited by John C. Norcross. New York: Oxford University Press.

Norton, Sally A., Maureen Metzger, Jane Deluca, Stewart C. Alexander, Timothy E. Quill and Robert Gramling. 2013. "Palliative Care Communication: Linking Patients' Prognoses, Values, and Goals of Care." *Research in Nursing and Health* 36.6: 582–90.

Parry, Ruth, Victoria Land and Jane Seymour. 2014. "How to Communicate with Patients about Future Illness Progression and End of Life: A Systematic Review." *BMJ Supportive & Palliative Care* 4.4: 331–41.

Quevedo, Francisco J. Leal. 2003. "La Palabra Y El Silencio En La Comunicación Médico-Paciente." *Arch Argent Pediat* 101.1: 54–56.

Quyen, Ngo-Metzger, Kristin August, Malathi Srinivasan and Solomon Liao. 2008. "End-of-Life Care: Guidelines for Patient-Centred Communication." *American Academy of Family Physicians* 2: 139–42.

Rodríguez-Prat, Andrea, Albert Balaguer, Andrew Booth and Cristina Monforte-Royo. 2017. "Understanding Patients' Experiences of the Wish to Hasten Death: An Updated and Expanded Systematic Review and Meta-Ethnography." *BMJ Open*: e016659. doi: 10.1136/bmjopen-2017-016659.

Saunders, Cicely. 1965. "The Last Stages of Life." *American Journal of Nursing* 65.3: 70–75.

Sinuff, Tasnim, Peter Dodek, John J. You, Doris Barwich, Carolyn Tayler, James Downar, Michael Hartwick, Christopher Frank, Henry T. Stelfox and Daren K. Heyland. 2015. "Improving End-of-Life Communication and Decision Making: The Development of a Conceptual Framework and Quality Indicators." *Journal of Pain and Symptom Management* 49.6: 1070–80.

Sleeman, K.E. 2013. "End-of-Life Communication: Let's Talk about Death." *Journal of the Royal College of Physicians of Edinburgh* 43.3: 197–99.

Szasz, Thomas. 1988. *The Myth of Psychotherapy: Mental Healing as Religion, Rhetoric and Repression*, Syracuse, NY: Syracuse University Press.

Trice, Elizabeth D. and Holly G. Prigerson. 2009. "Communication in End-Stage Cancer: Review of the Literature and Future Research." *Journal of Health Community* 14.1: 95–108.

van Wijngaarden, Else, Carlo Leget and Anne Goossensen. 2016. "Disconnectedness from the Here-and-Now: A Phenomenological Perspective as a Counteract on the Medicalisation of Death Wishes in Elderly People." *Medicine, Health Care and Philosophy* 19.2: 265–73.

Vassilas, Christopher A. and Julia Donaldson. 1998. "Telling the Truth: What Do General Practitioners Say to Patients with Dementia or Terminal Cancer?" *British Journal of General Practice* 48.428: 1081–82.

Walter, Tony. 1994. *The Revival of Death*. London; New York: Routledge.

Wong, Geoff, Trish Greenhalgh, Gill Westhorp, Jeanette Buckingham and Ray Pawson. 2013. "RAMESES Publication Standards: Meta-Narrative Reviews." *Journal of Advanced Nursing* 69.5: 987–1004.

Zuehlke, T.E. and J.T. Watkins. 1975. "Psychotherapy with the Dying Patients an Exploratory Study." *Journal of Clinical Psychology* 31.4: 729–32.

Zuehlke, T.E. and J.T. Watkins. 1977. "Psychotherapy with Terminally Ill Patients." *Psychother-Theor-Res* 14.4: 403–10.

Index

Page numbers in *italics* denote figures.

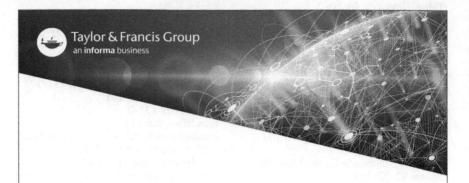